CLINICAL DECISIONS IN
Glaucoma

CLINICAL DECISIONS IN

Glaucoma

ELIZABETH HODAPP, M.D.

Associate Professor

RICHARD K. PARRISH II, M.D.

Associate Professor

DOUGLAS R. ANDERSON, M.D.

Professor

Bascom Palmer Eye Institute
Department of Ophthalmology
University of Miami School of Medicine
Miami, Florida

with **91** *illustrations and* **12** *color plates*

Mosby

St. Louis Baltimore Boston Chicago London Philadelphia Sydney Toronto

Mosby
Dedicated to Publishing Excellence

Editor: Laurel Craven
Assistant Editor: Lauranne Billus
Project Manager: Karen Edwards
Production Editor: James W. Russell
Designer: Gail Morey Hudson
Production Assistant: Jeanne Genz
Manufacturing Supervisor: John Babrick

Printed in the United States of America

Mosby–Year Book, Inc.
11830 Westline Industrial Drive
St. Louis, Missouri 63146

Library of Congress Cataloging–in–Publication Data

Hodapp, Elizabeth.
Clinical decisions in glaucoma / by Elizabeth Hodapp, Richard K. Parrish II, Douglas R. Anderson.
p. cm.
Includes bibliographical references and index.
ISBN 0-8016-6799-2
1. Glaucoma—Handbooks, manuals, etc. I. Parrish, Richard K. II. Anderson, Douglas R., 1938– . III. Title.
[DNLM: 1. Glaucoma—diagnosis. WW 290 H687c 1993]
RE871.H57 1993
617.7'41—dc20
DNLM/DLC
for Library of Congress 93-12006
CIP

96 97 GW/MY 9 8 7 6 5 4 3

Preface

This book aims to help the ophthalmologist care for patients who have or may have glaucoma. It is not a textbook—fine, comprehensive textbooks already exist. It is a management manual, and we address some of the common glaucoma management questions that arise in the clinical practice of ophthalmology. In a clinical situation, "What do I do today with this person who has a pressure of 26 mm Hg?" is a more immediate question than is "How, precisely, does high pressure damage the optic nerve?" Also, a list of the things to do today (and next month and next year) helps more than does a classification of disease or a discourse on pathophysiology. We want to present common glaucoma as a chronic condition, one that is managed for many years in most patients.

We present first the general principles underlying our approach to glaucoma care and our overall glaucoma management scheme (Chapter 1). Next, we detail what to do in the common clinical presentations suggestive of glaucoma. We do not present every possible situation, nor do we discuss every possible permutation of those situations we do present. Rather, we emphasize the common conditions and conditions for which there exists specific treatment.

The most common situation suggesting glaucoma arises when a patient is found to have elevated intraocular pressure (IOP). Most such people lack symptoms, and we first outline the evaluation of a patient with asymptomatic elevated IOP (Chapter 2). We do not go into great detail as to how to perform an examination, but instead present our mental checklists of what to look for at various steps of the examination. Most symptom-free patients with elevated IOP will either have primary open-angle glaucoma (POAG) or will be POAG suspects. So the prototype for management of chronic glaucoma is POAG and suspected POAG, the managements of which we describe in detail (Chapters 3 through 5). We then present our approach to patients with normal pressure whose clinical presentations suggest that they have glaucoma or are at higher-than-normal risk to develop glaucoma (Chapters 6 and 7). Next we deal with acutely symptomatic elevated pressure (Chapter 8) and then with elevated pressure occurring in conjunction with uveitis (Chapter 9) and with surgical and accidental trauma (Chapter 10). For each situation, we describe how to figure out what is going on and how to care for the patient. Quite a number of conditions will, after diagnosis or after some particular diagnosis-specific intervention, turn out to be managed very much like POAG. We review the particular management points for the more common secondary glaucomas and miscellaneous conditions associated with glaucoma in our final chapter (Chapter 11).

We have chosen to dispense with extensive explanations and exhaustive discussions of the various alternatives for treatment. We will not enter into all the possible theroretic complexities of clinical diagnosis and decision making. Conflicting literature regarding glaucoma abounds and is available to all. We have elected to describe what we currently think is best, based on our experience and on previously published information, and we try to be as explicit as possible. As guidelines we have chosen to list numbers and percentages and precise follow-up intervals. The numbers and intervals are arbitrary, but we have based them on our own clinical sense and consider them reasonable. We use the imperative voice frequently in line with our perception of this as a management manual.

Elizabeth Hodapp
Richard K. Parrish II
Douglas R. Anderson

Contents

1

General Precepts

Intraocular pressure (IOP) relates to, but does not define, glaucoma. Many conditions in the group "glaucoma" have an IOP sufficiently elevated that it may produce ocular symptoms such as visual loss or pain. Also included in the "glaucoma" category are cases with characteristic glaucoma-like optic nerve damage without elevated pressure. Except when the pressure is sufficiently elevated to produce symptoms, the goal of long-term management is to prevent visual loss related to optic nerve damage.

Independent of the cause for any chronic pressure elevation, most types of glaucoma appear to damage the eye in the same manner. The pathophysiology of chronic glaucomatous damage has received much attention but remains unexplained. If in time it is understood, it may be possible to treat specifically the various elements that participate with the IOP to produce optic nerve damage. Currently, however, treatment is simply aimed at lowering the IOP sufficiently that optic nerve damage halts or is slowed.

Our management scheme for glaucoma is based on these general precepts:

1. The higher the pressure, the greater the risk of glaucomatous damage.
2. There are factors other than pressure that contribute to optic nerve damage and determine an individual's susceptibility to harm from pressure, but they are unknown.
3. In patients with glaucoma, lowering the IOP decreases the rate of glaucomatous damage, but there is no way to know with certainty at what pressure level glaucomatous damage ceases or will be acceptably slow for a given person.
4. Every method of lowering pressure causes side effects, costs money, and involves risk to the patient.
5. The goals of treatment for glaucoma are to lower pressure enough to preserve good vision for the lifetime of the patient while causing as few side effects and incurring as few costs as possible.

Few dispute the importance of decreasing the IOP in patients with glaucoma. However, the relationship between the height of the pressure and the rate of damage varies from person to person, and hence the benefit of lowering the pressure varies among individuals. For each patient, the benefit of lower pressure should outweigh the risks and costs of treatment.

Our two fundamental management requirements are derived from the general precepts and the chronic nature of glaucoma:

1. **Glaucoma management involves balancing the risks and benefits of lowering the IOP in each patient individually.**
2. **Glaucoma management depends on the ability to recognize change in status over time.**

Simply recognizing the presence of glaucomatous damage, particularly the earliest signs of damage, helps little in the chronic care of a patient who has, may have, or may develop glaucoma. It is the *rate* of damage that is important. We recommend managing patients with findings suggestive of glaucoma by taking the following steps:

1. Treat any treatable conditions, such as pupillary block or proliferative retinopathy, that contribute to elevated pressure. Also treat conditions, such as a narrow angle that closes with dilation, that are likely to cause elevated pressure, and will have a better outcome if trouble is avoided rather than dealt with after it arises.
2. Establish a baseline by quantifying the degree of damage. Determine and record for the future the status of the patient at the time he or she is seen.
3. Decide if therapy is indicated now; if so, set a pressure goal. This is the intellectually difficult step.
4. Treat the patient to achieve your goal. If treatment proves difficult, evaluate the certainty of the need to achieve the goal.
5. Follow the patient's course to see both if the goal is maintained and if the degree of damage remains stationary.
6. Modify goals as indicated by the patient's course.

2

The Asymptomatic Patient with Elevated Pressure

Elevated intraocular pressure—not visual symptoms—first identifies most patients who have glaucoma. Not everyone with high pressure has glaucoma, but the doctor should evaluate patients with high eye pressures and should follow up on their future courses, regardless of whether the evaluation reveals glaucoma. No sharp boundary separates *elevated* from *normal* pressure. It may not be sensible to arbitrarily divide eyes into those with "normal" or "high" pressure at a sharp cutoff point, but simply to recognize that the higher the IOP, the greater the patient's likelihood to have or to develop glaucomatous optic nerve damage. As an arbitrary point at which to become suspicious, the traditional definition of elevated pressure as a pressure of 22 mm Hg or greater (two standard deviations above the mean) serves as well as any other. Of course, we recommend that every complete ocular examination be performed with the possibility of glaucoma firmly in mind (always evaluate the optic nerve and anterior chamber), but we recommend an expanded evaluation, including gonioscopy and formal visual field assessment, for those patients whose pressure is 22 mm Hg or greater.

Although almost any of the glaucomas *may* be observed first as an asymptomatic pressure elevation, most patients who are found to have high pressure on routine examinations have one of the following conditions:

- Primary open-angle pressure elevation (glaucoma or glaucoma suspect)
- Chronic angle closure glaucoma (the term *glaucoma* is traditionally used for this condition, even if there is no nerve damage)
- Pseudoexfoliation with elevated pressure (glaucoma or suspect)
- Pigmentary dispersion with elevated pressure (glaucoma or suspect)

The most important aspect of the evaluation of an asymptomatic individual who has elevated pressure is to identify any cause of pressure elevation for which something particular can or should be done. First, identify specifically treatable causes of elevated pressure. Then determine if the person belongs to a diagnostic group that is treated differently from primary open-angle glaucoma suspects. The less important aspect of this *initial* evaluation is deciding if glaucomatous damage already exists.

DETERMINING THE CAUSE OF ELEVATED IOP

With a complete eye examination (including gonioscopy), clinicians can distinguish the various likely causes of high pressure and identify the occasional patient with an unusual cause. In the ordinary course of an evaluation, the history and refraction, as well as external, pupillary, motility, and anterior segment examinations, precede tonometry. When the pressure is elevated, it may be necessary to obtain additional history and reexamine the eye to look for subtle findings that may aid differential diagnosis. The salient points from each part of the evaluation follow.

History

There are two types of historical information to obtain: history related to diagnosis and history related to management decisions.

DIAGNOSTIC POINTS

Corticosteroid use. Oral or topical (for example, to the skin of the face) corticosteroids may elevate the IOP.

Injury. Trauma may cause damage to the outflow system which, years later, results in elevated pressure. If the patient had recent trauma or has had intraocular surgery, refer to Chapter 10.

MANAGEMENT POINTS

Family history. Glaucoma is often hereditary. If any of the patient's relatives have glaucoma, determine the severity of their disease. A family history of severe glaucoma increases the suspicion that a patient may have a similarly severe course. The opposite, a family history of mild disease, is not as reliable a predictor in our experience.

Medical history. Patients who are allergic to sulfa drugs or who have renal disease are relatively poor candidates for carbonic anhydrase inhibitor use. Congestive heart failure and asthmatic respiratory problems may worsen during β-blocker use. Vasospastic disease (migraine, Raynaud's phenomenon) and low blood pressure may increase a patient's susceptibility to pressure-induced damage. A past hemodynamic crisis may explain optic nerve damage that is related to previous changes in perfusion of the optic nerve rather than to the present IOP.

Examination

REFRACTION

Always use the best refraction and an appropriate add for perimetry. Axial myopia probably makes the eye more susceptible to pressure-induced damage, and accompanying retinal degeneration may confound visual field evaluation. Highly hyperoptic eyes are prone to develop primary angle closure glaucoma.

SLIT LAMP EXAMINATION

Pigmentary glaucoma, pseudoexfoliation, asymptomatic inflammation, and remote and forgotten trauma may all have slit lamp findings. Examine the cornea for a Krukenberg spindle and check carefully for anterior segment inflammation. Look for iris transillumination defects, neovascularization (unusual in this setting), and the residua of trauma, such as iris sphincter rupture. After the pupil is dilated, examine the lens for pseudoexfoliation.

If the patient has had cataract surgery, especially if an anterior chamber intraocular lens was implanted, note whether a patent iridectomy is present.* Also record the orientation of the implant if one is present, because mobile lens implants may cause both inflammation and elevated IOP. Increased IOP in the early and late postoperative period may be related to the surgery and is discussed in Chapter 10. However, individuals who have recovered from cataract surgery may have elevated pressure on subsequent examinations, and their evaluation generally proceeds as does that of phakic patients.

Tonometry

Applanation tonometry is standard; record the time of measurement. The pressure in the two eyes rarely differs by more than 2 mm Hg in normal eyes, but moderate asymmetry of pressure is common in primary open-angle glaucoma. Widely disparate readings, especially if only one reading is above normal, suggest one of the secondary unilateral glaucomas. In an asymptomatic patient with unilateral elevated IOP, pseudoexfoliation and old trauma are the most common diagnoses.

Gonioscopy

First determine if the angle is open or closed. If the angle is open, then look for such findings as heavy pigmentation, angle recession, neovascularization, developmental anomalies, or blood in Schlemm's canal. These findings suggest particular diagnoses. If the angle is closed, determine the type of angle closure. Perform compression gonioscopy if unable to clearly determine the details of the iris insertion. The three general mechanisms of angle closure, illustrated in Figure 2-1, are pupillary block (common), anterior pulling (occasional), and posterior pushing (rare). Additional variants on pupillary block in aphakic or pseudophakic patients are described in Chapter 10.

The distinction among different types of angle closure proceeds by first noting if there is either inflammation or some other obvious cause of angle closure other than pupillary block. Unless another diagnosis, such as an iridocorneal endoethelial syndrome, rubeosis iridis, or uveitis with peripheral anterior synechiae (PAS), is clear, perform an iridectomy because it is otherwise difficult to rule out pupillary block. For the same reason, perform an iridectomy if the angle is open but very narrow in what appears to be a pupillary block mechanism. (Management of narrow angles in individuals with normal IOP is discussed in Chapter 7.)

After the iridectomy, reexamine the eye with the gonioprism. If pupillary block was present, the angle should be open or PAS should be visible. If pupillary block was absent, completion of the examination generally clarifies the cause. When the pupil is dilated, reexamine the angle and check the pressure to rule out plateau iris, which is discussed in Chapter 8.

The anterior segment examination provides the information necessary to satisfy the first two goals of the evaluation of elevated IOP, to identify specifically treatable causes of elevated pressure and to recognize if a person belongs to a particular diagnostic group. Chart 2-1 summarizes the differential diagnostic steps, as detailed below.

---

*The term *iridectomy* is used throughout this book to refer to a hole in the iris. Unless *surgical* iridectomy is specified, we assume that an iridectomy (if recommended) will be performed with a laser unless it accompanies another intraocular procedure.

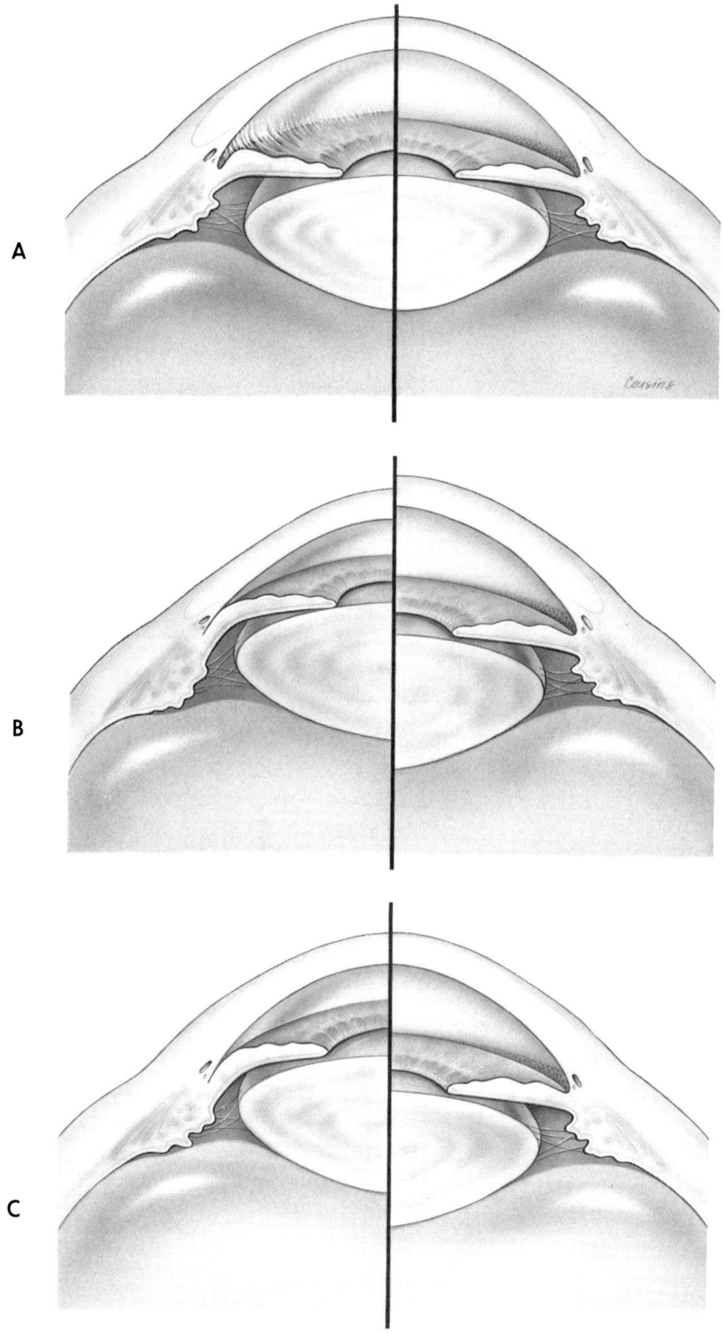

FIG. 2-1 **A,** Anterior pulling angle closure, *left*; normal for comparison, *right*. Aqueous humor flows freely from the posterior to the anterior chamber. The central anterior chamber depth does not change as a result of the angle closure. **B,** Pupillary block angle closure, *left*; normal for comparison, *right*. Because of resistance to aqueous humor flow between the posterior and anterior chambers, pressure in the posterior chamber rises and aqueous humor pushes the peripheral iris forward. The anterior lens surface does not move forward, but, as shown, primary pupillary block glaucoma usually develops in smaller-than-average eyes with shallow central anterior chambers. **C,** Posterior pushing angle closure, *left*; normal for comparison, *right*. The lens moves forward and pushes the iris over the trabecular meshwork. The central anterior chamber is shallowed.

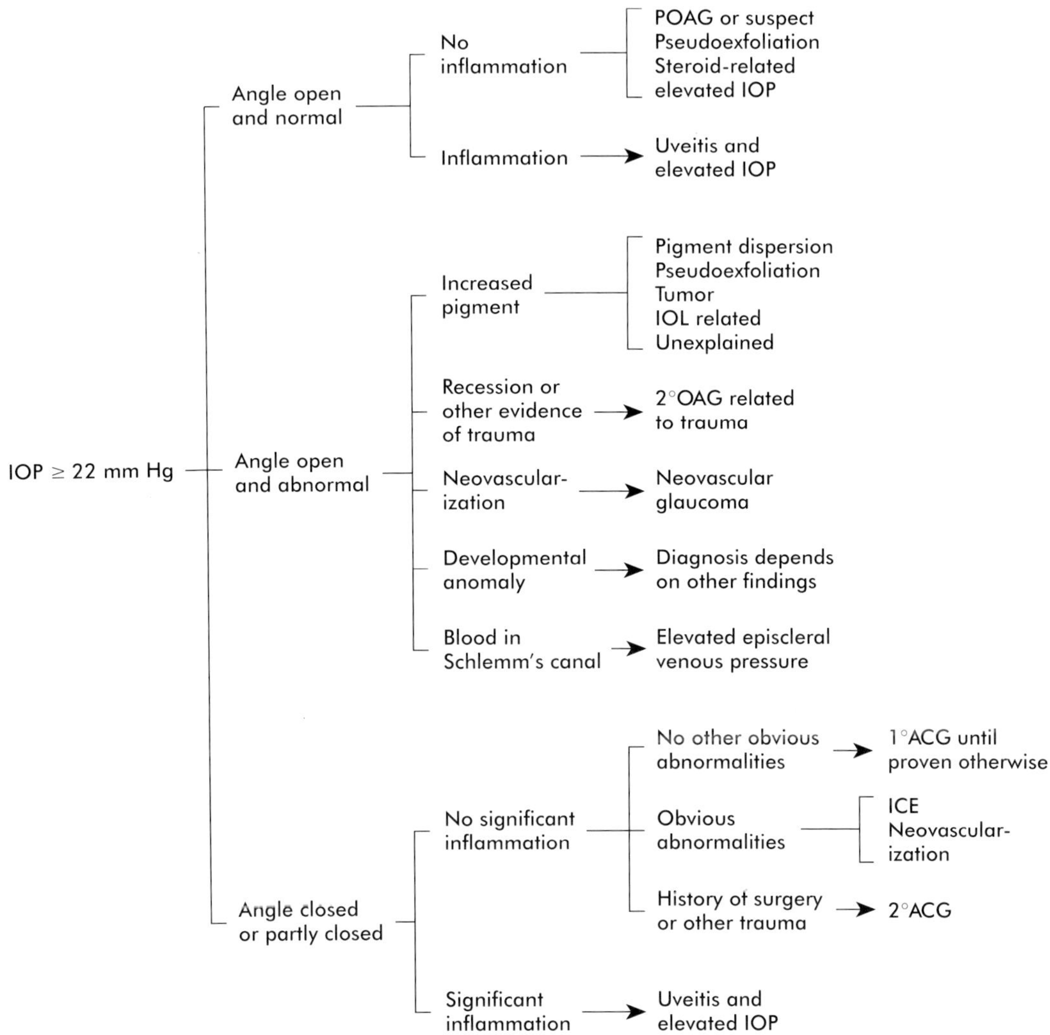

CHART 2-1 Differential diagnosis of elevated pressure in an asymptomatic eye. The majority of patients belong to one of these groups.

◆ *IOP ≥ 22 mm Hg—Angle open and normal*

In a quiet eye with normal pigment and no obvious abnormalities, the most likely diagnosis is primary open-angle pressure elevation. Pseudoexfoliation with elevated pressure also generally presents in this way. It is managed the same as primary pressure elevation with a few special considerations mentioned in Chapter 11. The angle appears normal in individuals with corticosteroid-induced pressure elevation, which is also discussed in Chapter 11. If there is anterior segment inflammation, evaluate and manage the patient as described in Chapter 9.

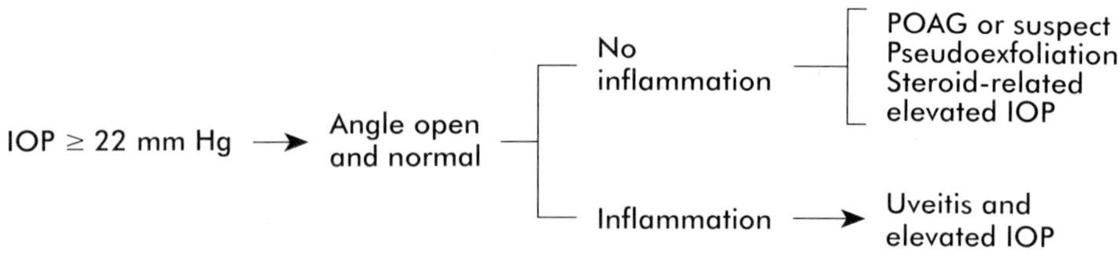

◆ ***IOP ≥ 22 mm Hg—Angle open and abnormal***

Increased pigmentation in an open angle usually indicates either the pigment dispersion syndrome or pseudoexfoliation. Pigmentary dispersion typically occurs in young myopic individuals, usually men, who also have Krukenberg spindles and iris transillumination defects. Pseudoexfoliation develops in older people, and the diagnosis depends on finding pseudoexfoliative material on the pupillary border and lens capsule. Both conditions are treated almost identically to primary open-angle pressure elevations and are discussed in Chapter 11. A secondary type of pigment dispersion occasionally develops in eyes with lens implants that chafe the posterior iris. Rarely, an intraocular tumor—typically a melanoma—sheds pigmented cells into the angle. If no other explanation for pigmentation is found, examine the eye carefully for tumor, especially if the pigmentation is uniocular.

Angle recession or other evidence of trauma (subluxed lens, choroidal rupture) is most often noted in patients with unilateral elevated pressure. The management of glaucoma following trauma resembles that of primary open-angle glaucoma with differences discussed in Chapter 11.

Neovascularization of the anterior segment rarely causes elevated IOP without symptoms. The evaluation and management of neovascularization are discussed in Chapter 8.

Developmentally abnormal angles are occasionally noted in individuals with elevated pressure. Many patients' findings fall into the Axenfeld/Rieger group,

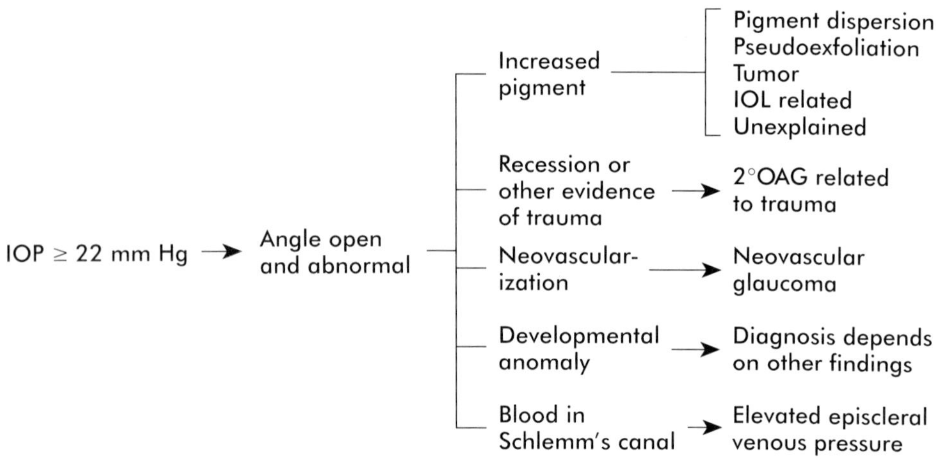

but others have findings such as high iris insertion, multiple iris processes, or peculiar iris stroma that do not "fit" a specific syndrome. In the Axenfeld/Rieger group, gonioscopy may show peripheral iris atrophy, heavy uveal meshwork, and iris strands that bridge the angle and attach to or in front of Schwalbe's line, which is often thickened and anteriorly displaced. Slit lamp findings include iris atrophy and pupillary irregularity. Adult patients seen with these findings are treated as those with primary open-angle pressure elevation or fully developed glaucoma.

Blood in Schlemm's canal in an eye with elevated IOP indicates elevated episcleral venous pressure. The most common causes are congenital anomalies, such as the Sturge-Weber syndrome, which are associated with other visible vascular anomalies, but in some individuals high pressure related to acquired asymptomatic arteriovenous shunts may develop. High pressure associated with elevated episcleral venous pressure is discussed in Chapter 11.

◆ *IOP ≥ 22 mm Hg—Angle closed, no inflammation or other obvious abnormality*

When an asymptomatic person has angle closure and elevated IOP in an unoperated eye without inflammation, the most common cause is primary chronic angle closure related to pupillary block. The first step in management is to perform an iridectomy. If the pressure falls (even if not to normal) after relief of pupillary block, an asymptomatic person with chronic angle closure is managed as described in Chapter 8 (chronic management of primary angle closure glaucoma). If the pressure does not decrease in an asymptomatic patient with chronic angle closure glaucoma, evaluation and treatment are almost identical to primary open-angle pressure elevation, with specific differences discussed in Chapter 11. Angle closure without other obvious abnormality that is not relieved by iridectomy is evaluated as described in Chapter 8. Angle closure in an eye that has had recent surgery is discussed in Chapter 10.

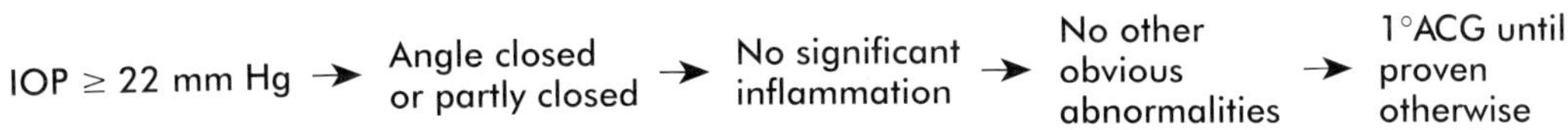

◆ *IOP ≥ 22 mm Hg—Angle closed, obvious abnormality or previous surgery*

Several distinct syndromes are associated with angle closure and may be present in an asymptomatic person with elevated pressure.

The iridocorneal endothelial syndromes (essential iris atrophy, Chandler's syndrome, Cogan-Reese iris nevus syndrome) generally occur in one eye of young, usually female individuals. If typical iris findings—corectopia, iris atrophy, or nevus formation—are present, the diagnosis is easy. Iridectomy does not prevent progression of the angle closure, and management resembles that of open-angle glaucoma. Particular provisos are outlined in Chapter 11.

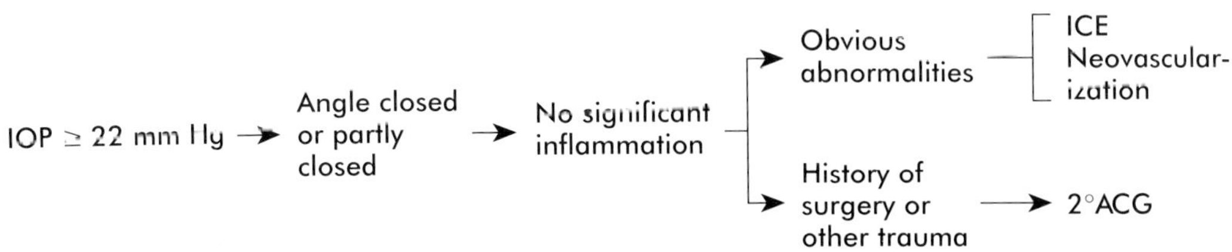

Neovascularization is rare in this setting. It is usually associated with at least mild inflammation and is usually associated with symptoms. It is evaluated and managed as described in Chapter 8.

Secondary angle closure after surgery is discussed in Chapter 10.

◆ *IOP ≥ 22 mm Hg—Angle closed, significant inflammation but no other obvious abnormality*

Inflammation causes angle closure by all three of the mechanisms described in Figure 2-1. Anterior segment inflammation can result in both peripheral anterior synechiae, which pull the iris anteriorly over the trabecular meshwork, and in posterior synechiae, which seal the pupil and cause pupillary block. In addition, posterior segment inflammation may precipitate angle closure by rotating the ciliary body and pushing the lens forward. Evaluation and treatment are discussed in Chapter 9.

IOP ≥ 22 mm Hg → Angle closed or partly closed → Significant inflammation → Uveitis and elevated IOP

At this point in the examination, the major treatable causes of IOP elevation will have been noted. Most patients will have had no anterior segment abnormality other than elevated pressure, and the pressure elevation is "primary" or "idiopathic." The final aspects of the initial examination, the fundus and visual field examinations, rarely contribute to the diagnosis of the type of pressure elevation, but they are the basis for establishing the stage or severity of the disease and the way in which management will proceed.

If glaucomatous damage exists in a person with elevated pressure, the patient is said to have glaucoma. If no damage is demonstrable, he or she is said to be a glaucoma suspect. Such people may have glaucoma, but if they do, it is as yet too mild to diagnose with certainty. Even in people who have obvious glaucoma, the degree of damage at the time of diagnosis is less important in guiding management than is the rate of future damage. Thus, regardless of whether abnormalities are found, both the fundus examination and the visual examination form the baseline examination that is crucial for future comparison.

EVALUATING THE OPTIC NERVE

Using a slit lamp beam and a fundus lens, examine the nerve at high magnification with the patient's pupils dilated. The slit beam defines contour better than does diffuse illumination. In the presence of a small pupil or media opacity, an indirect fundus lens, such as the 78D or 90D lens, may provide an easier view than does a direct lens. However, direct lenses, such as the Hruby lens or the fundus contact lens, provide better stereopsis than indirect lenses and we prefer them. Assess the color and the width of the neural rim, the size of the contour cup, and the presence or absence of notches and hemorrhages. Express to the nearest one tenth the ratio of the width of the cup, not the pallor, to the width of both the horizontal and vertical axes of the disc. The following findings strongly suggest pressure-related damage:

- Asymmetry between the two cups of 0.2 disc diameters or greater in either axis in discs of equal size (Plates 1 to 4).
- Vertical elongation of the cup such that the vertical cup measurement is greater than the horizontal (Plate 5).

- A thinner rim of tissue in a vertical pole of the disc than elsewhere (Plate 6).
- Distinct local notching of the nerve tissue (Plate 7).
- Disc margin hemorrhage (Plate 8).

Although none of these findings alone defines glaucoma, each suggests acquired damage. After examining the disc, evaluate the fundus for evidence of other disease. In particular, look for old branch retinal vessel occlusions or other retinal lesions that might correspond with any field defects present.

The optic nerves should be photographed for the sake of future comparison. The most useful photographs are stereoscopic and magnified (2× standard fundus magnification). Photographs provide a permanent color record that can be taken with the patient if he or she moves. Few clinicians can accurately capture the disc appearance on a drawing, and even the best hand drawings are less satisfactory than photographs because of the mobility of patients and the mobility and mortality of physicians. Other methods of recording and later comparing the optic nerve head topography are currently being investigated and marketed. None is readily available to most ophthalmologists, and none has been shown to be better than visual comparison of two photographs by the clinician.

Nerve fiber layer photographs are available in some institutions. Experienced observers can recognize early glaucomatous changes in the nerve fiber layer. It is unclear, however, how often such recognizable defects occur without an evident abnormality of the optic nerve photographs or visual field. Nor is it known whether serial nerve fiber layer photographs allow the recognition of perceptible changes over time better than do serial nerve photographs or serial visual fields.

EVALUATING THE VISUAL FIELD

All complete eye examinations include some assessment of the visual field. For the many patients who are not under particular suspicion of glaucoma or other condition affecting the field, confrontation fields suffice, but patients with elevated IOP should have formal visual fields. It is preferable to obtain fields before ocular manipulation (tonometry, gonioscopy, or pupillary dilation). Thus, in an initial evaluation when tonometry and gonioscopy have already been completed, the fields are better tested on a separate date. If this is unrealistic, wait at least an hour to allow the corneal epithelium to recover.

We strongly recommend automated static threshold perimetry. It is possible to provide good care for patients with manifest or suspected glaucoma without using an automated static threshold perimeter. However, automated instruments make it much easier to care for patients, and they also allow better care. Static threshold perimetry generally yields less variable results than kinetic perimetry, and it permits high-quality perimetry to be performed by technicians with less extensive training. Static threshold perimeters give numerical data, which allows for averaging of more than one baseline examination and automated comparison with subsequent data. It also allows for computerized analysis of visual fields done in different offices. Patients who move from place to place can carry their fields with them on a computer disc.

We currently use a Humphrey perimeter equipped with the Statpac 2 program. All illustrations in this text are from that instrument. Extensive details about testing strategies and printout options on this and other perimeters are beyond the scope of this book but are available in standard perimetric texts. Figures 2-2 through 2-6 briefly describe the standard test program and data presentations used in this book.

Text continued on page 16.

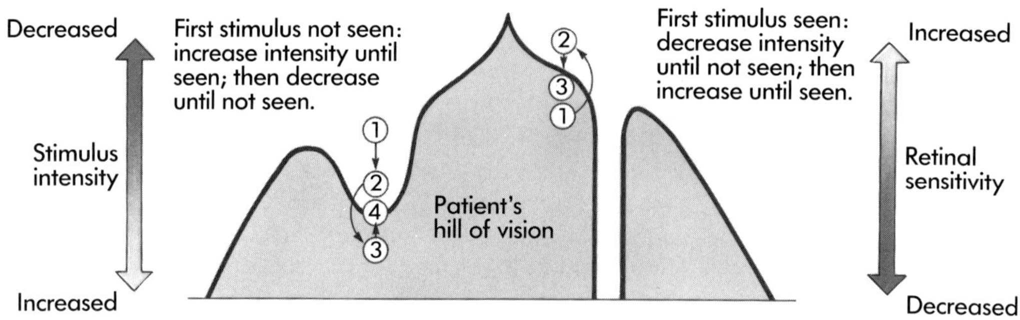

FIG. 2-2 Typical strategy of threshold determination on automated static threshold perimeter. Most perimeters increase or decrease the stimulus intensity in 4 dB steps until threshold is crossed and then move back in 2 dB steps until it is crossed again. (1 db = 0.1 log unit of attenuation of the maximum stimulus.) (Adapted from The Field Analyzer Primer.)

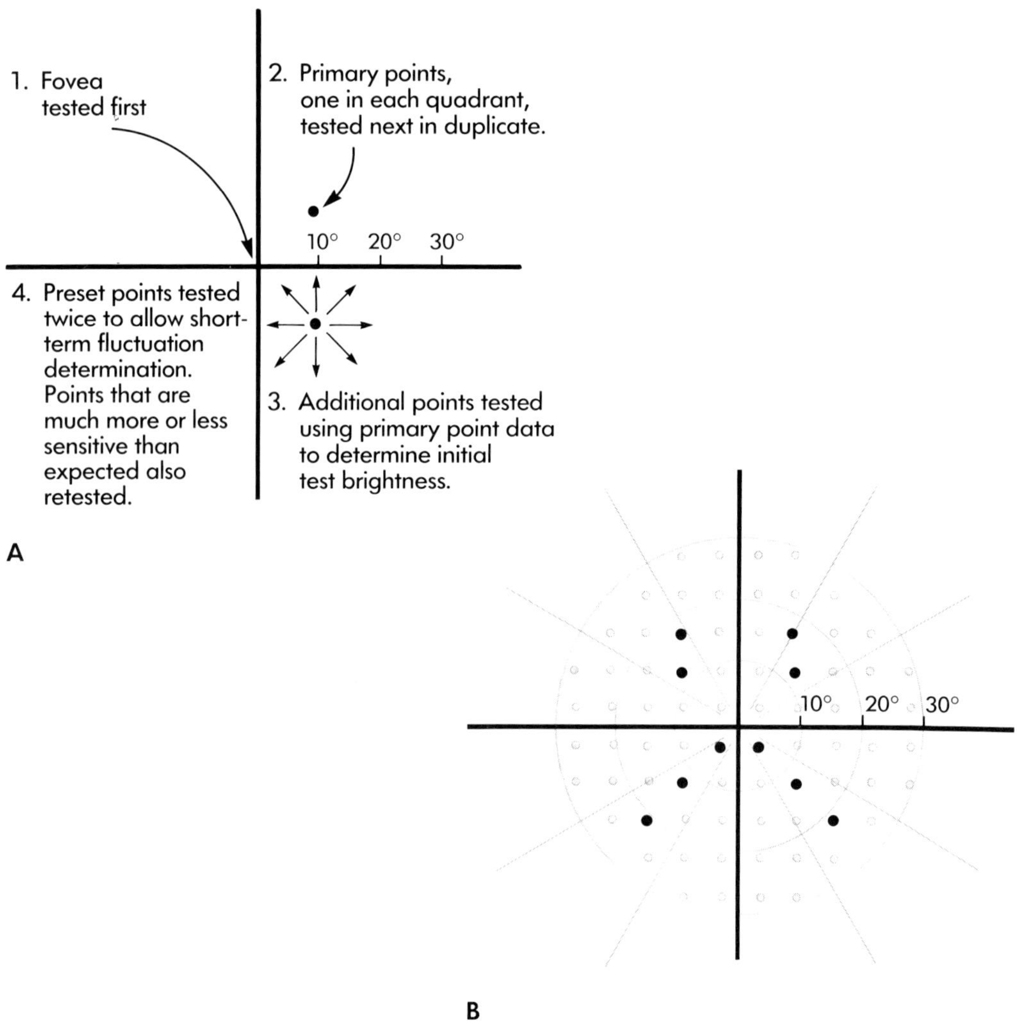

FIG. 2-3 Field algorithm. **A,** General testing sequence for threshold programs on the Humphrey perimeter. **B,** Test points on the 30-2 program; double-determined points that determine the short-term fluctuation are shown in solid circles.

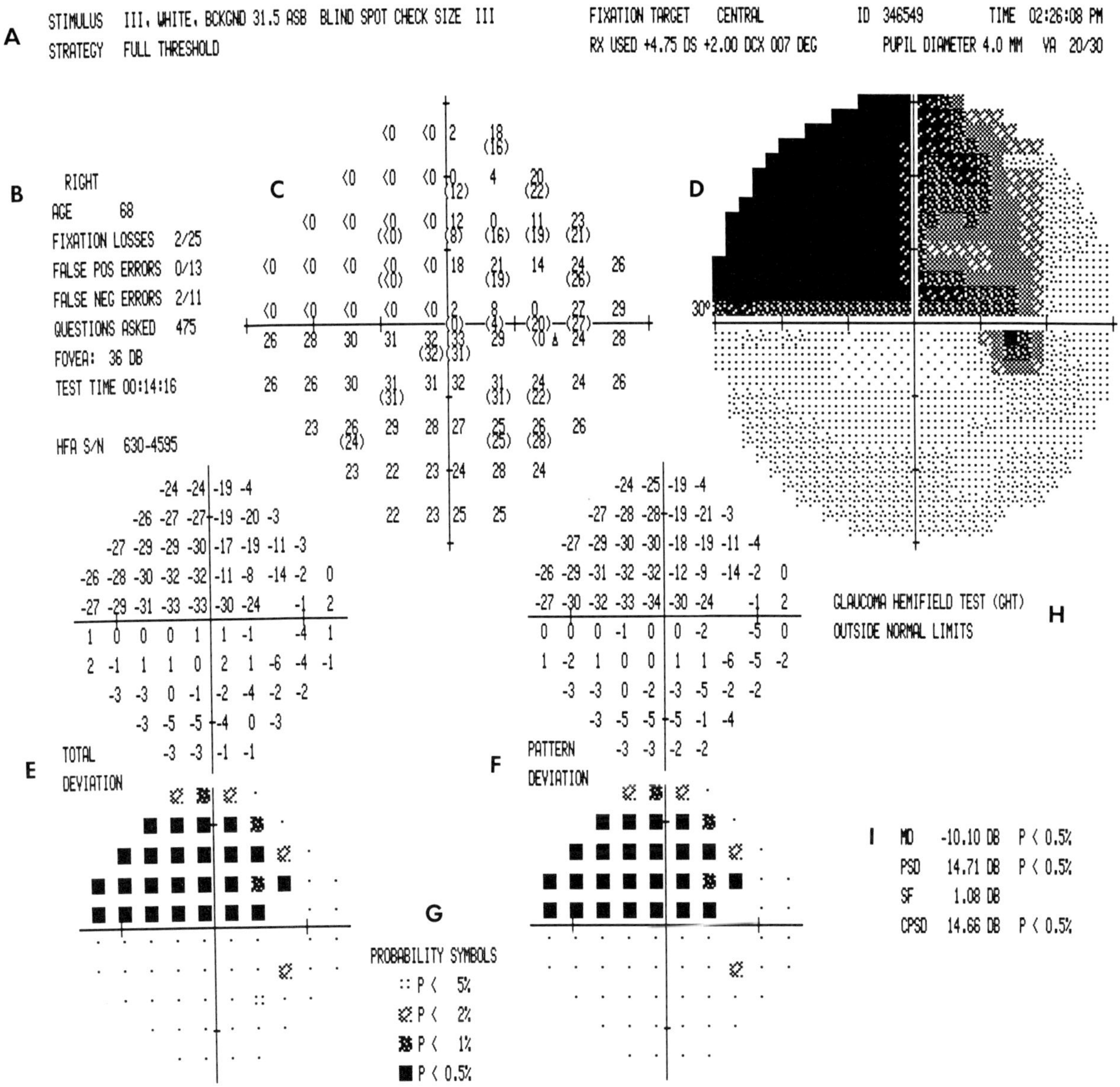

FIG. 2-4 Humphrey 30-2, single-field analysis. **A,** Patient information and test conditions. **B,** Reliability parameters. Fixation losses, false-positive errors, and false-negative errors are discussed in the text. **C,** Test results in dB. The higher the number, the greater the visual sensitivity. Numbers in parentheses refer to the second result of a separate threshold determination. **D,** Grey scale. **E,** Total deviation. The difference from normal in dB *(top)* and the likelihood that the results occurred by chance *(bottom)*. **F,** Pattern deviation. The total deviation, corrected for the overall height of the hill of vision to minimize the effect of media opacity, in dB *(top)* and the likelihood that the results occurred by chance *(bottom)*. **G,** Key to probability symbols. **H,** Glaucoma hemifield test (see text p. 46). **I,** Global indices. The mean deviation *(MD)*, pattern standard deviation *(PSD)*, short-term fluctuation *(SF)*, and corrected pattern standard deviation *(CPSD)* are discussed in the text.

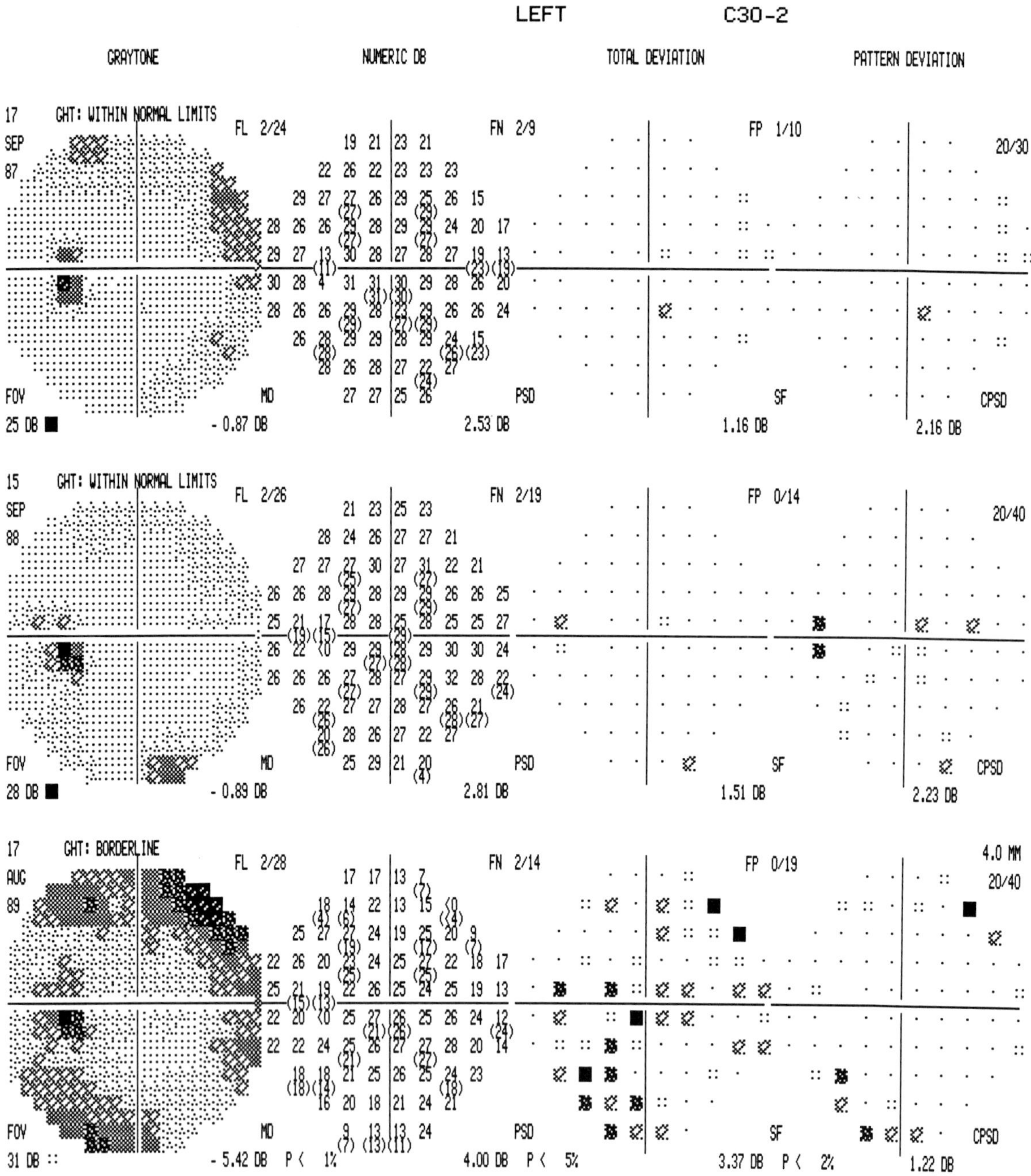

FIG. 2-5 Overview. This condensed printout of a series of fields includes most of the information from the single-field analysis.

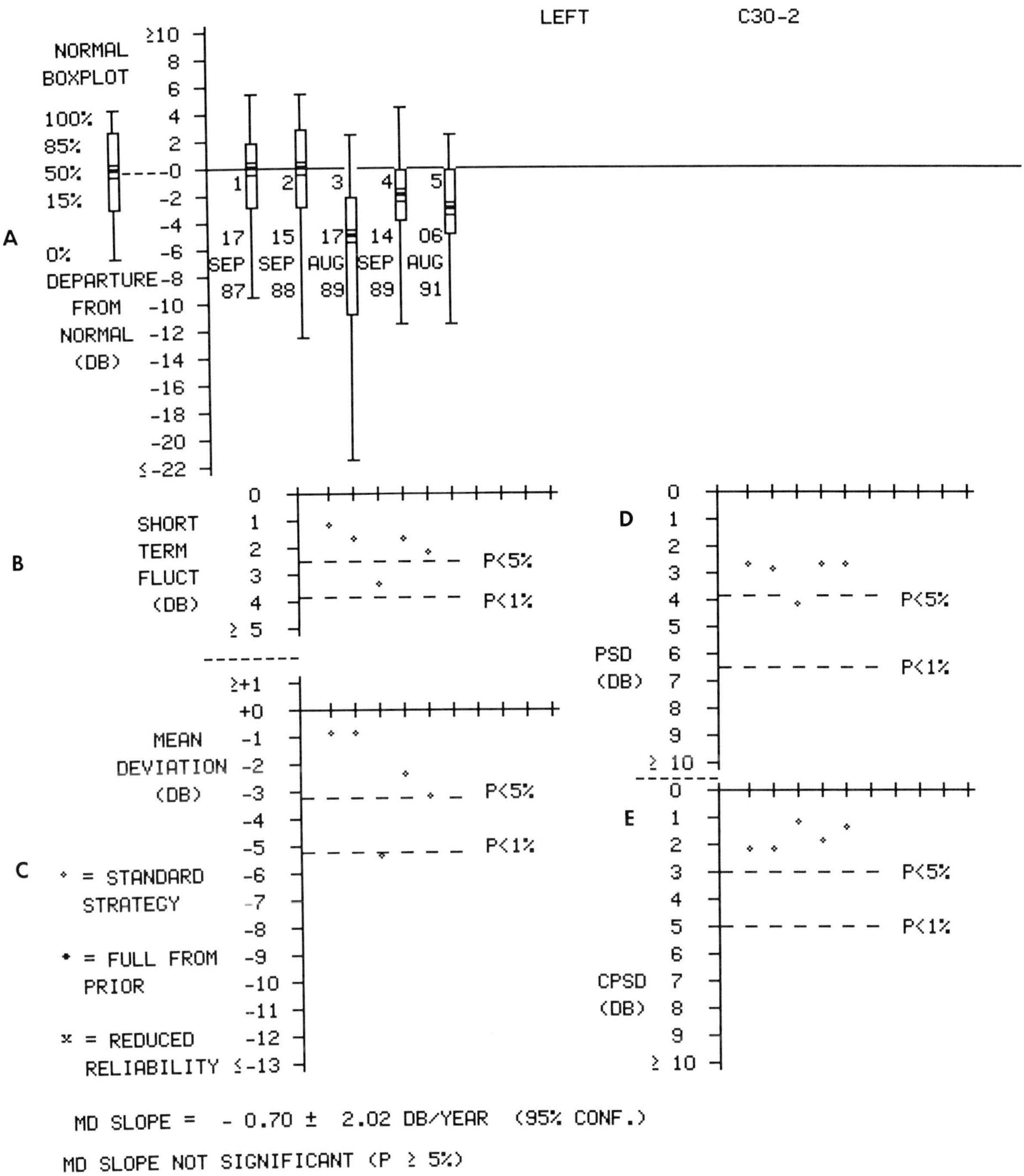

FIG. 2-6 Change analysis. **A,** Boxplot. The normal boxplot on the left shows the distribution of differences from normal of the test points. A normally shaped boxplot, even if it is depressed relative to normal, indicates a consistent depression. The longer the tail of the boxplot, the more focal is likely to be damage. **B,** Short-term fluctuation summary. **C,** Mean deviation summary. If there are five or more fields, the slope of the deviation will be figured and presented as will a statement about the likelihood that it occurred by chance. **D,** Pattern standard deviation summary. **E,** Corrected pattern standard deviation summary.

Baseline Visual Field Examination

Future therapeutic decisions depend on the relation between the baseline fields and subsequent fields; the more accurate the initial field baseline, the easier it is to determine in the future if a patient's condition is stable or changing. Patients with elevated pressure should have threshold tests. Although suprathreshold testing may be quite sensitive for identifying all but the most subtle defects, threshold testing permits much better comparison in the future.

We consider two fields to be the minimum baseline, although for some individuals, more fields may be necessary. Fields vary from day to day, and multiple tests give a more accurate measurement than one and provide a sense of the variability to be expected on different days in the patient. The time course for obtaining baseline fields is somewhat dependent on the patient's other findings. The more severe the damage, the more pressing the need to define the patient's position at the time of diagnosis and to proceed to therapy. We routinely obtain a Central 30-2 threshold test as the first field examination and perform a second Central 30-2 field examination within 1 or 2 months. If the first field is very depressed or constricted, we proceed as described on page 25. Depending on the similarity between the first two fields, additional early tests may be obtained to complete the baseline. (Patients whose disc and first field examination clearly show glaucomatous damage may start treatment while their field baseline is completed.) This toilsome baseline effort improves the clinician's future ability to make accurate judgments. Henceforth, when the term *baseline* is used in relation to fields, we refer to at least two fields with the baseline determined as described below.

FIRST TWO FIELDS VERY SIMILAR, ROUTINE BASELINE

If the first two fields are consistent and do not show a substantial learning effect (<2 dB mean deviation (MD) difference), we use them as a baseline for future comparison (Fig. 2-7).

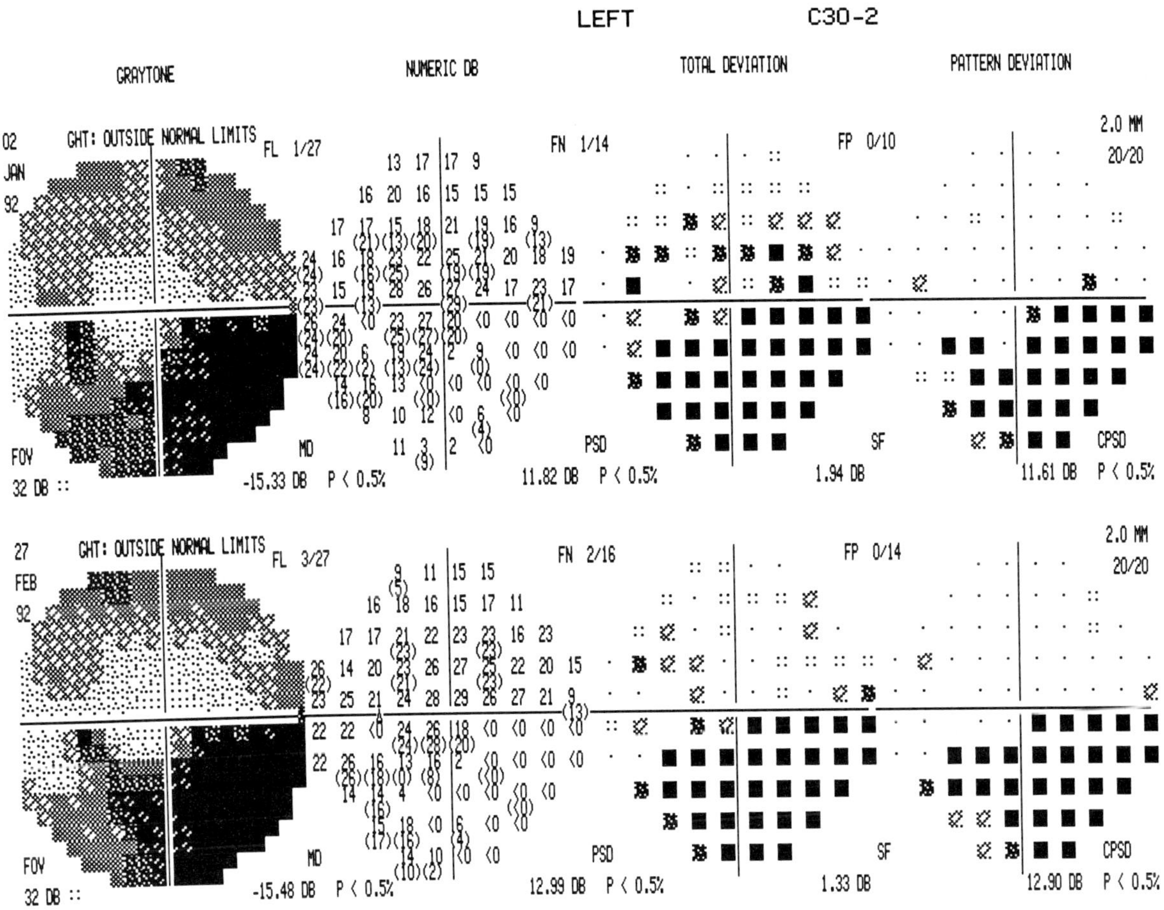

FIG. 2-7 Baseline pair of visual fields. The patient's first two fields are almost identical and together serve as the baseline for future comparison.

FIRST TWO FIELDS VARY, NONROUTINE BASELINE

The three common explanations for a marked difference between the first and second field are learning effect, marked true variability in the field, and poor patient reliability. Obtaining a third field helps to sort these and will, in most cases, complete the baseline studies.

Learning effect. Many people test better during perimetry after their first field. Some people improve a great deal, and in these individuals the baseline should exclude the first field. If the third field is similar to the second, use the second and third as a baseline (Figs. 2-8 and 2-9). Occasionally a patient continues to improve with subsequent fields beyond the second (Fig. 2-10). This makes establishment of a baseline difficult and frustrating, but the fields should be repeated fairly frequently until a consistent result is obtained. The severity of the other findings will guide the clinician in the timing of fields for the sake of a baseline—the more severe the disease, the more frequently the field should be tested until it stabilizes. Use the two or three most consistent fields as a baseline.

True variability or poor reliability. If the first three fields show random variation, attempt to determine if the patient is reliable and the field is truly variable, or if the patient is not reliable. The assessment of reliability is reviewed on page 36. If the patient seems to be reliable but the fields vary substantially, we may use an average of three fields as a baseline by creating a Master field (Figs. 2-11 and 2-12).

If the fields vary widely and apparently randomly, and if it seems that the patient is unreliable, attempt to reeducate the patient as to how to perform perimetry. If this does not help, at some point it may be determined that threshold fields will not be useful (Fig. 2-13). This is one instance when it is appropriate to try a suprathreshold field; if test length contributes to the patient's unreliability, suprathreshold testing may be better than nothing. If the patient simply cannot perform reliable field examinations, then he or she may be followed as described on pages 82 and 120.

Text continued on page 25.

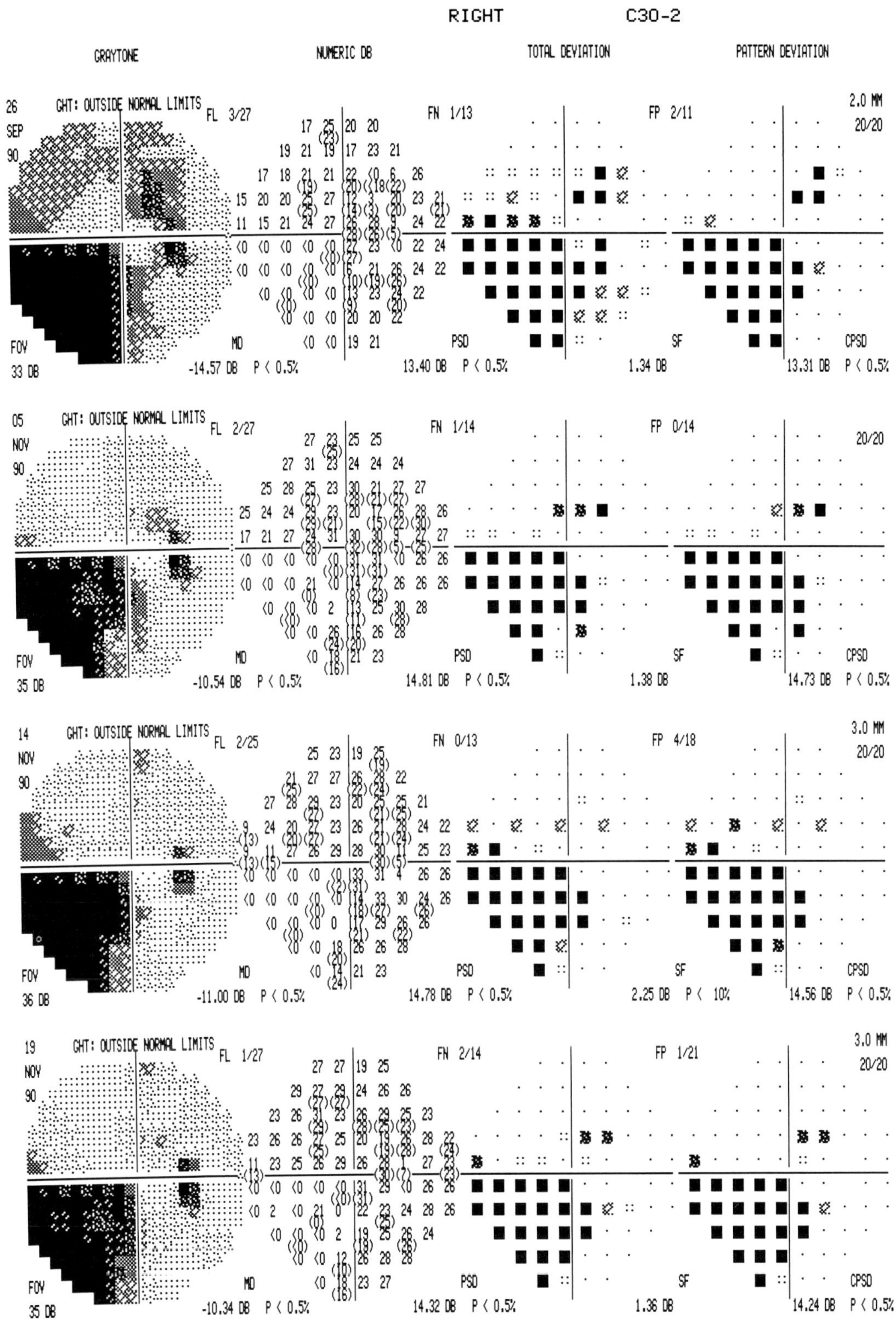

FIG. 2-8 Learning effect. The first four fields were obtained within 2 months. The first underestimated the patient's visual field and should not be part of the baseline for future comparison.

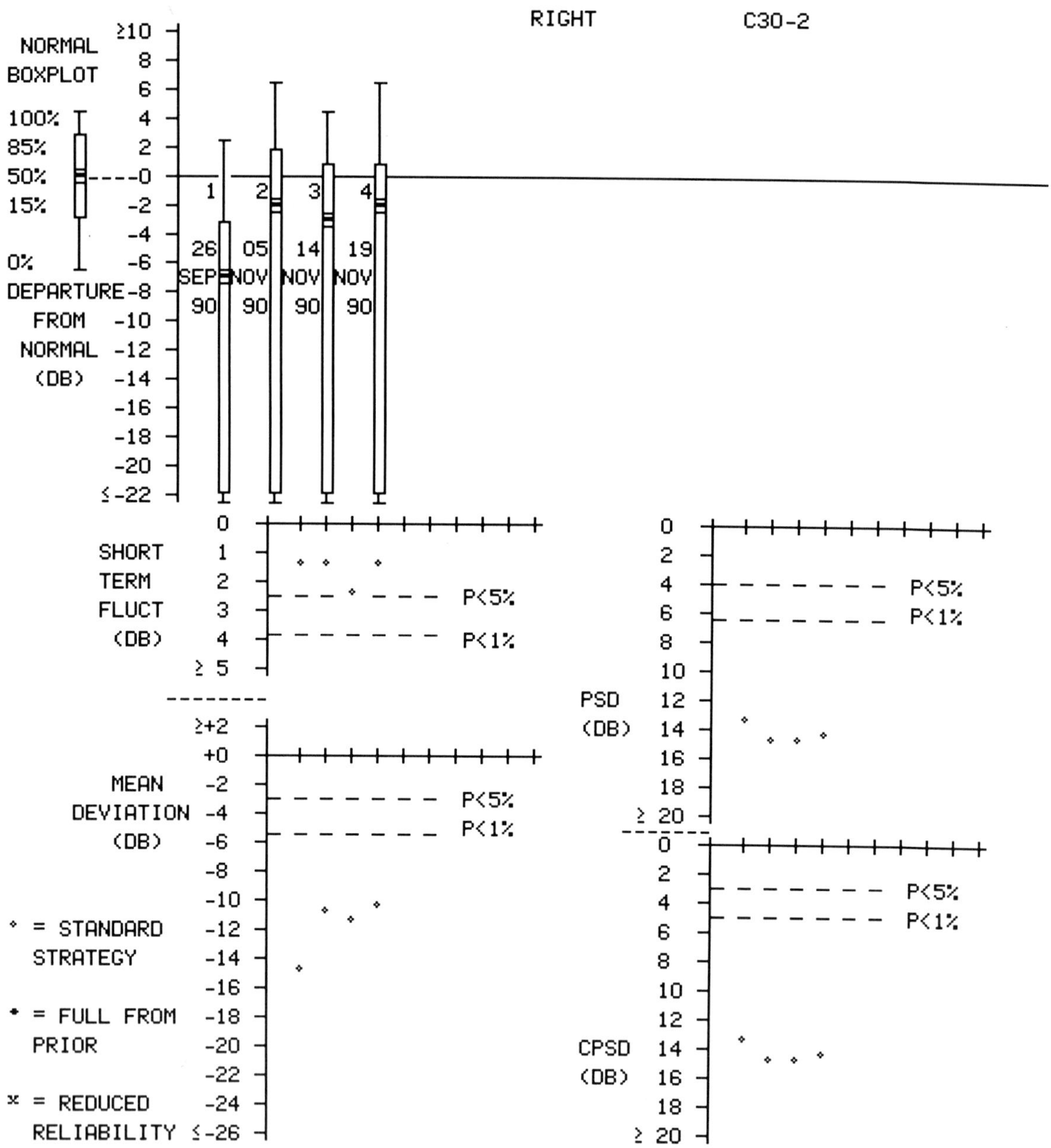

FIG. 2-9 Learning effect. Change analysis printout corresponding to Fig. 2-8.

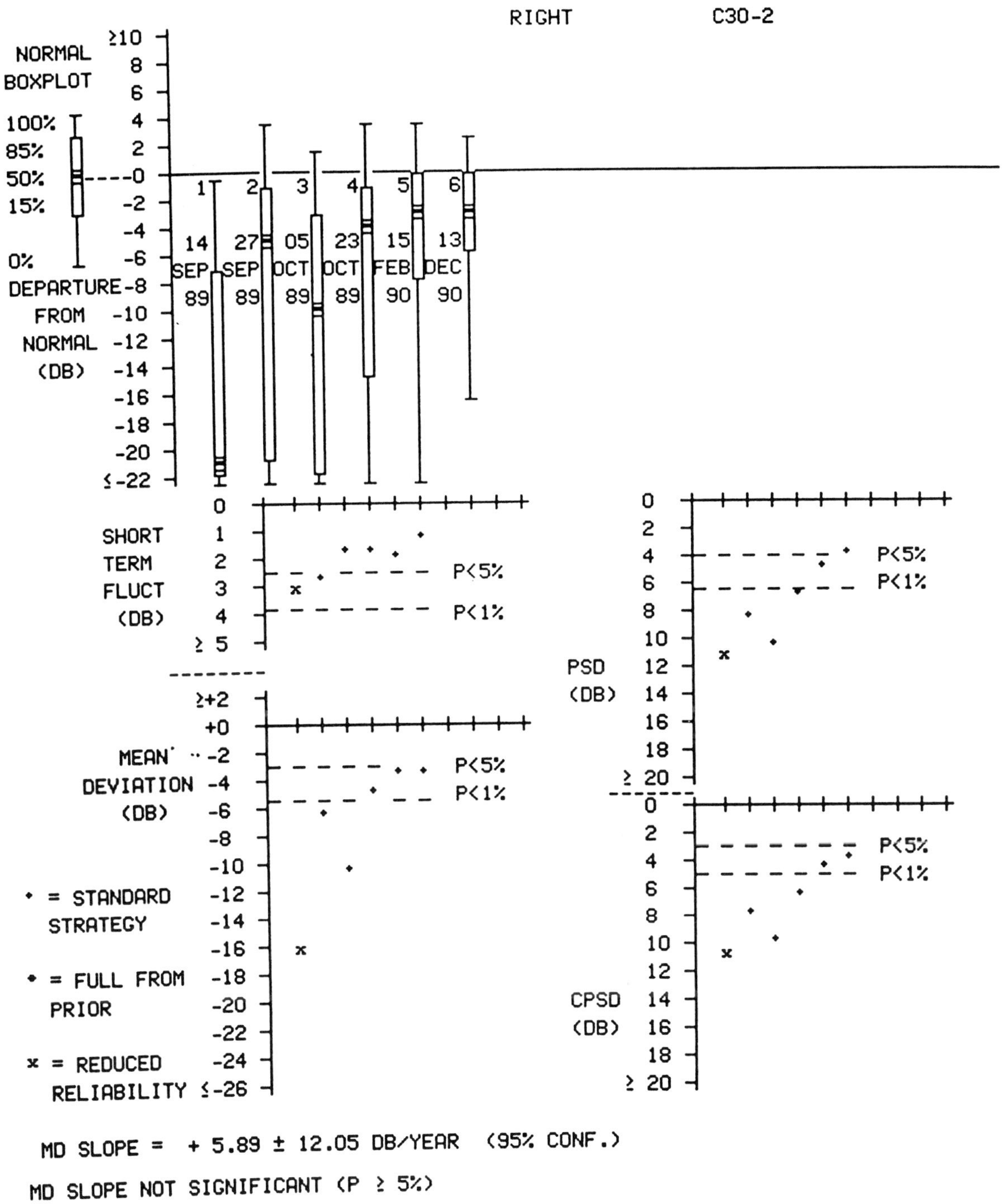

FIG. 2-10 Learning effect over multiple examinations. Until the learning curve levels, it is difficult to determine progression.

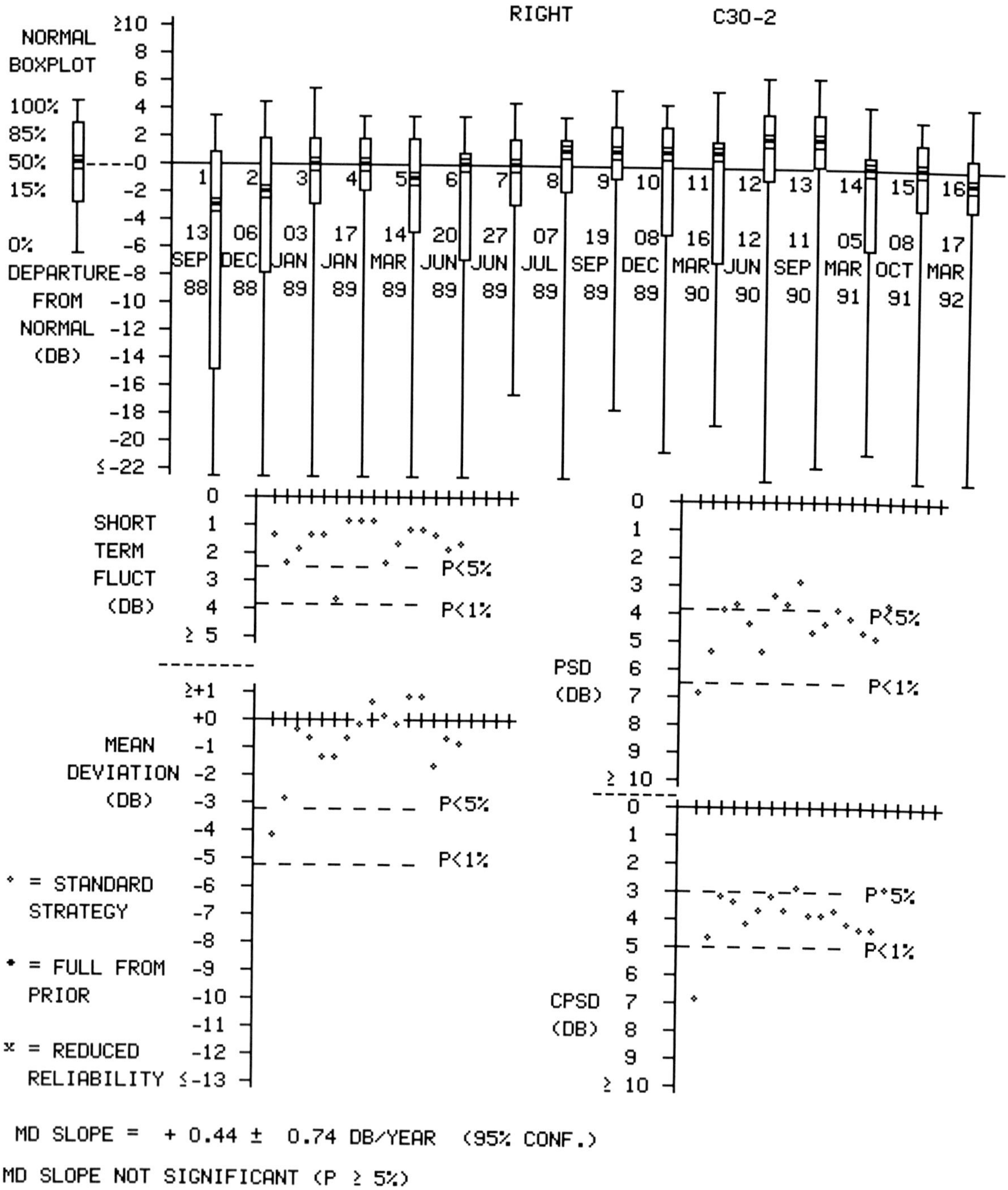

FIG. 2-11 Variable fields. This patient with early glaucoma had a learning effect and demonstrated ongoing variability. Her third, fourth, and fifth fields provide a reasonable averaged baseline.

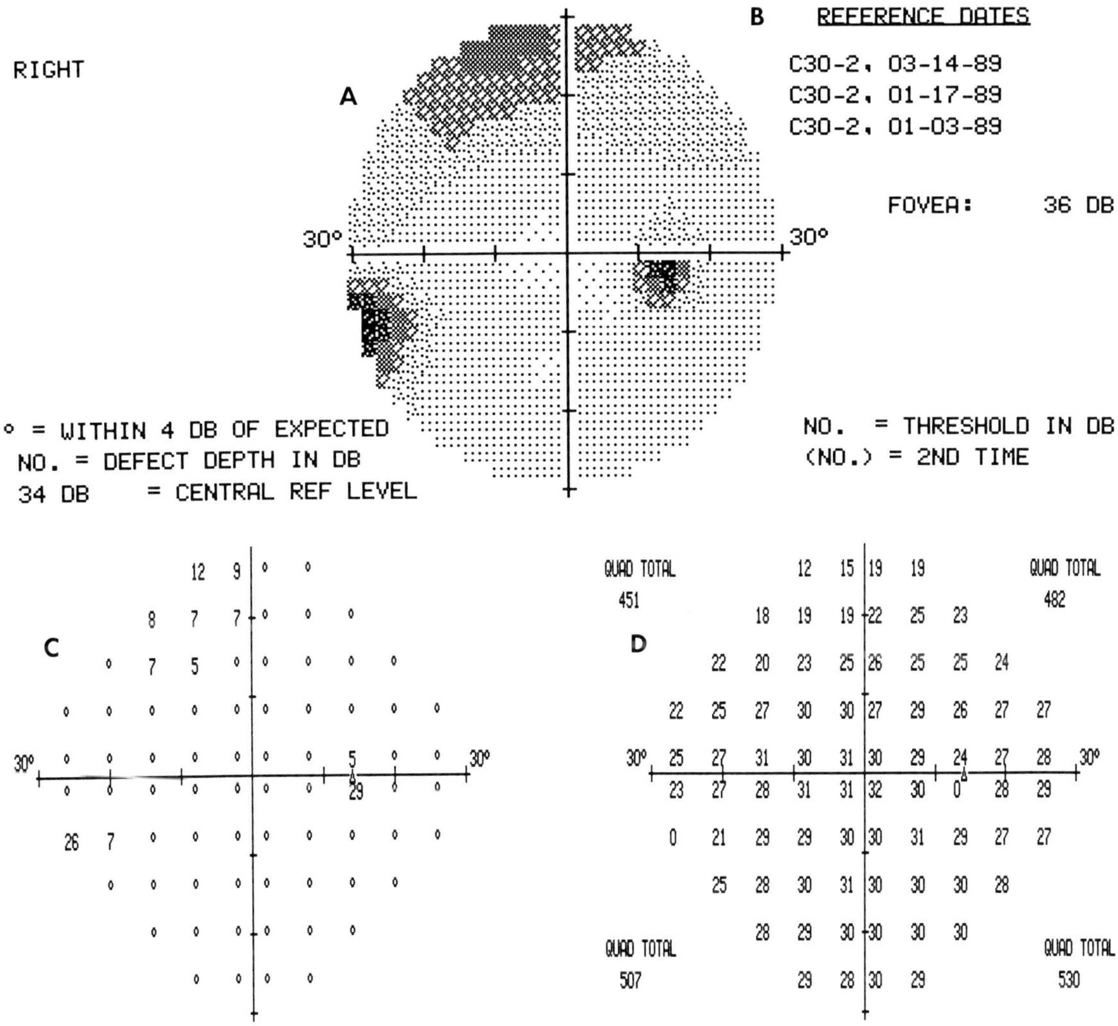

FIG. 2-12 Master file of fields 3, 4, and 5 from Fig. 2-11. **A,** Greyscale. **B,** List of fields combined to form Master. **C,** Defect depth plot. Numbers represent the defect depth of points that are at least 5 dB depressed compared to the overall height of the patient's hill of vision. *o* refers to points that are within 4 dB of expected. **D,** Average threshold values at each point.

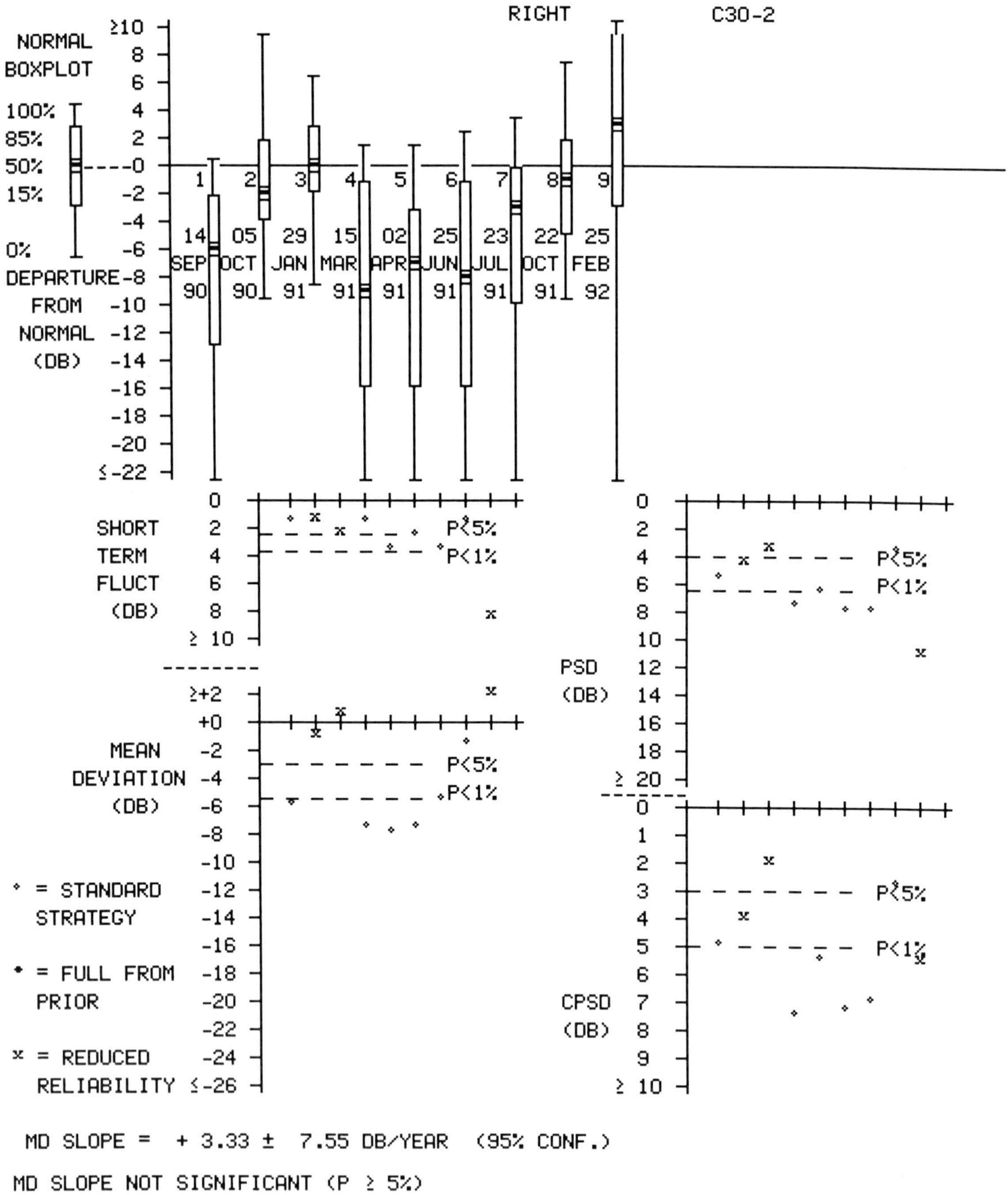

FIG. 2-13 Widely variable fields without a stable baseline.

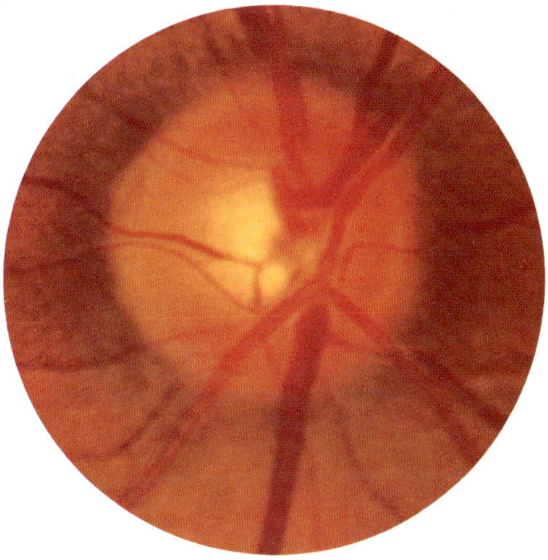

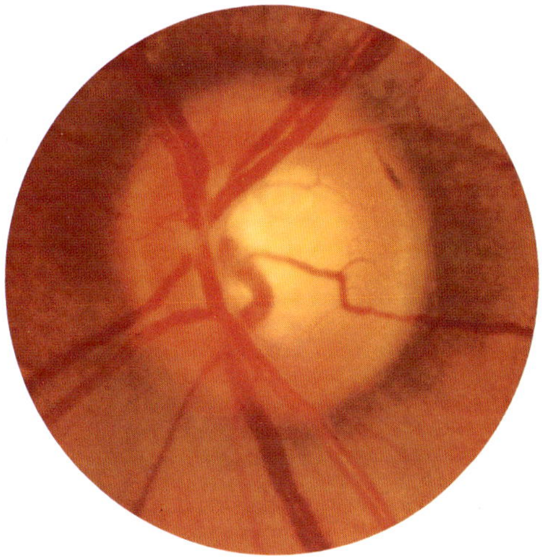

PLATES 1 and 2 Cup asymmetry in nerves of equal size. The patient has early glaucoma.

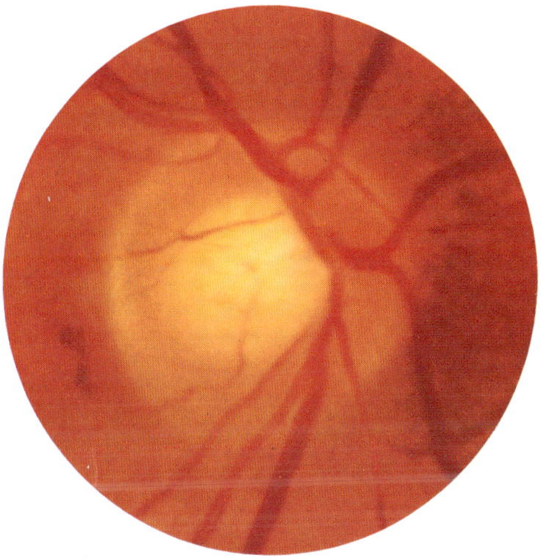

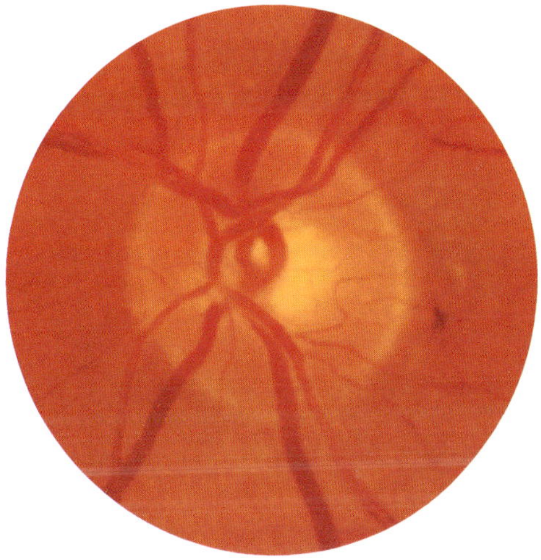

PLATE 3 and 4 Cup asymmetry in nerves of different size. The patient does not have glaucoma.

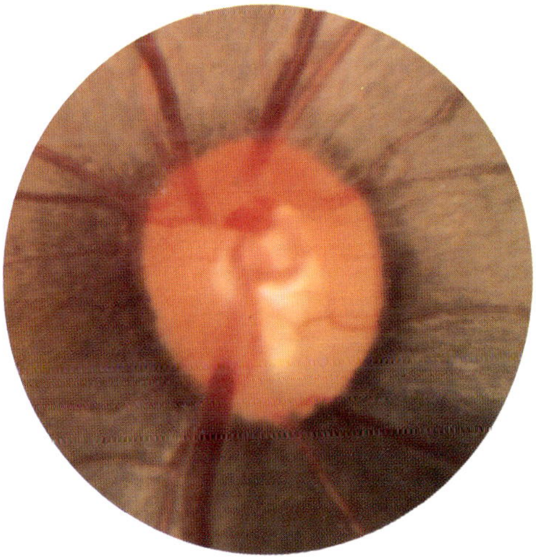

PLATE 5 Vertical elongation of the cup.

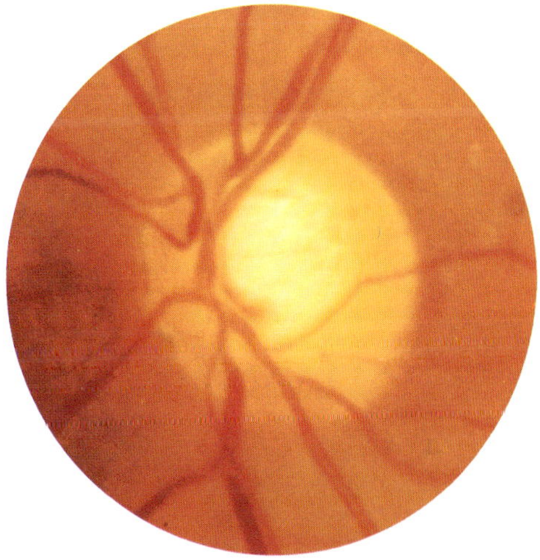

PLATE 6 Thinning of the rim at the superior pole of the disc.

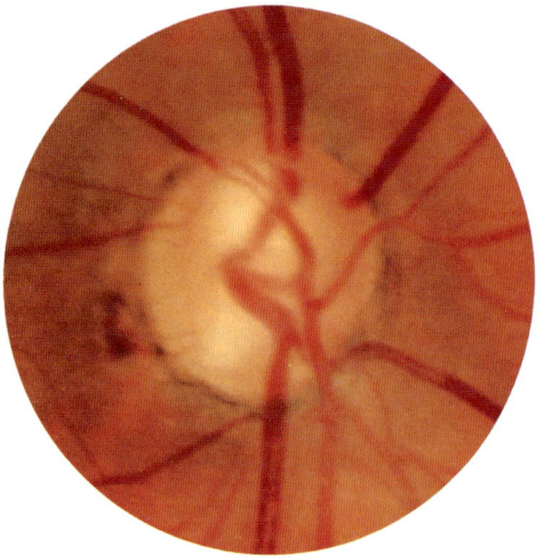

PLATE 7 Notching of the neuroretinal rim both superotemporally and inferotemporally.

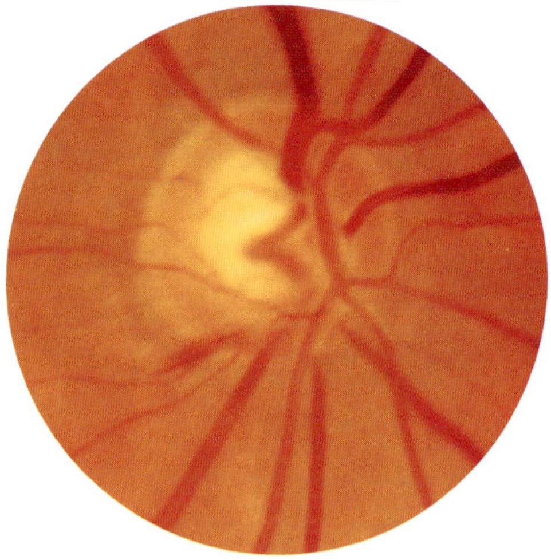

PLATE 8 Disc margin hemorrhage.

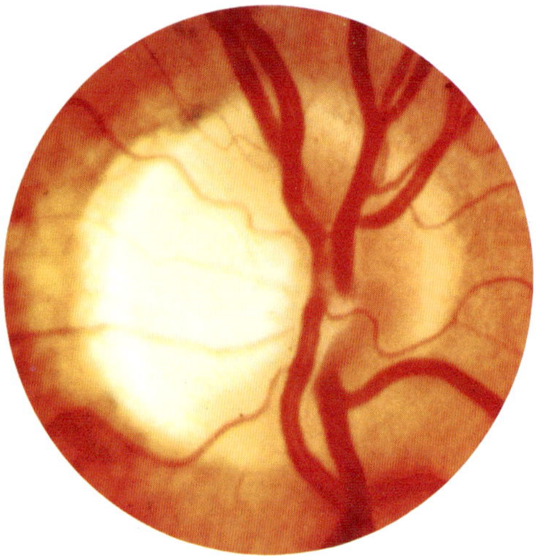

PLATE 9 Pallor out of proportion to cupping in a patient with dominant optic atrophy and a field defect. (Photo courtesy Joel Glaser, M.D.)

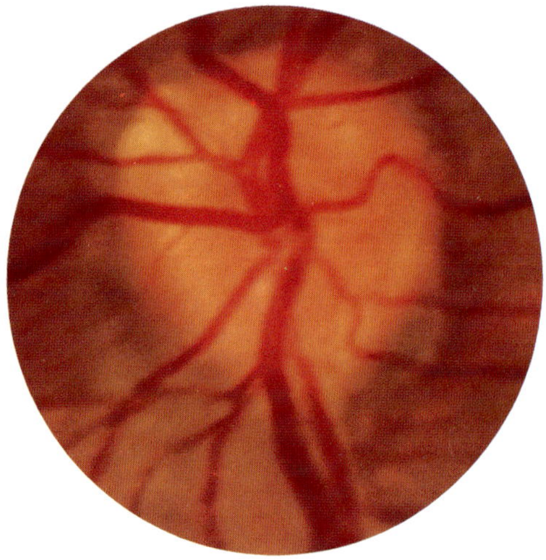

PLATE 10 Drusen of the disc associated with an arcuate field defect.

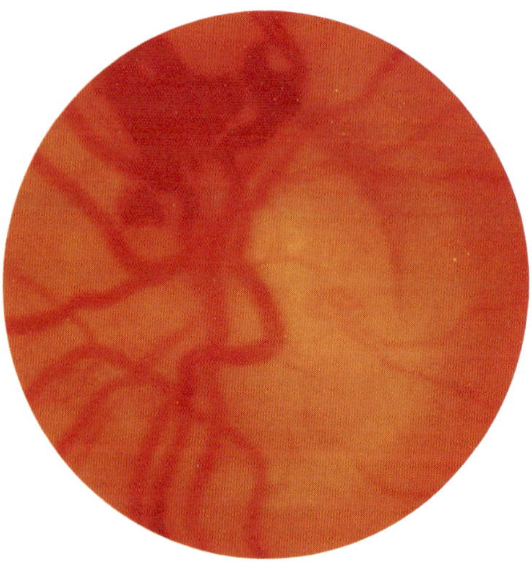

PLATE 11 Shunt vessels in a patient with a field defect and a previous central retinal vein occlusion.

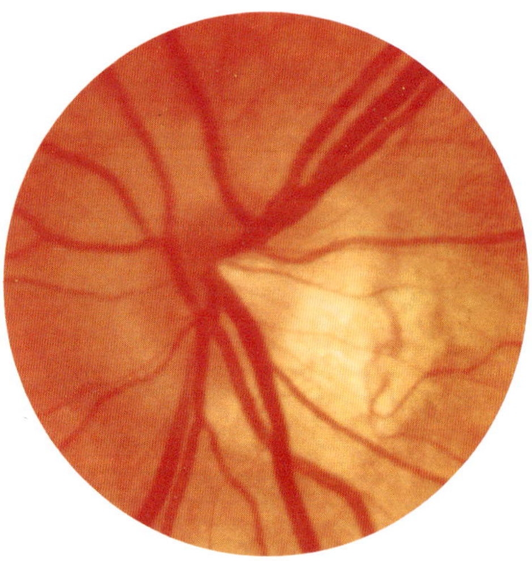

PLATE 12 Hypoplastic disc in a patient with a field defect. (Photo courtesy Joel Glaser, M.D.)

FIRST FIELD VERY DEPRESSED OR CONSTRICTED

Depression. The higher the threshold values and the more points seen, the better the basis to recognize changes. The standard 30-2 program uses a size 3 (4 mm^2) target. Retesting a very depressed field using a size 5 (64 mm^2) target may provide much more useful data (Figs. 2-14 and 2-15). The Statpac single-field analysis (to help determine if the field is normal or not) is not available for size 5. However, the decision to use size 5 presumes that the field is clearly abnormal; a baseline against which to judge progression is being produced. The overview printout is available for size 5 (Figs. 2-16 and 2-17).

Marked constriction. If the majority of points seen on the 30-2 threshold test fall within the central 10°, it is better to obtain a set of baseline 10-2 threshold tests. This program tests only the central 10° using points separated by 2° (Figs. 2-18 and 2-19). If the field is both depressed and constricted, a 10-2 program using a size 5 test object may be useful (Figs. 2-20 and 2-21).

Text continued on page 34.

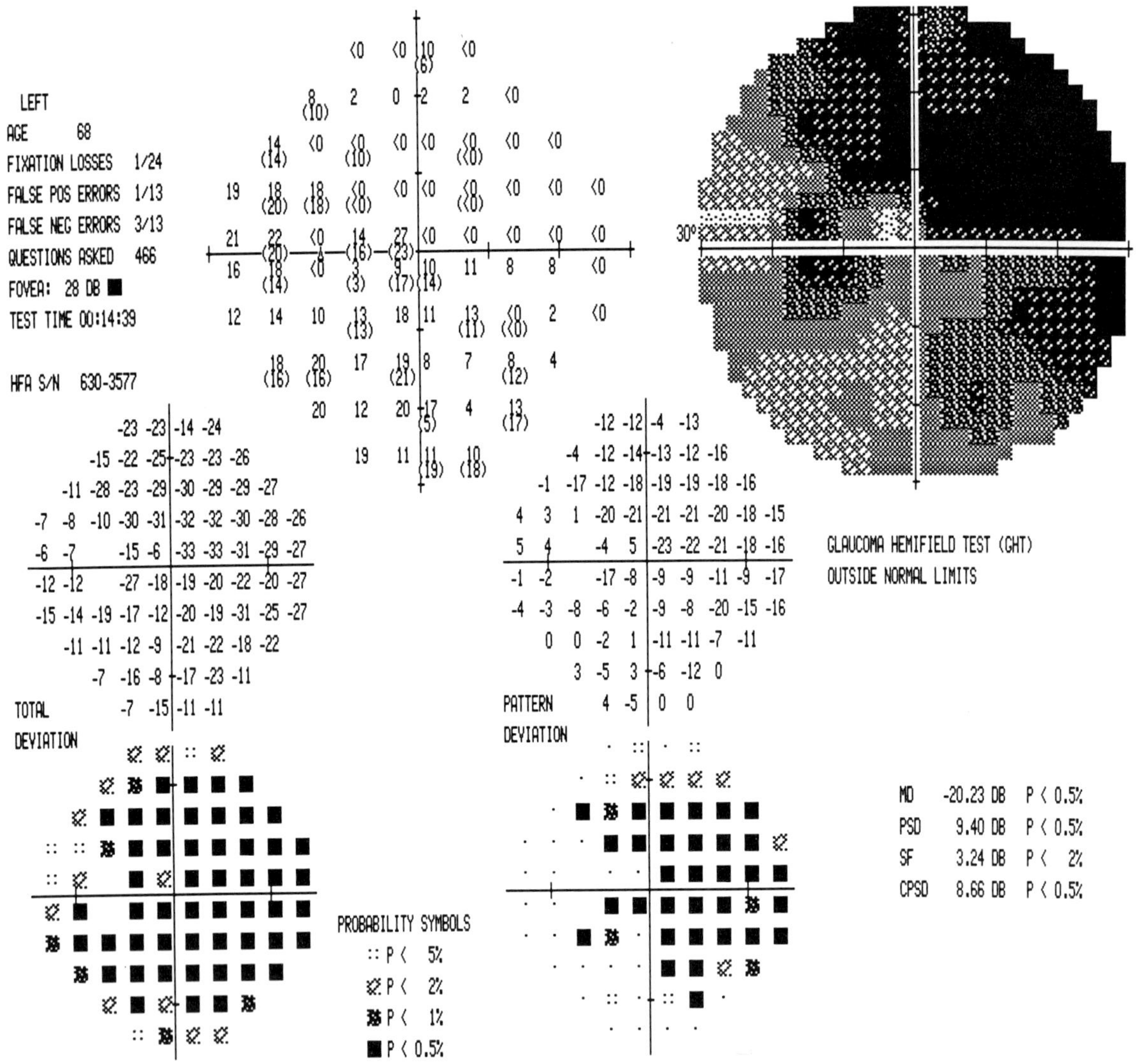

FIG. 2-14 Depressed field, size 3 target. Threshold values are so depressed that progressive deterioration will be impossible to judge well. The patient's field with a size 5 target is shown in Fig. 2-15.

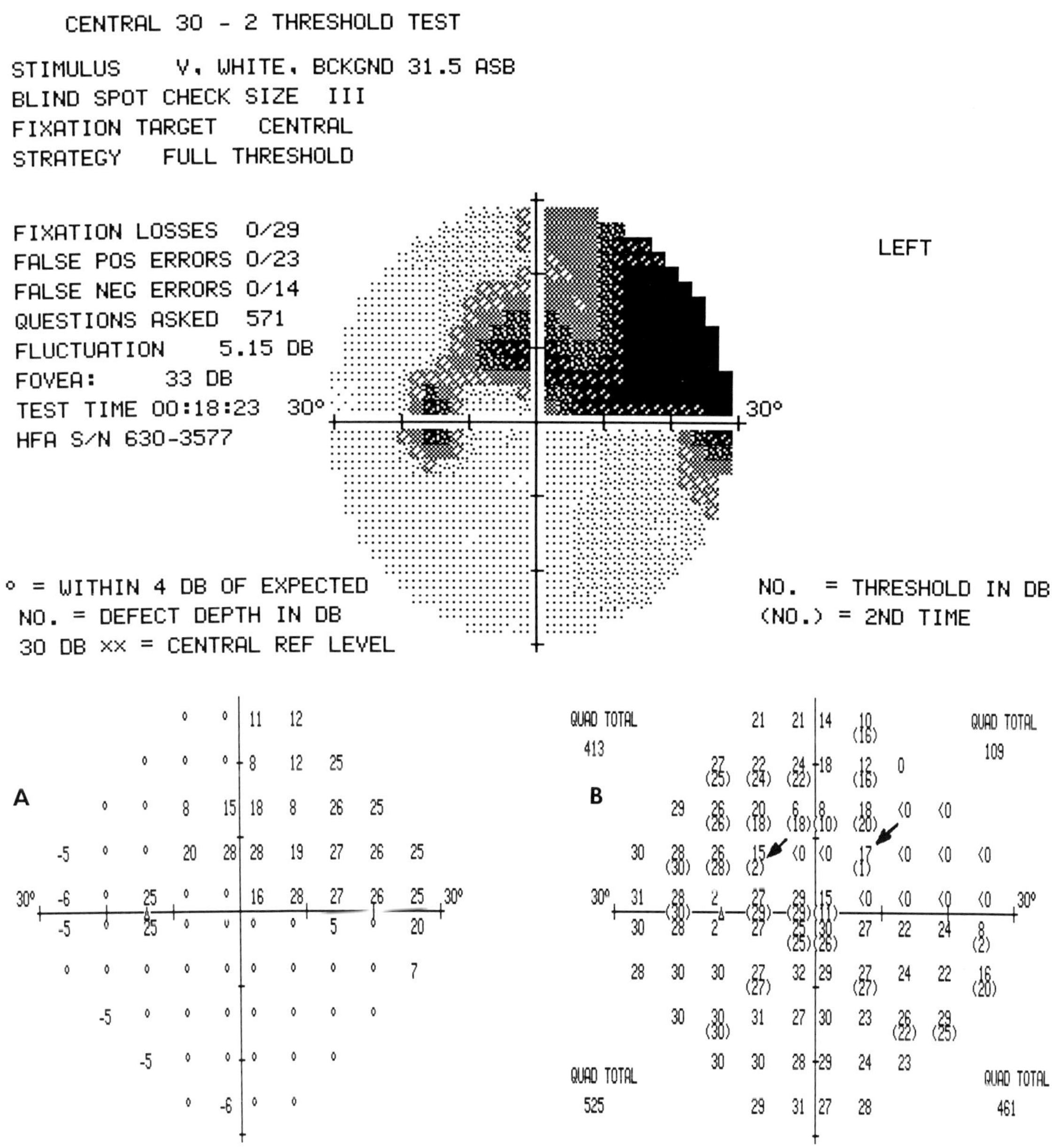

FIG. 2-15 Depressed field, size 5 target. **A,** The defect depth plot highlights points that are particularly depressed relative to the overall field. **B,** Threshold values. These sensitivities are high enough to follow. The high short-term fluctuation (5.15 dB) reflects the variability of two points on the border of an absolute scotoma *(arrows)*. In the less abnormal areas, the patient responded consistently.

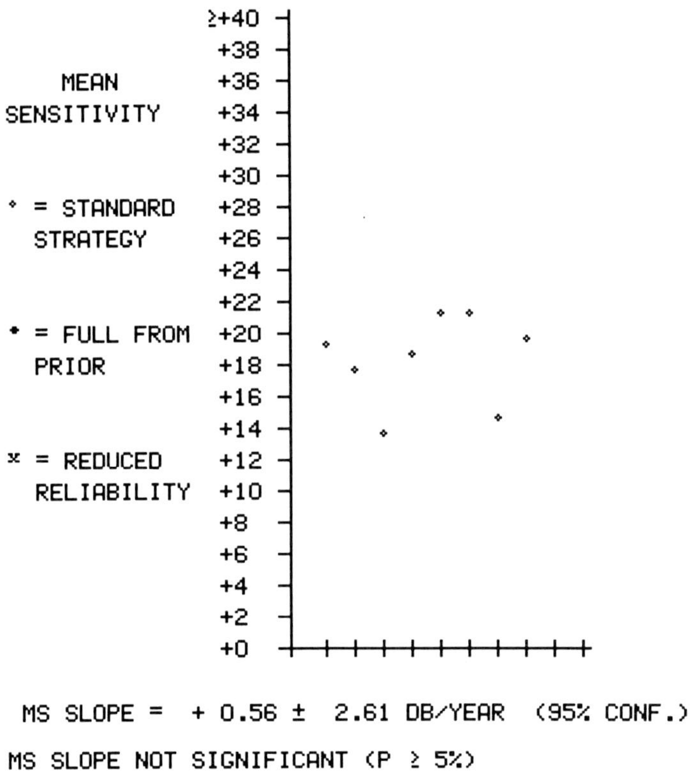

FIG. 2-16 Size 5 overview. Mean sensitivity of the series of fields chosen.

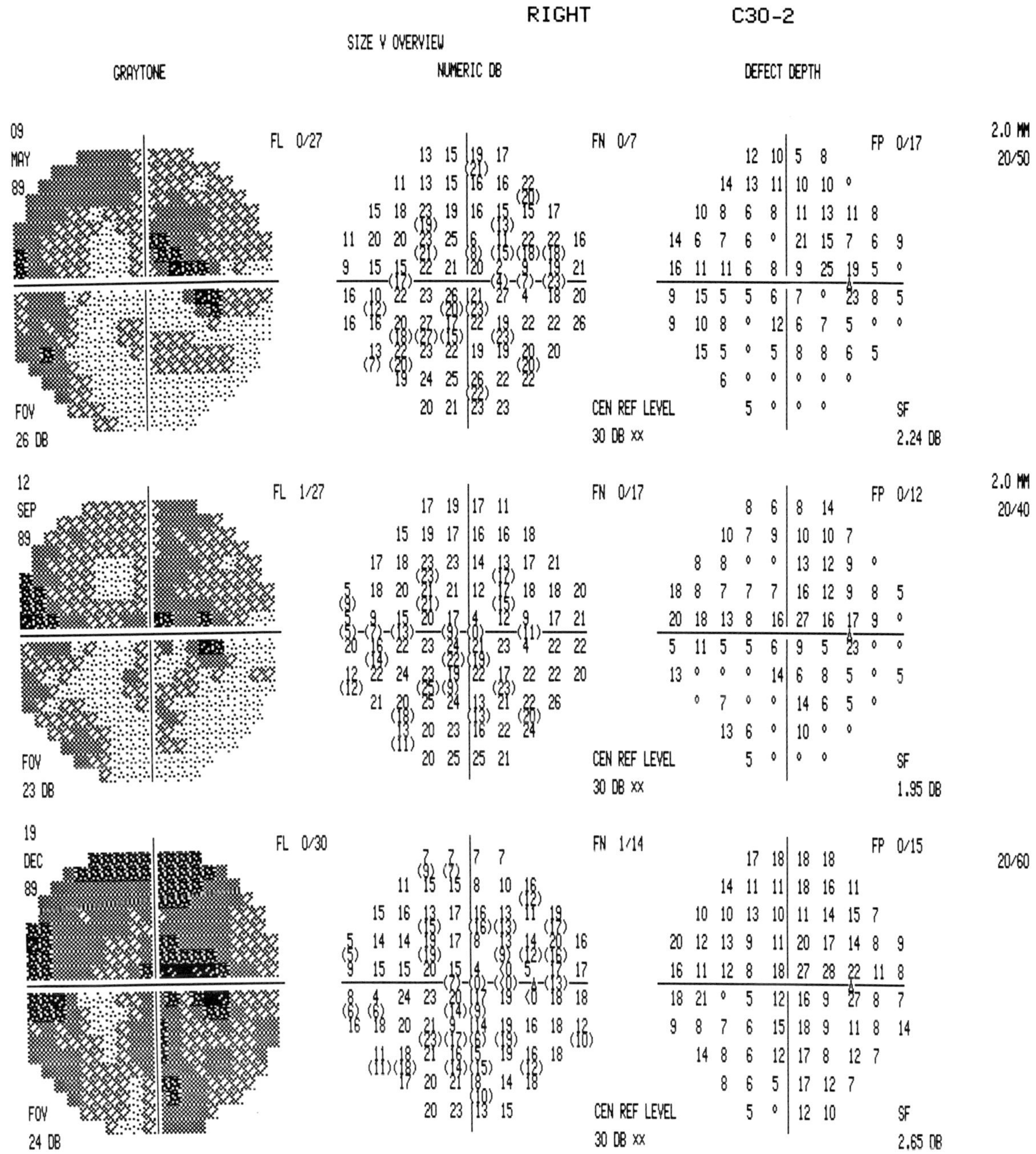

FIG. 2-17 Size 5 overview. Condensed printout. The defect depth plot refers to points that are particularly depressed compared to the patient's hill of vision.

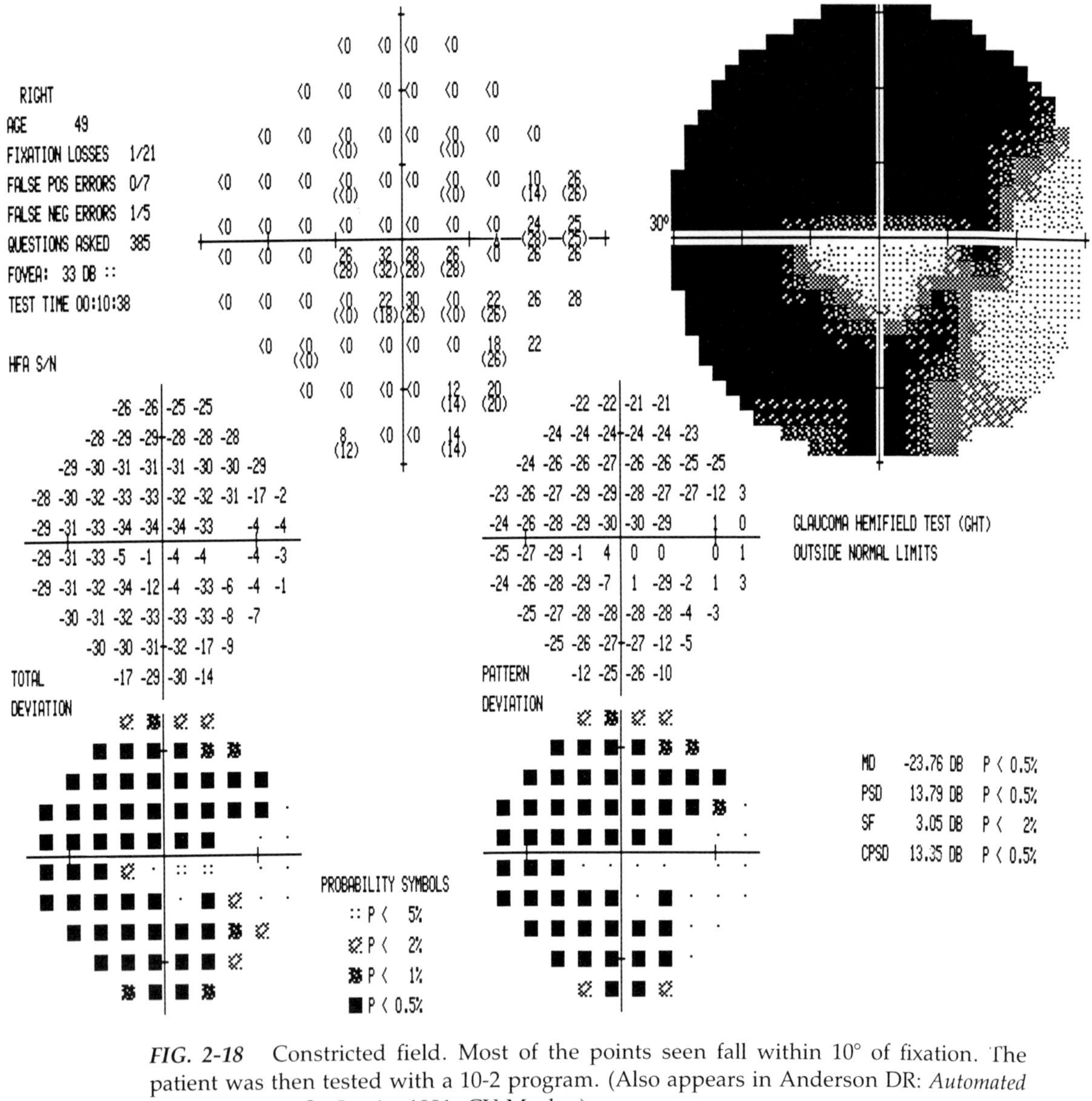

FIG. 2-18 Constricted field. Most of the points seen fall within 10° of fixation. The patient was then tested with a 10-2 program. (Also appears in Anderson DR: *Automated static perimetry*, St. Louis, 1991, CV Mosby.)

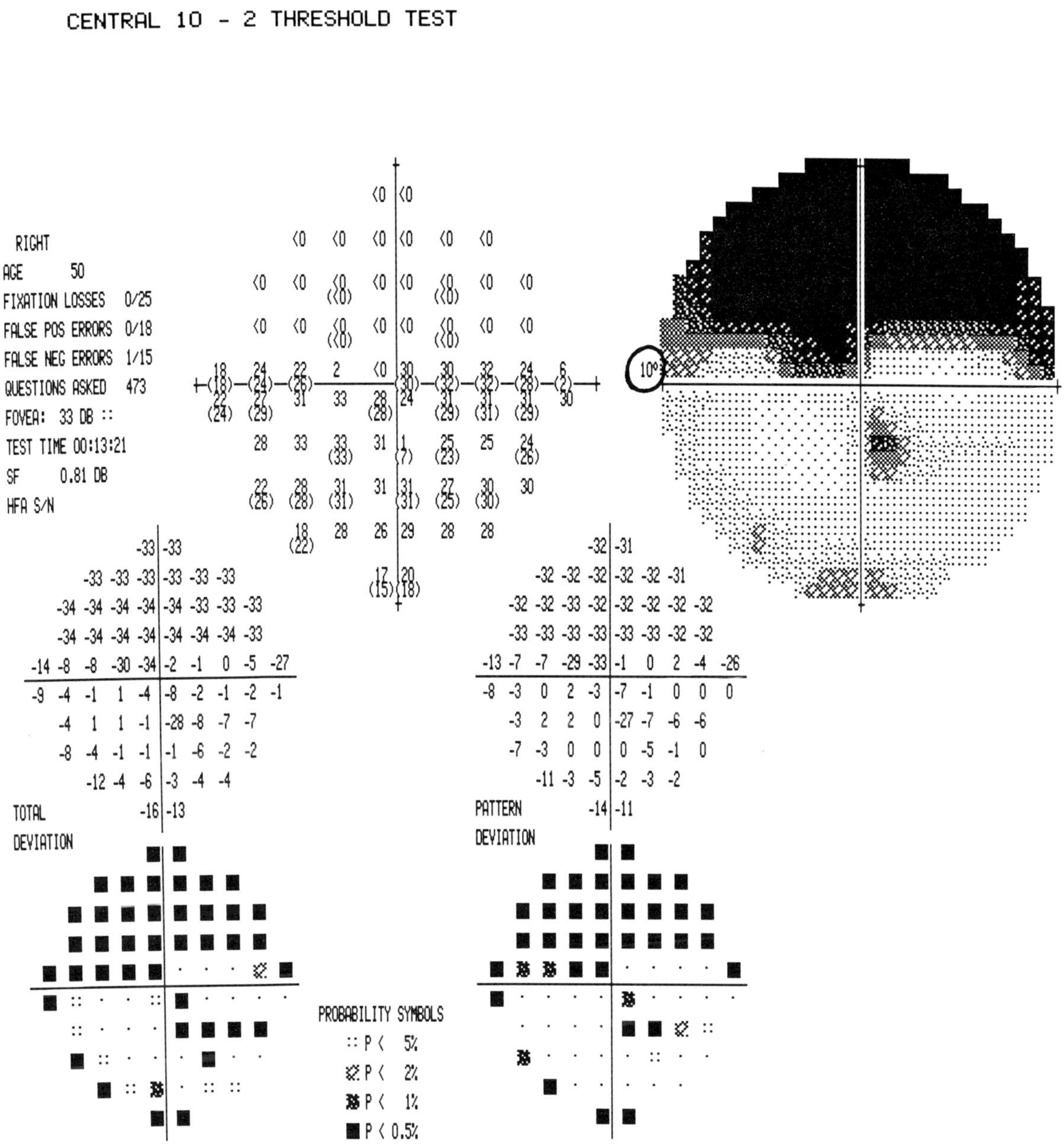

FIG. 2-19 The 10-2 test on the patient illustrated in Fig. 2-18 provides a larger number of test points to follow in the future; multiple fields can be printed in an overview. (Also appears in Anderson DR: *Automated static perimetry*, St. Louis, 1991, CV Mosby.)

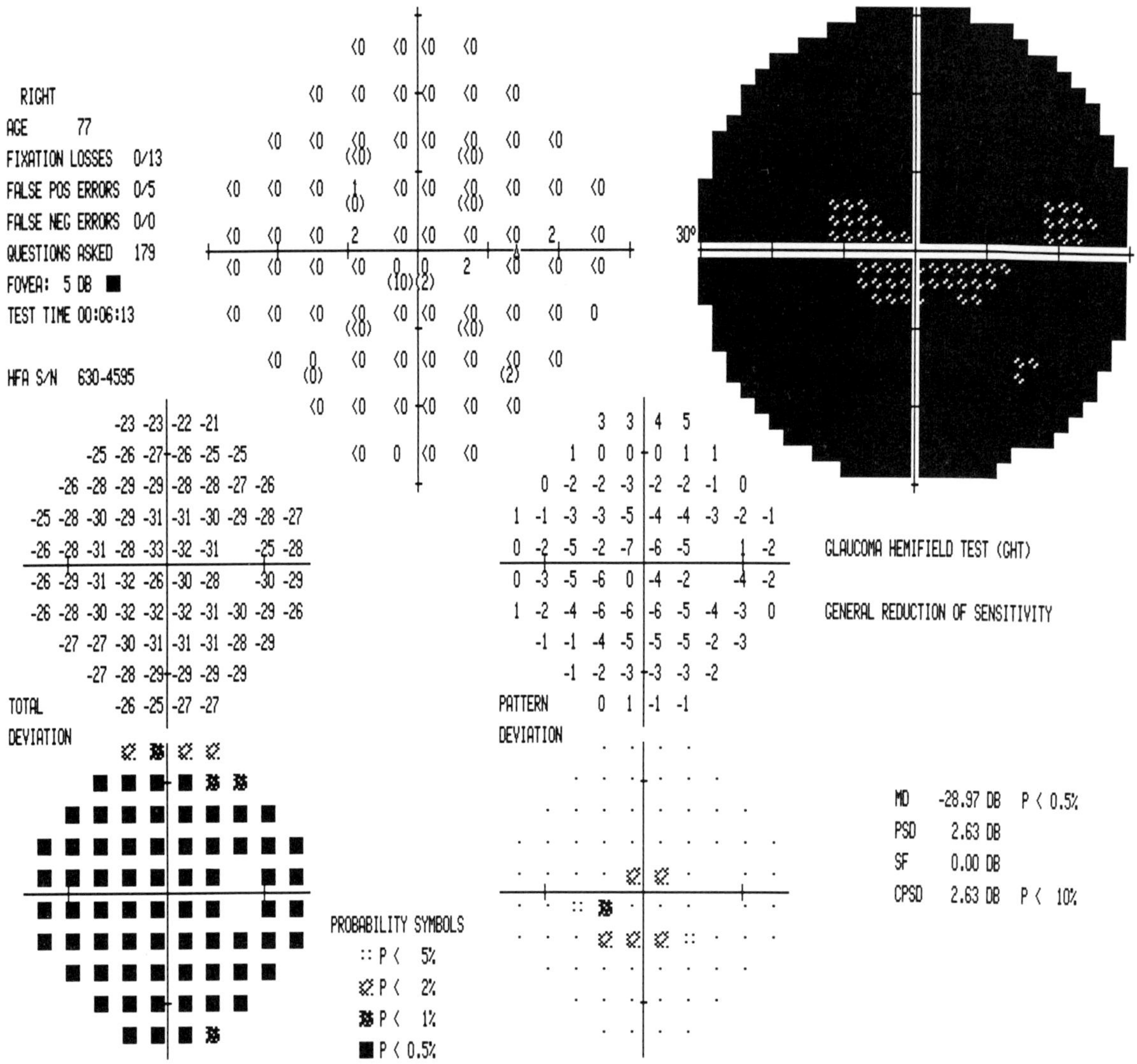

FIG. 2-20 Depressed and constricted field. 30-2 program with the size 3 (4 mm^2) target.

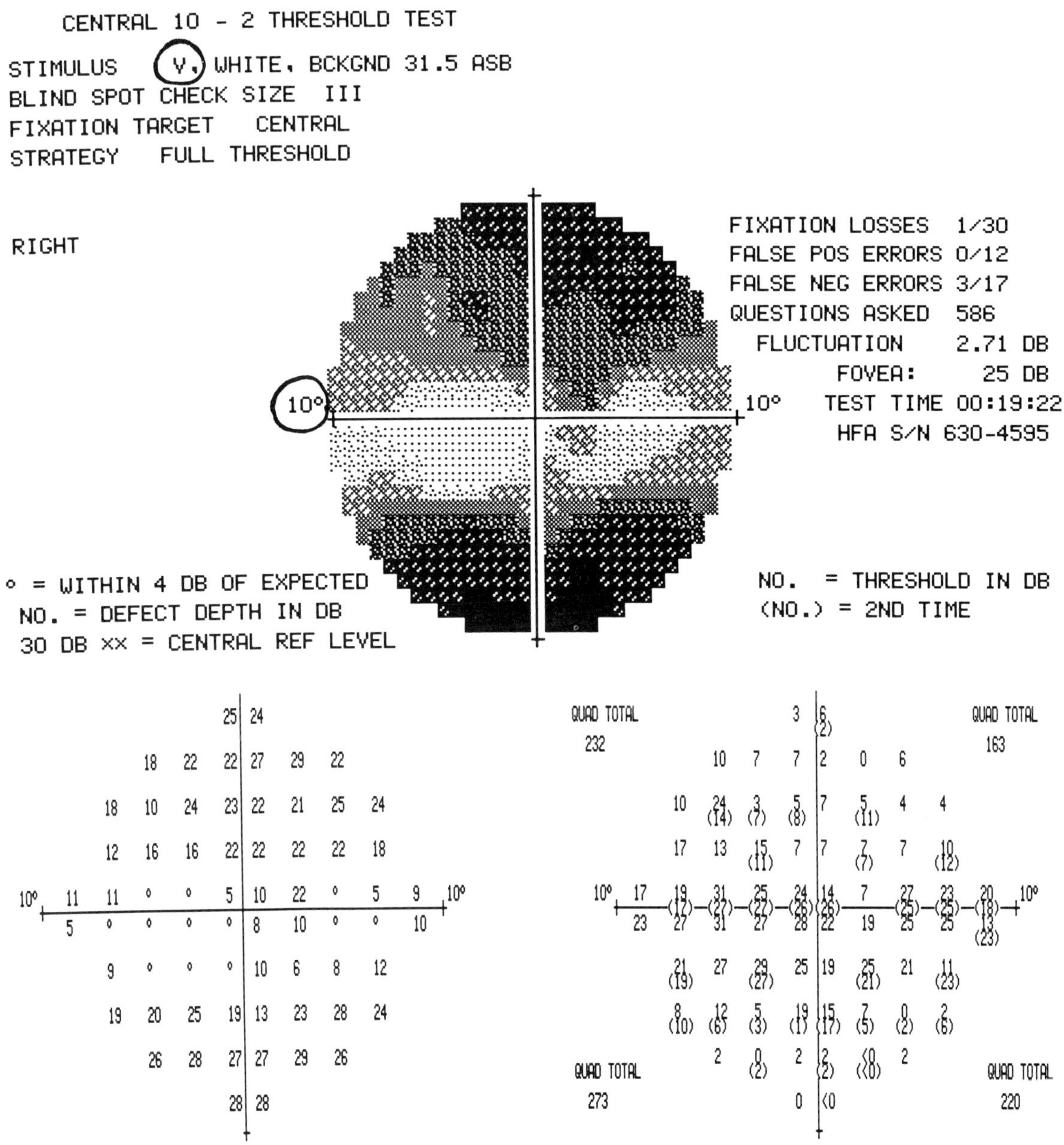

FIG. 2-21 10-2 program with the size 5 (64 mm^2) target on the patient illustrated in Fig. 2-20. The size 3 target was seen in only a few points.

Visual Field Interpretation

The interpretation of a visual field involves three steps—recognition of artifact, determination of reliability, and assessment for evidence of damage.

ARTIFACT

Two common field artifacts are those caused by the upper lid and the lens rim artifact. The lid artifact is always superior and thus easier to recognize (Fig. 2-22). A lens rim artifact appears if a corrective lens is either too far from the eye or is not centered. In either case the rim of the lens projects into the central 30°. Lens rim artifacts are usually sharply demarcated absolute defects (Fig. 2-23).

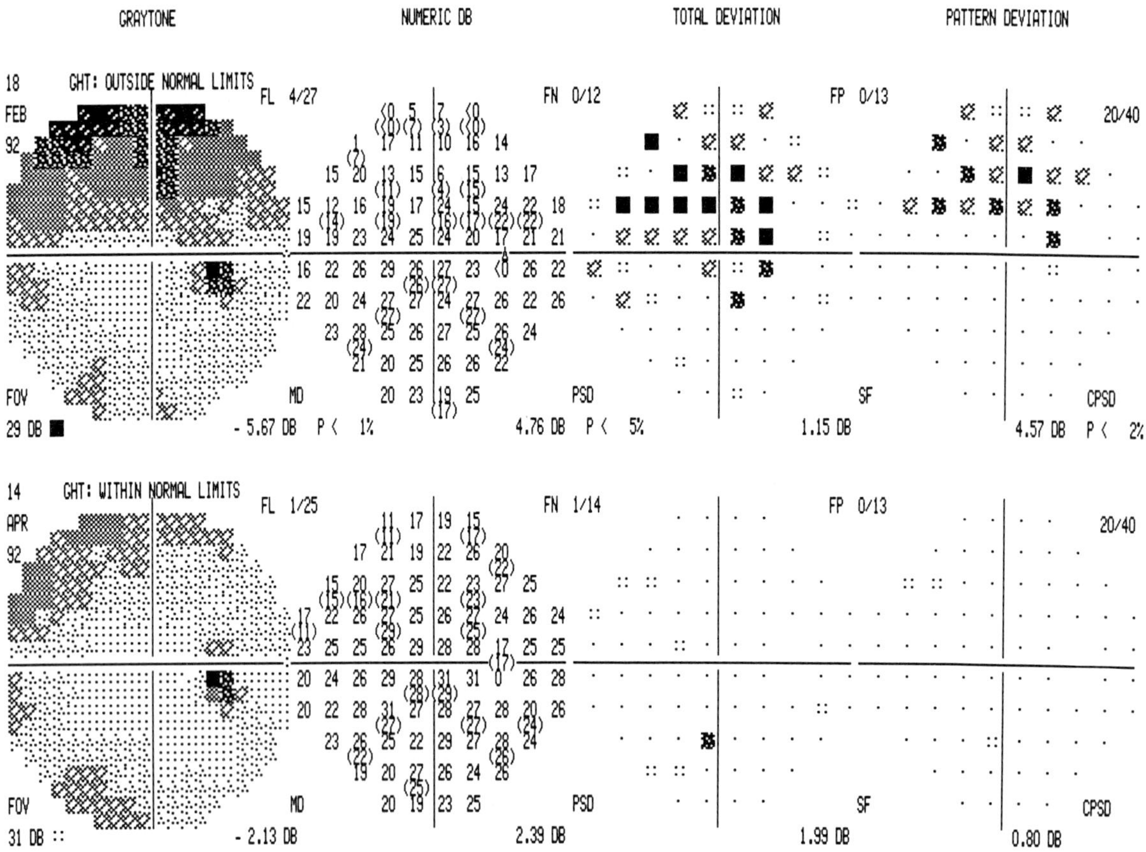

FIG. 2-22 Lid artifact. Between the first and second field, the patient had ptosis surgery.

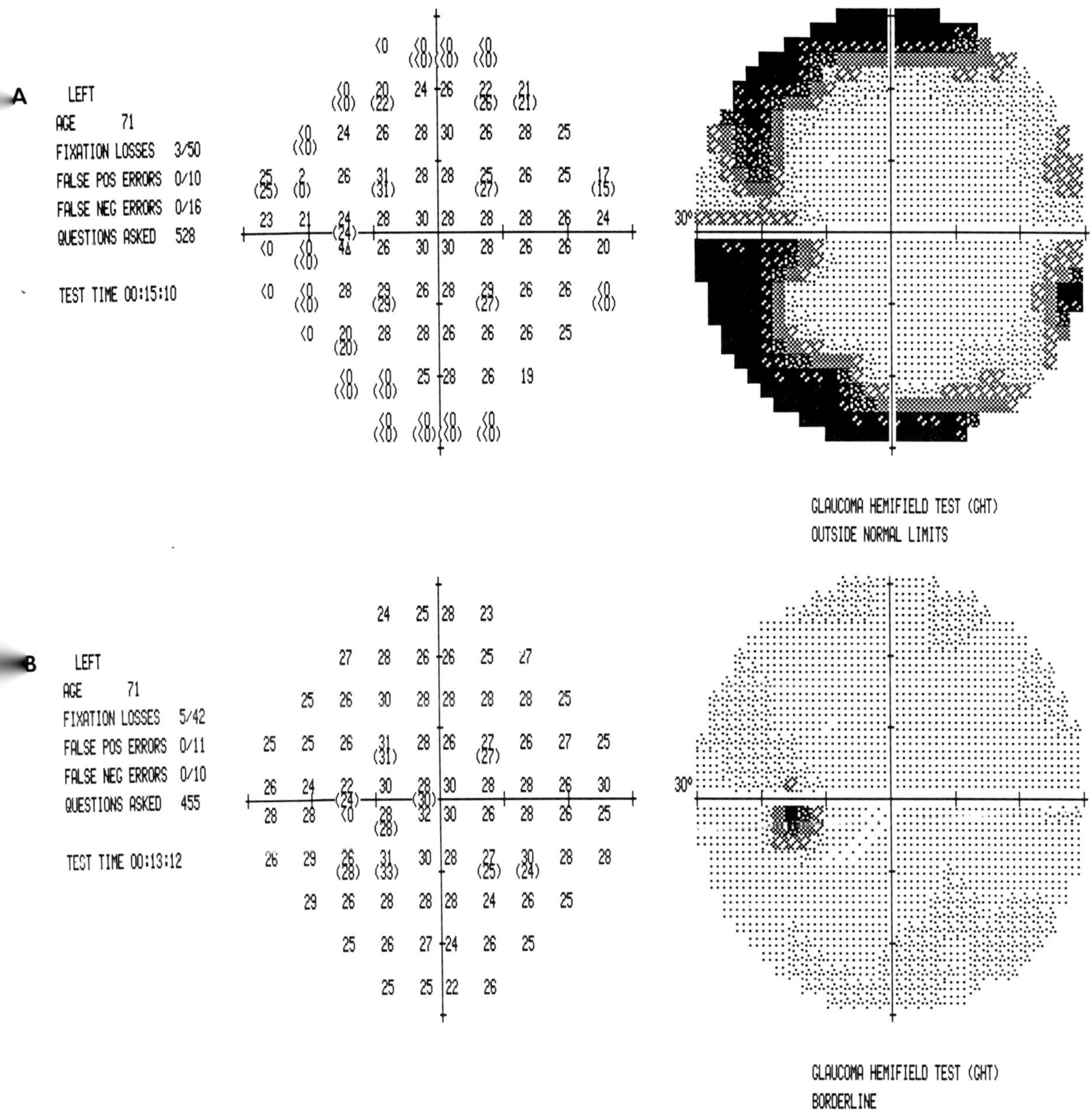

FIG. 2-23 Lens rim artifact. These fields were obtained 9 days apart. **A,** Typical absolute defect at the periphery of the field. **B,** Field obtained with lens centered and close to the eye.

RELIABILITY

Reliability estimates depend on four main signs: false-positive rate, false-negative rate, fixation loss rate, and short-term fluctuation. The clinician should determine the reliability of each field. In the context of beginning long-term management, however, it is reasonable to interpret the baseline fields together.

False positives. If the patient responds when the perimeter makes a noise but does not present a stimulus, the machine records a false-positive response. False-positive responses do not increase in damaged visual fields, and a field with more than one false-positive response is usually unreliable. The perimeter will signal low reliability if the false-positive rate is ≥33% (Fig. 2-24), but we regard fields with even one false-positive response with suspicion, and two or more as a sign of likely unreliability. Usually reliable fields can be obtained by educating the patient to be reasonably certain of seeing the stimulus, not to respond in haste (no need to respond while the stimulus is still on), and to expect stimuli that he or she cannot see. In such cases, the baseline examinations should be obtained after the education (Figs. 2-25 and 2-26). If educating a patient does not result in a more reliable field, then fields may simply not be helpful in that patient.

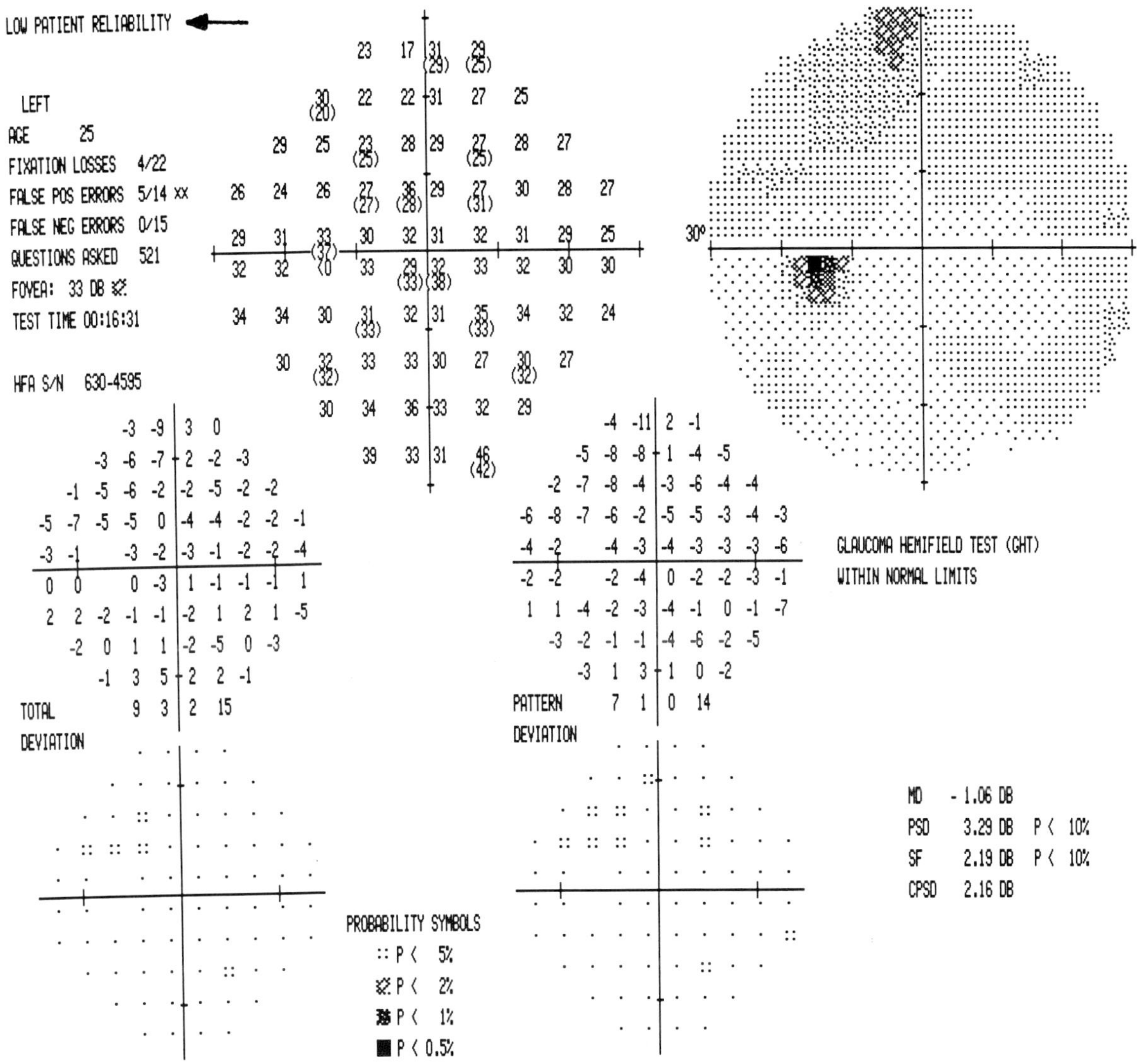

FIG. 2-24 High false-positive rate. This patient's false-positive rate just exceeds the 33% limit to prompt the unreliability message *(arrow)*.

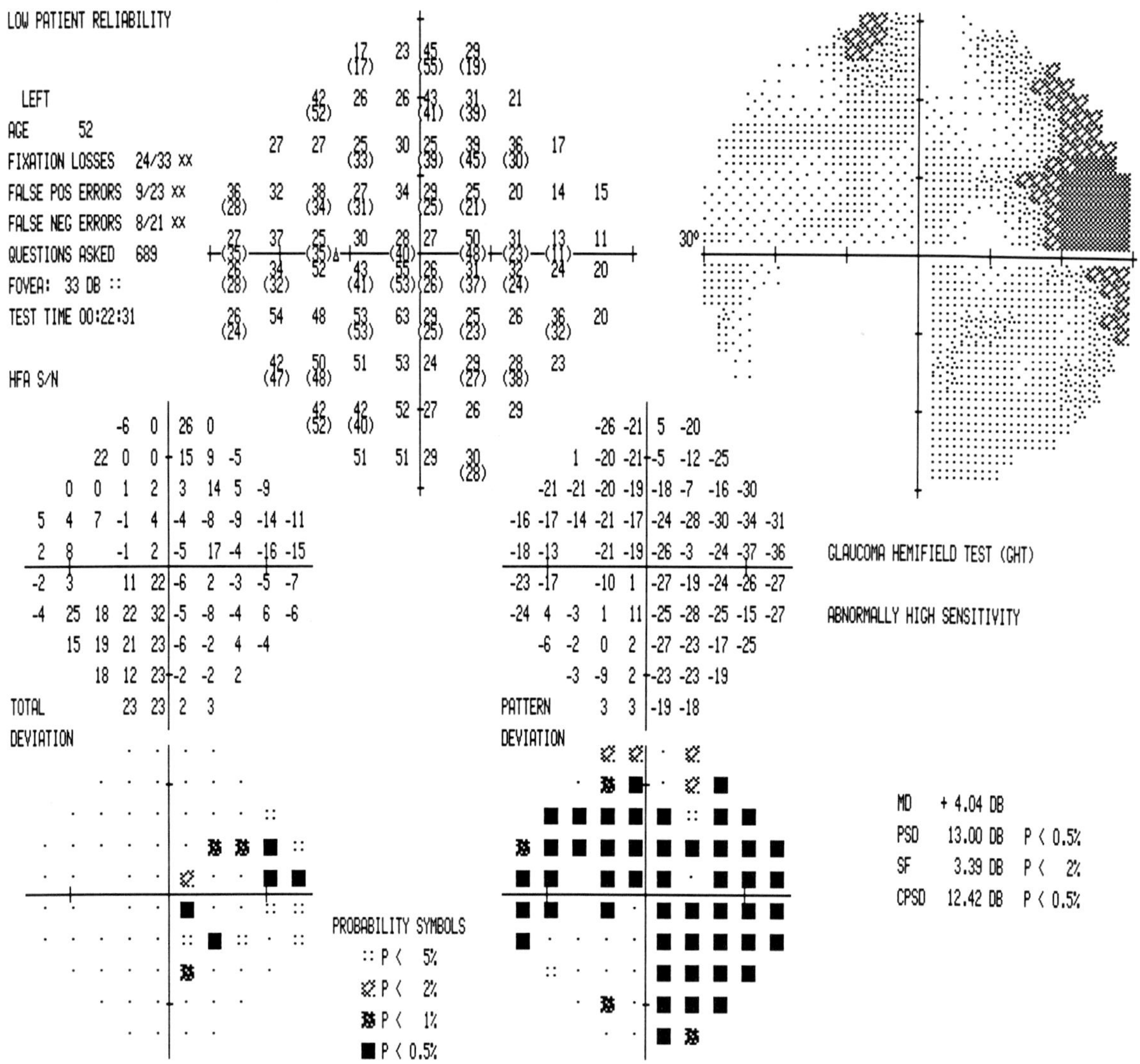

FIG. 2-25 High false-positive rate. The field is so abnormal that the clinician might be tempted to entirely abandon perimetry. However, the patient was educated in how to respond and, 3 weeks later, performed the field examination shown in Fig. 2-26. (Also appears in Anderson DR: *Automated static perimetry*, St. Louis, 1991, CV Mosby.)

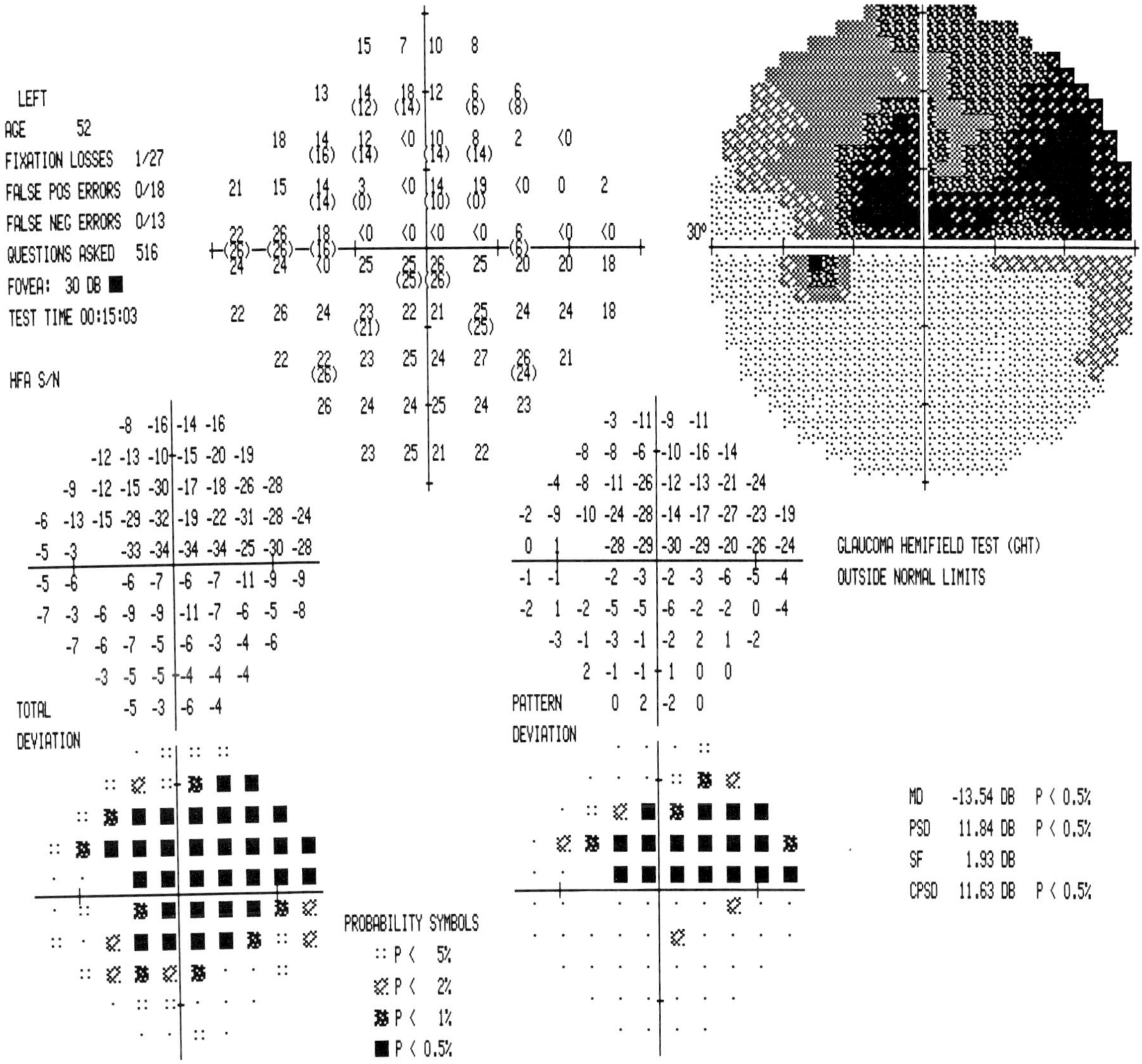

FIG. 2-26 High false-positive rate, after education. Same patient as in Fig. 2-25. (Also appears in Anderson DR: *Automated static perimetry*, St. Louis, 1991, CV Mosby.)

False negatives. False-negative responses—a failure to respond to a stimulus 9 dB brighter than one previously seen at the same location—do not necessarily indicate unreliable fields. Inconsistent responses characterize regions of depressed sensitivity, and a brighter stimulus may truly not be visible on second presentation (Fig. 2-27). Conversely, a tired patient may fail to respond to a stimulus that was previously visible to him or her; in this situation the field test is unreliable. Interpret fields with many false-negative responses in light of the entire clinical picture.

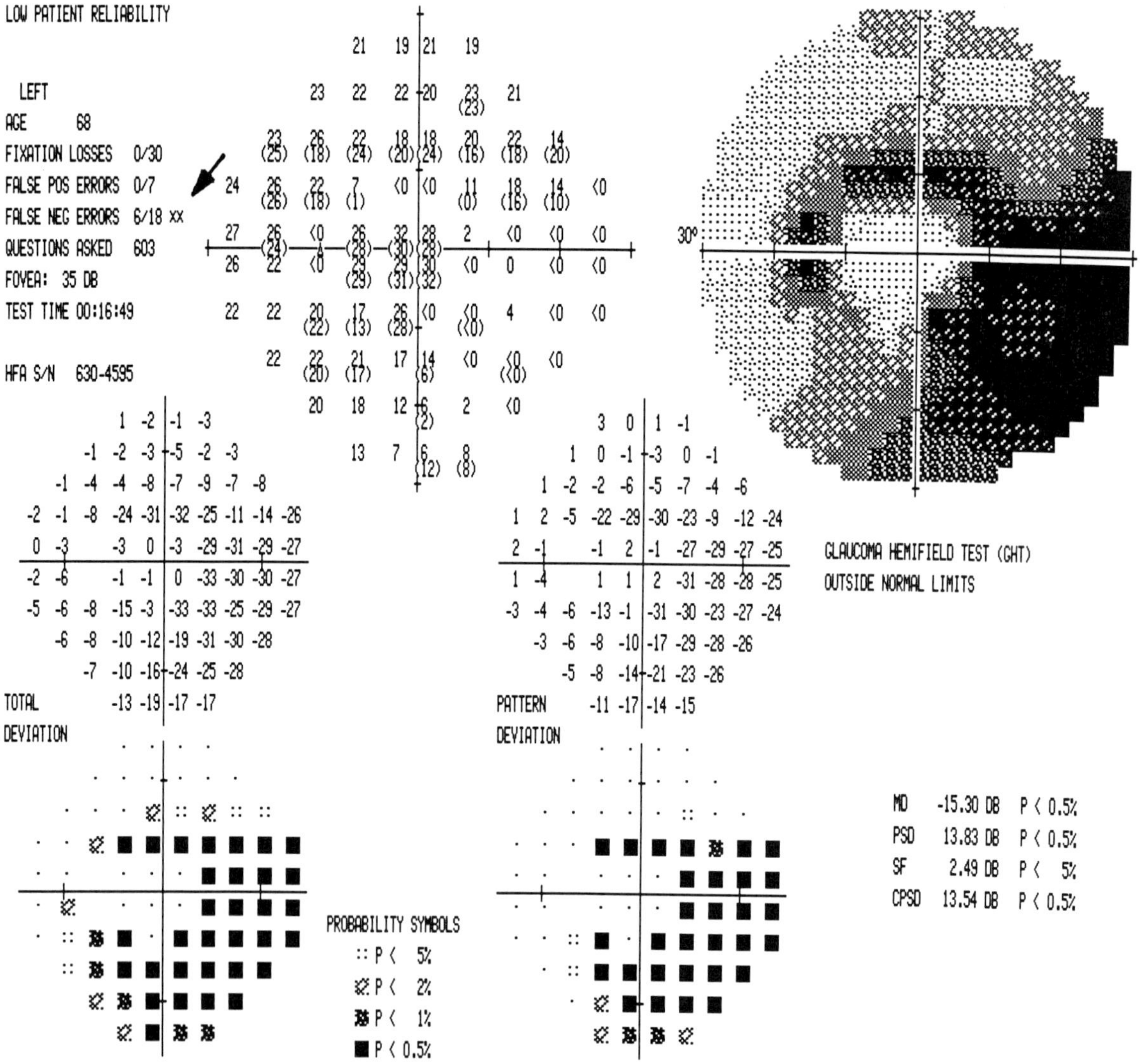

FIG. 2-27 High false-negative rate. In this widely damaged field, the false-negative rate *(arrow)* is probably related to true variability. There are no fixation losses, no false positives, and a short-term fluctation that is not high for a severely damaged field.

One characteristic field defect seen in people with high false-negative rates related to fatigue is the cloverleaf field in which the patient responds to the early test points but then fails to respond (Fig. 2-28). A variant of this field is the apparently constricted field shown in Figure 2-29, in which the patient failed to respond to the points tested last which were, because of the test logic, the peripheral points.

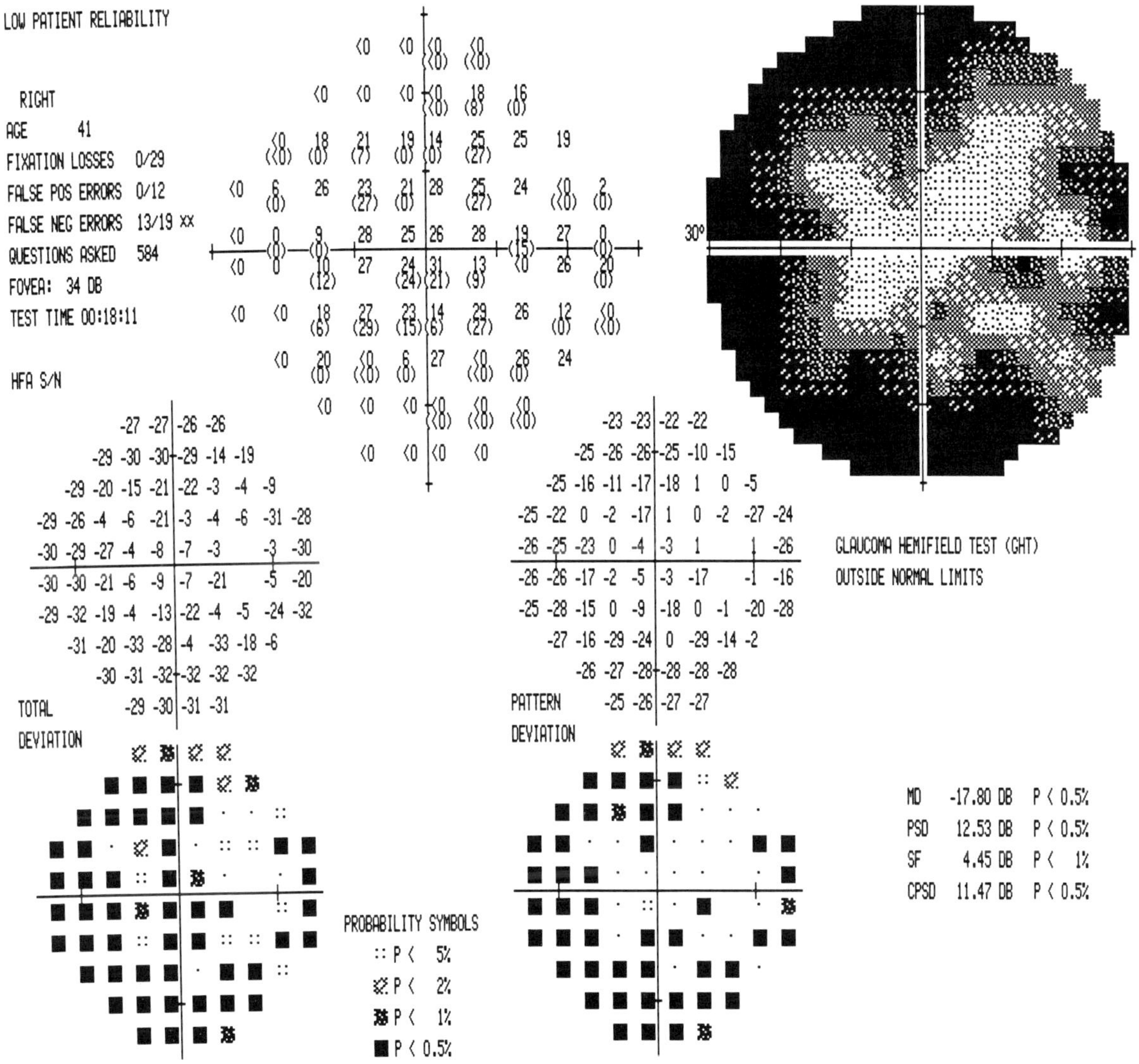

FIG. 2-28 Cloverleaf field (see text).

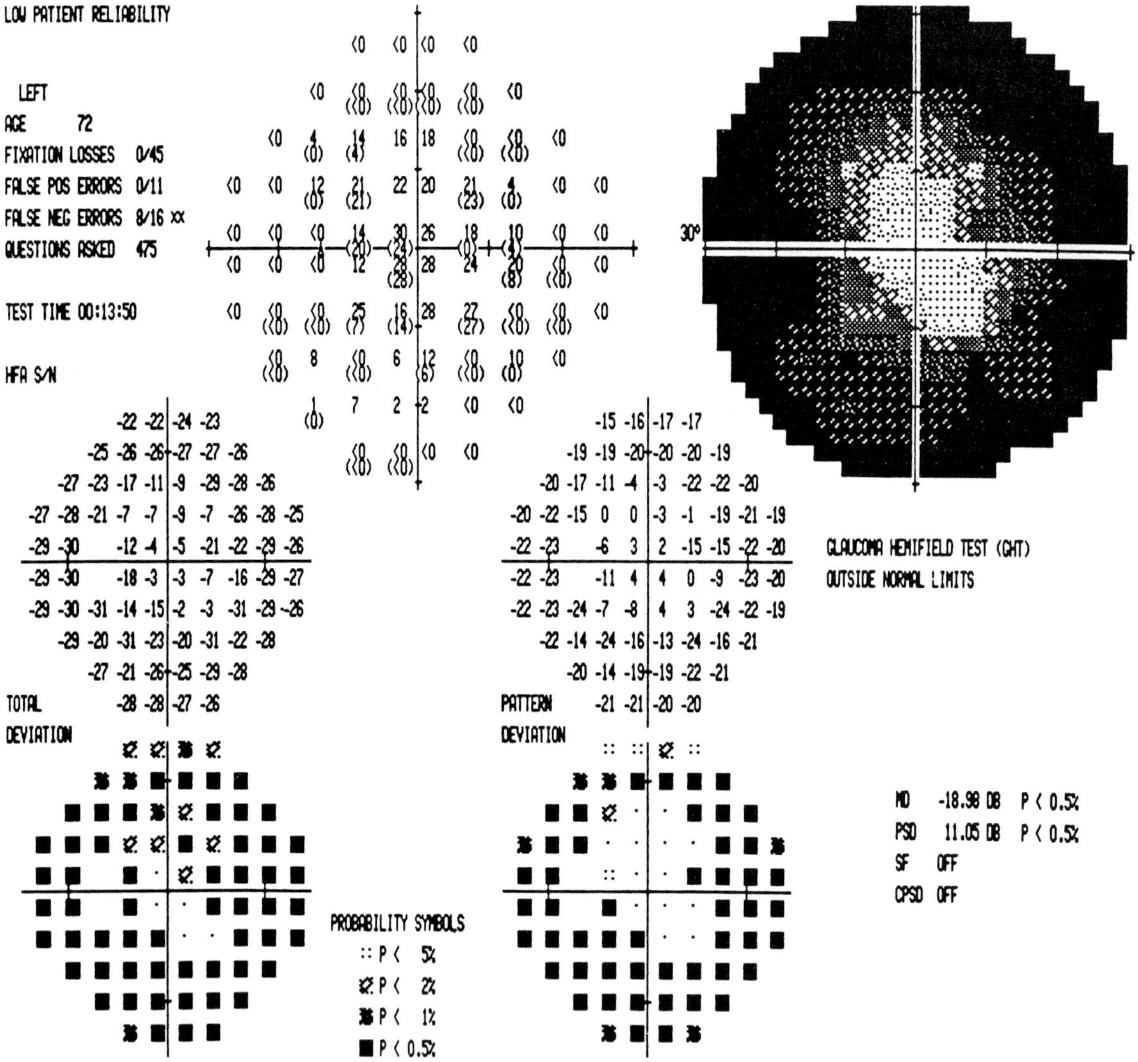

FIG. 2-29 Pseudocentral island related to rapid fatigue in a normal individual.

Fixation losses. Not all fixation losses represent true loss of fixation. The Humphrey perimeter monitors fixation by first quickly locating the blind spot and then projecting an occasional maximum stimulus into it. If the patient responds to the stimulus, the machine records a fixation loss. A high number of fixation losses may thus indicate that the center of the blind spot was slightly mislocated. A high false-positive rate will give a high fixation loss rate as well (Fig. 2-25). If the false-positive and false-negative rates are low and if the short-term fluctuation is low, we discount a high fixation loss rate. We also discount it if the two baseline fields are very similar (Fig. 2-30).

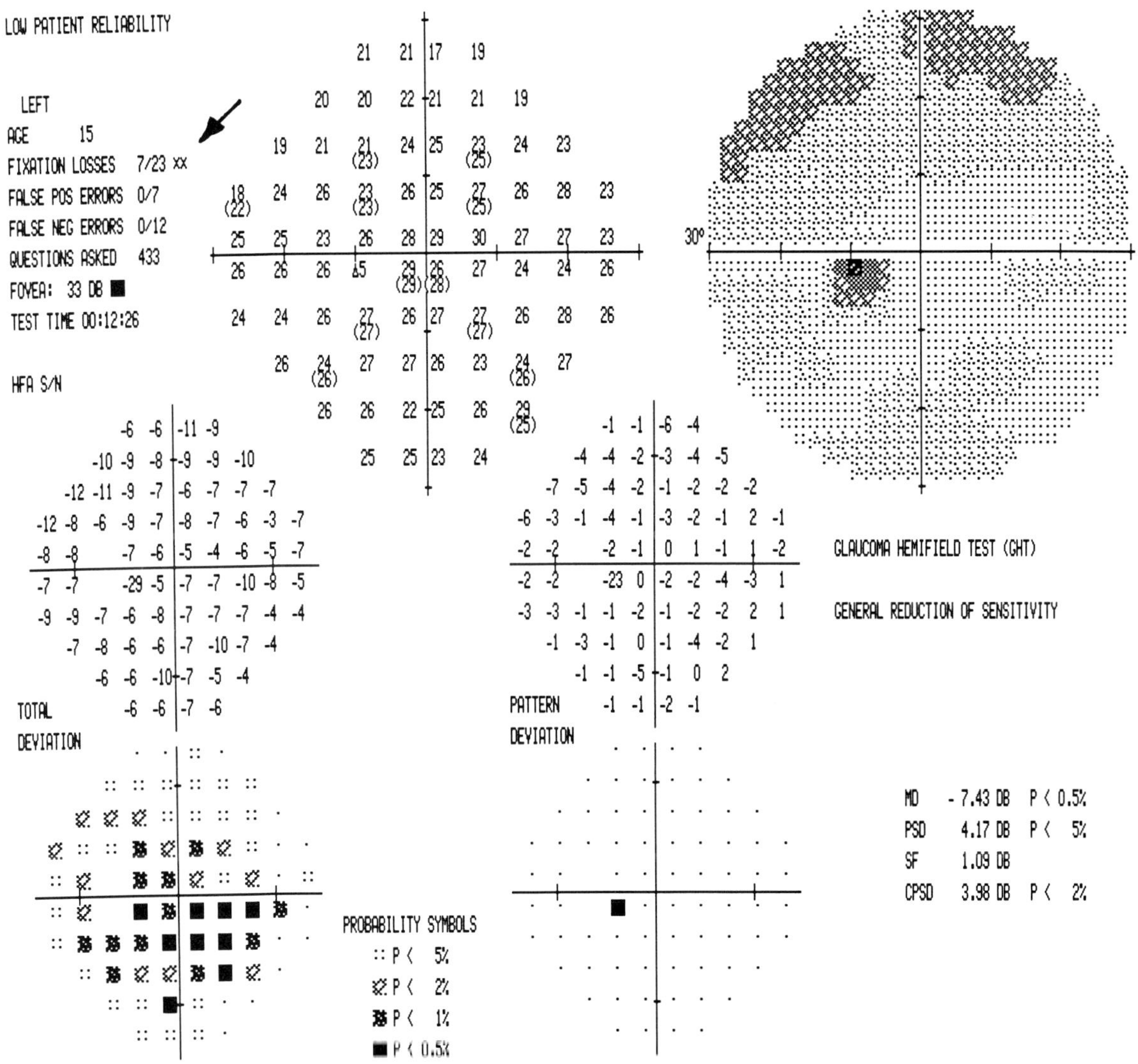

FIG. 2-30 High fixation losses in a reliable field. The fixation losses *(arrow)* probably result from mislocation of the center of the blind spot. The patient's aphakic correction shifts her blind spot toward fixation. Other reliability parameters are excellent, and multiple fields are almost identical. Fig. 2-32 shows another reliable patient with a large number of fixation losses related to macular disease.

Short-term fluctuation. The short-term fluctuation (SF) is not called a reliability parameter; but it often gives useful reliability information. A low (≤2 dB) SF indicates good reproducibility on retests at 10 preset points and usually indicates a reliable field, one in which a retest gives a similar answer. A high (≥3 dB) SF indicates poorer reproducibility, which may relate either to poor patient reliability or to field damage with true variability. Damaged fields are more variable than normal fields. In addition, points on the edge of a scotoma

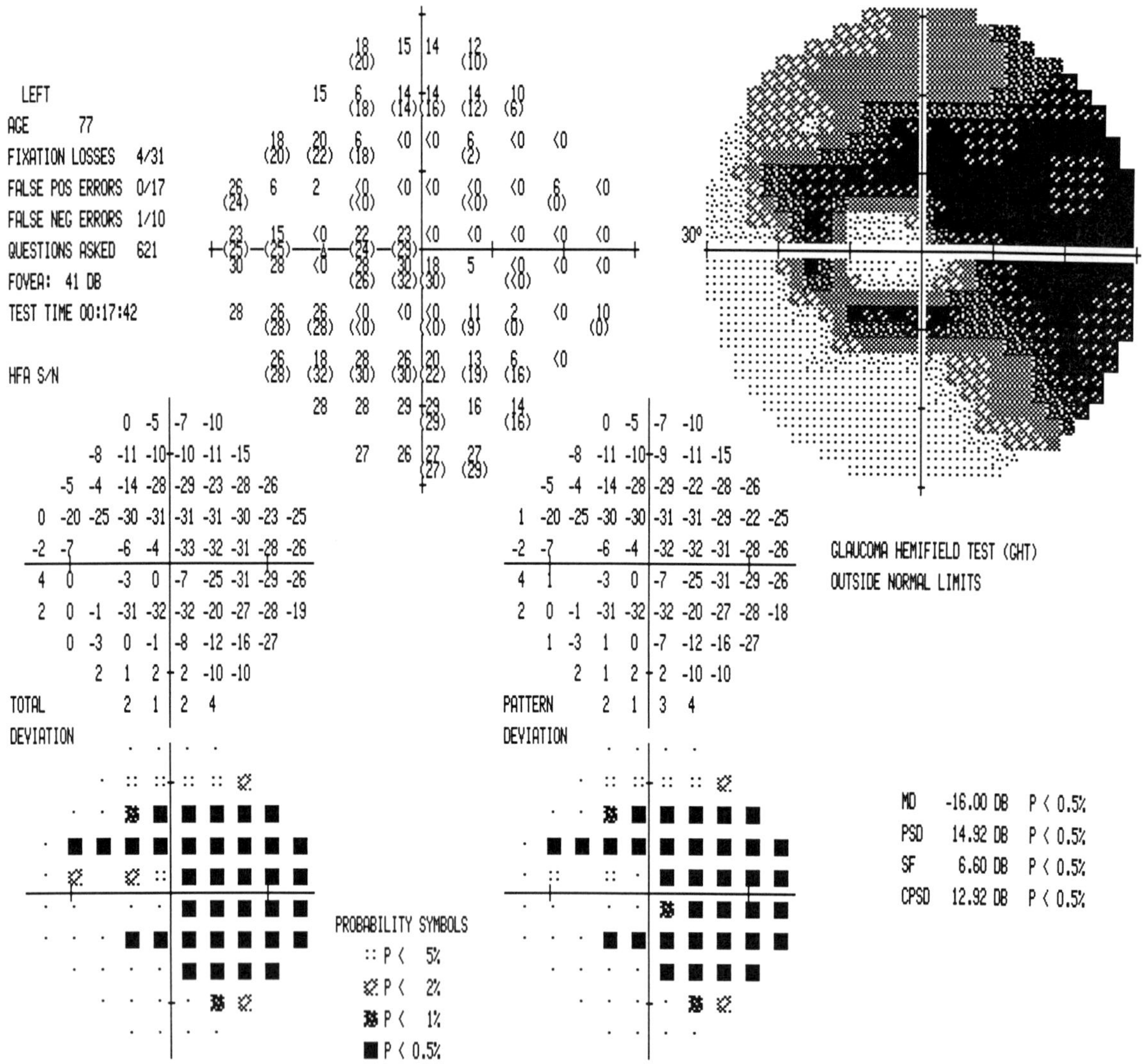

FIG. 2-31 High short-term fluctuation in a reliable patient. The patient's left eye has advanced glaucoma and a high SF of 6.60 dB. However, the points that do not fall near the edge of a scotoma are consistent on double determinations. The other eye is shown in Fig. 2-32.

vary widely, and if several such points are among the 10 that determine the SF, the value may be quite high in a reliable patient. Figures 2-31 and 2-32 show two eyes of the same individual, both of which have severe glaucoma, that have very different SF values. Always look on the numeric printout and determine whether the patient responded consistently in the areas of best vision. If a patient is reliable where he or she can see well, the person is probably reliable, even if not reproducible, where he or she sees poorly.

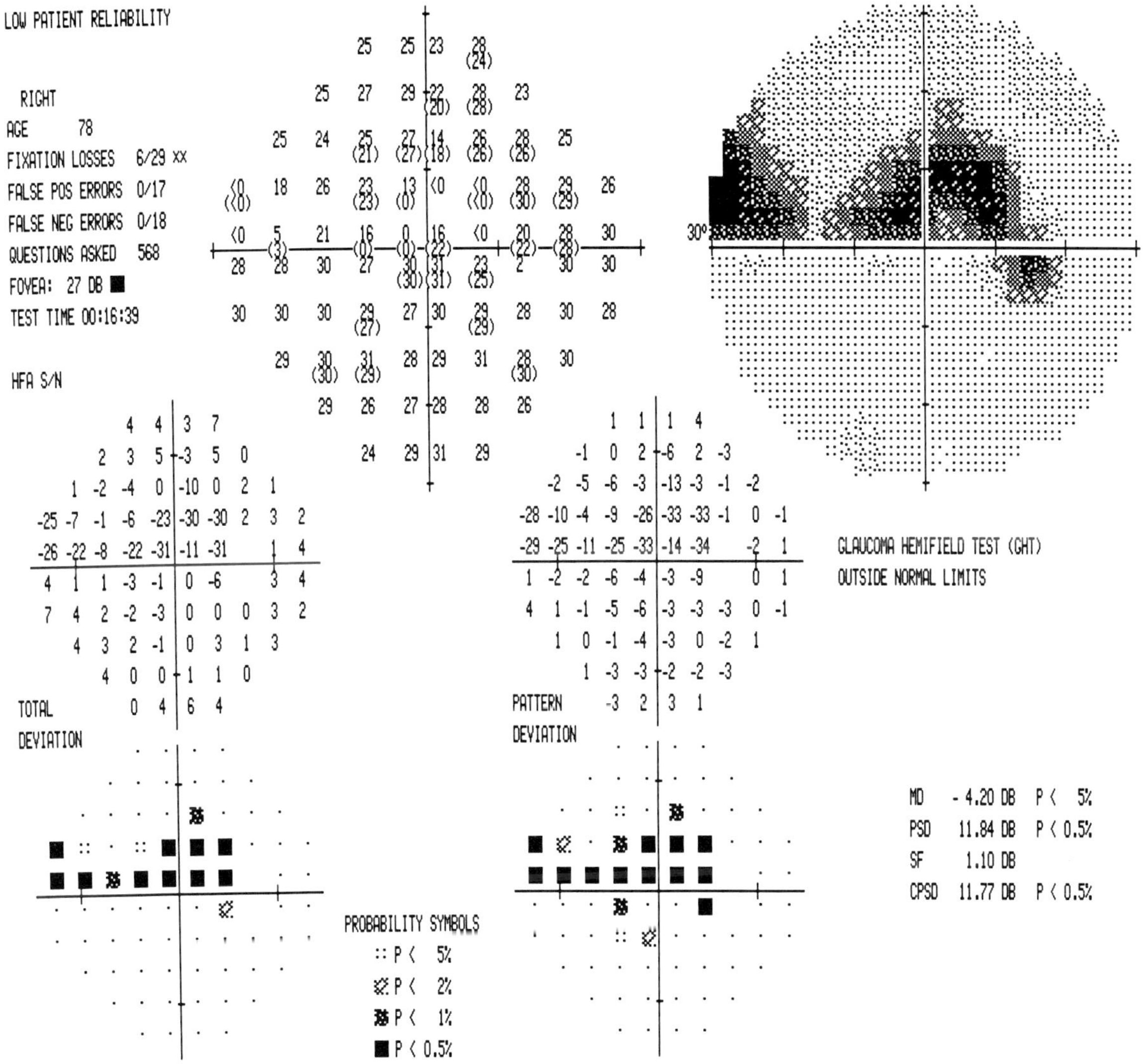

FIG. 2-32 The right eye of the same patient shown in Fig. 2-31 has more localized damage and a low short-term fluctuation. The patient also has macular disease and a visual acuity of 20/200, which contributes to her fixation losses.

NORMALITY AND ABNORMALITY

Despite the impossibility (and relative therapeutic unimportance) of classifying equivocal fields as normal or abnormal, both doctors and patients want to know if a field shows acquired damage. Obvious defects pose no diagnostic dilemmas. However, the earliest defects of glaucoma are often equivocal. A very good determinant of the presence of glaucomatous damage on a single field is the Glaucoma Hemifield Test (GHT), which compares corresponding areas in the superior and inferior hemifields (Figs. 2-33 and 2-34). This analysis relates only to glaucoma, and it always should be interpreted in light of the rest of the clinical picture. It does not, for example, analyze temporal nerve fiber bundle defects or vertical hemianopias (Fig. 2-35). In the absence of other cause for field abnormality and in the presence of a suspicion of glaucoma, a hemifield test outside normal limits on both (or on a minimum of two) baseline field examinations strongly suggests that the patient has glaucoma. Two other reliable indicators of acquired damage are (1) a cluster of three or more nonedge points in a location typical for glaucoma, all of which are depressed on the pattern deviation plot at a $p < 5\%$ level and one of which is depressed at a $p < 1\%$ level (Figs. 2-36 and 2-37), and (2) a corrected pattern standard deviation that occurs in less than 5% of normal fields (see box on p. 47 and Figs. 2-38 and 2-39).

Text continued on page 52.

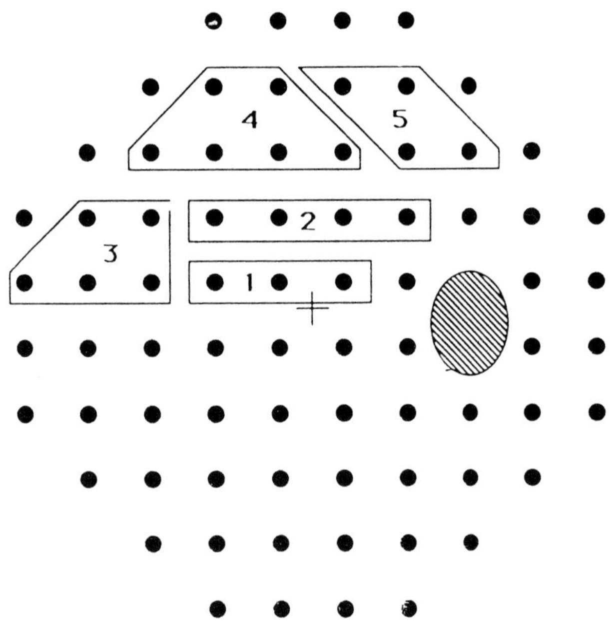

FIG. 2-33 Glaucoma hemifield test. The five numbered zones are compared to corresponding zones in the lower hemifield. The program also compares the overall height of the hill of vision compared to age-adjusted normal. (Reproduced from Statpac 2 Users Guide.)

Minimum Criteria for Diagnosing Acquired Glaucomatous Damage

- A Glaucoma Hemifield Test outside normal limits on at least two fields

or

- A cluster of three or more nonedge points in a location typical for glaucoma, all of which are depressed on the pattern deviation plot at a $p < 5\%$ level and one of which is depressed at a $p < 1\%$ level on two consecutive fields

or

- A corrected pattern standard deviation that occurs in less than 5% of normal fields on two consecutive fields

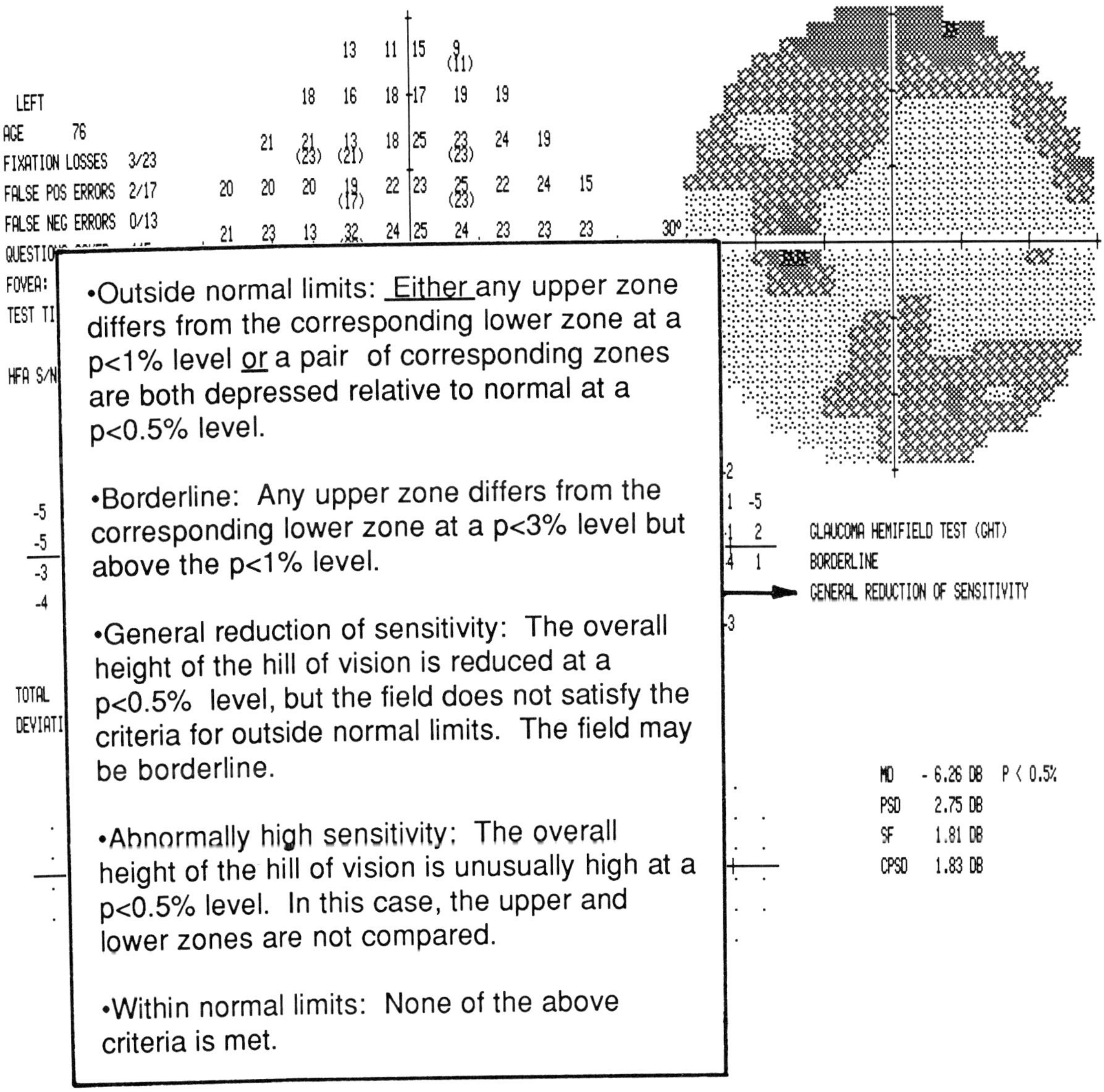

FIG. 2-34 Glaucoma hemifield test. Messages and their meanings.

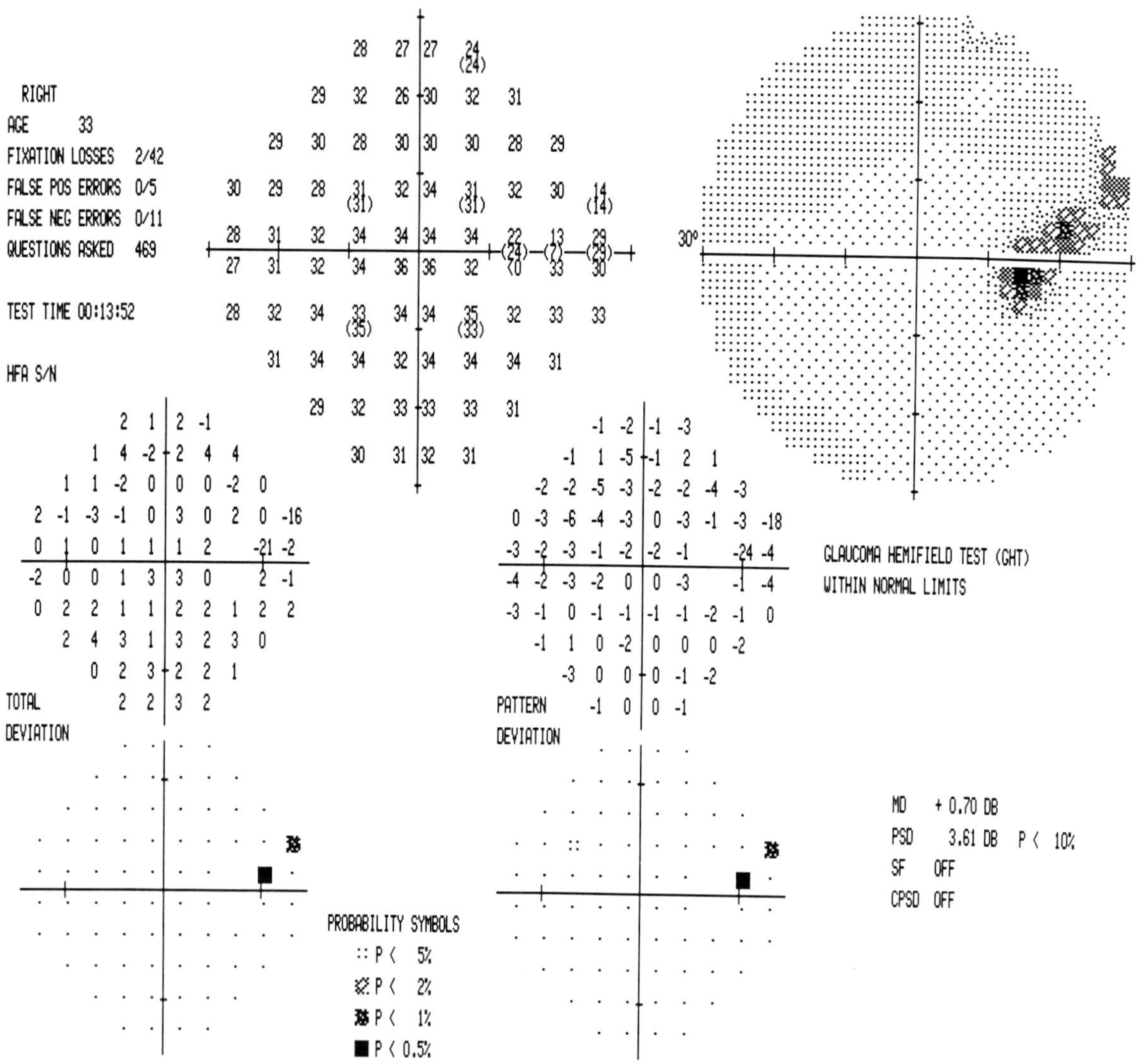

FIG. 2-35 Glaucoma hemifield test and temporal defect. The hemifield test does not deal with points temporal to the disc. This deep defect did not affect the hemifield results.

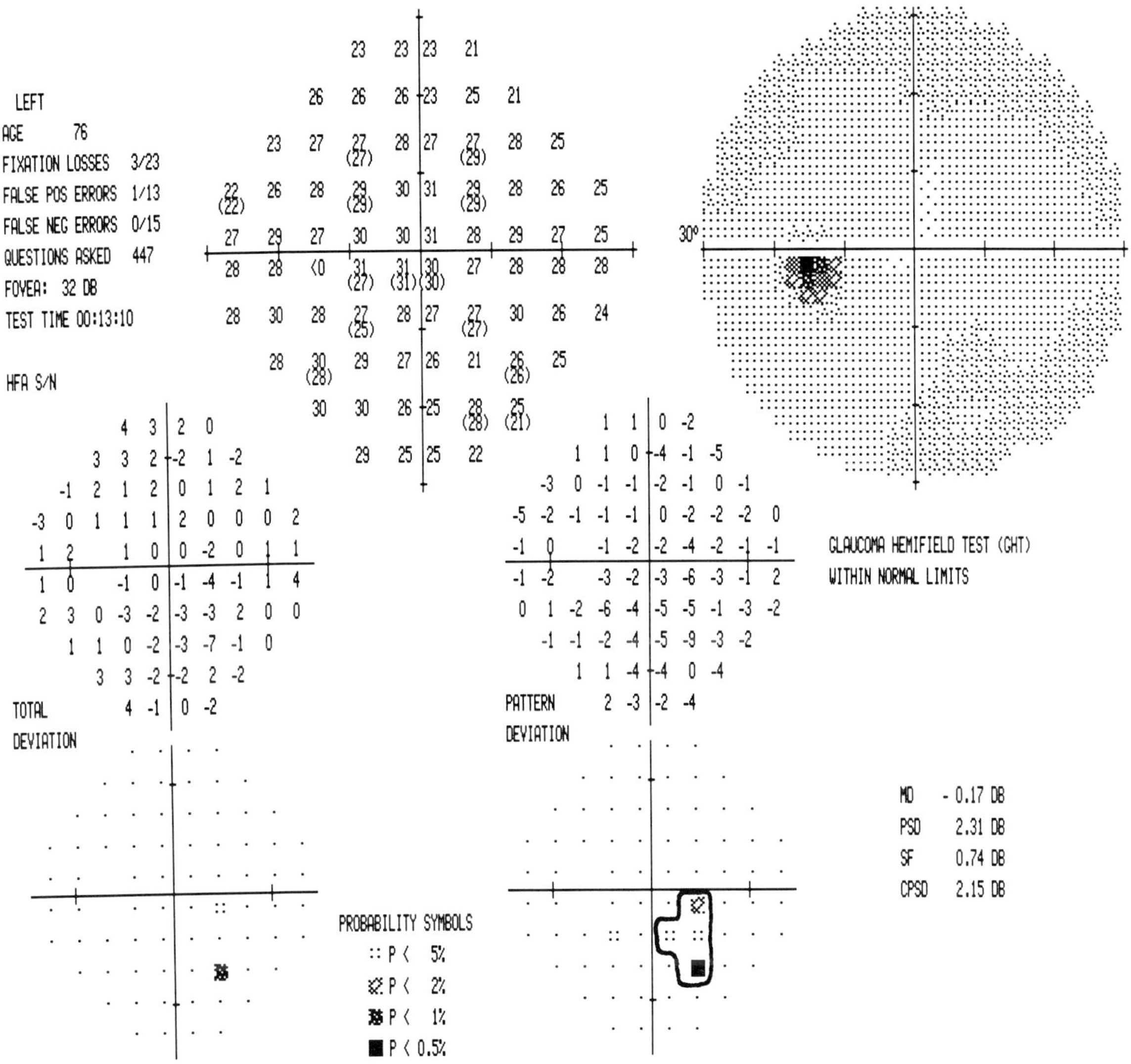

FIG. 2-36 Minimal pattern deviation criteria for acquired abnormality. At least three (here four, *circled*) clustered nonedge points each depressed at a 5% level and one at least at a 1% (here 0.5%) level. This defect was confirmed in repeated testing.

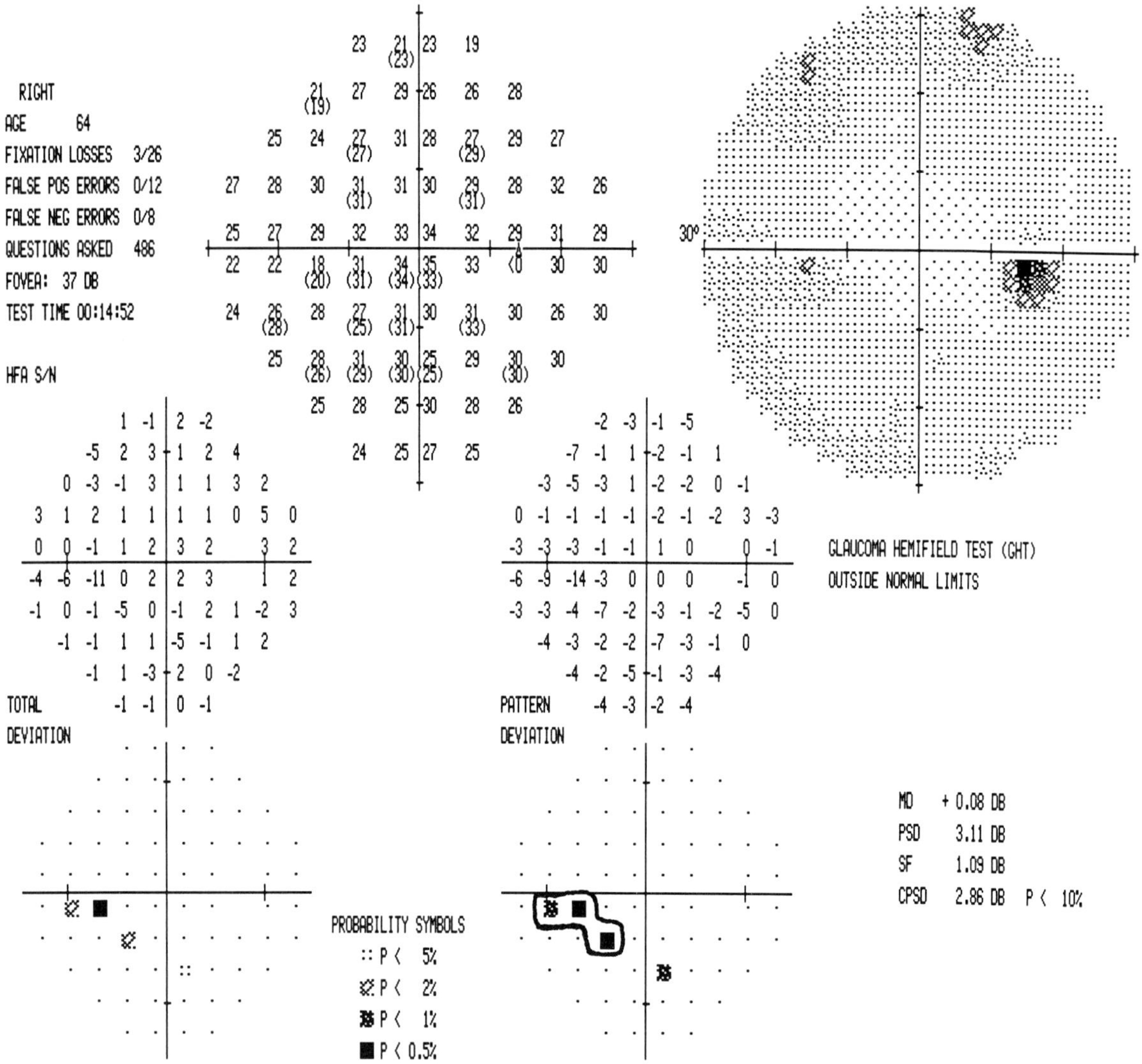

FIG. 2-37 Minimal pattern deviation criteria for acquired abnormality.

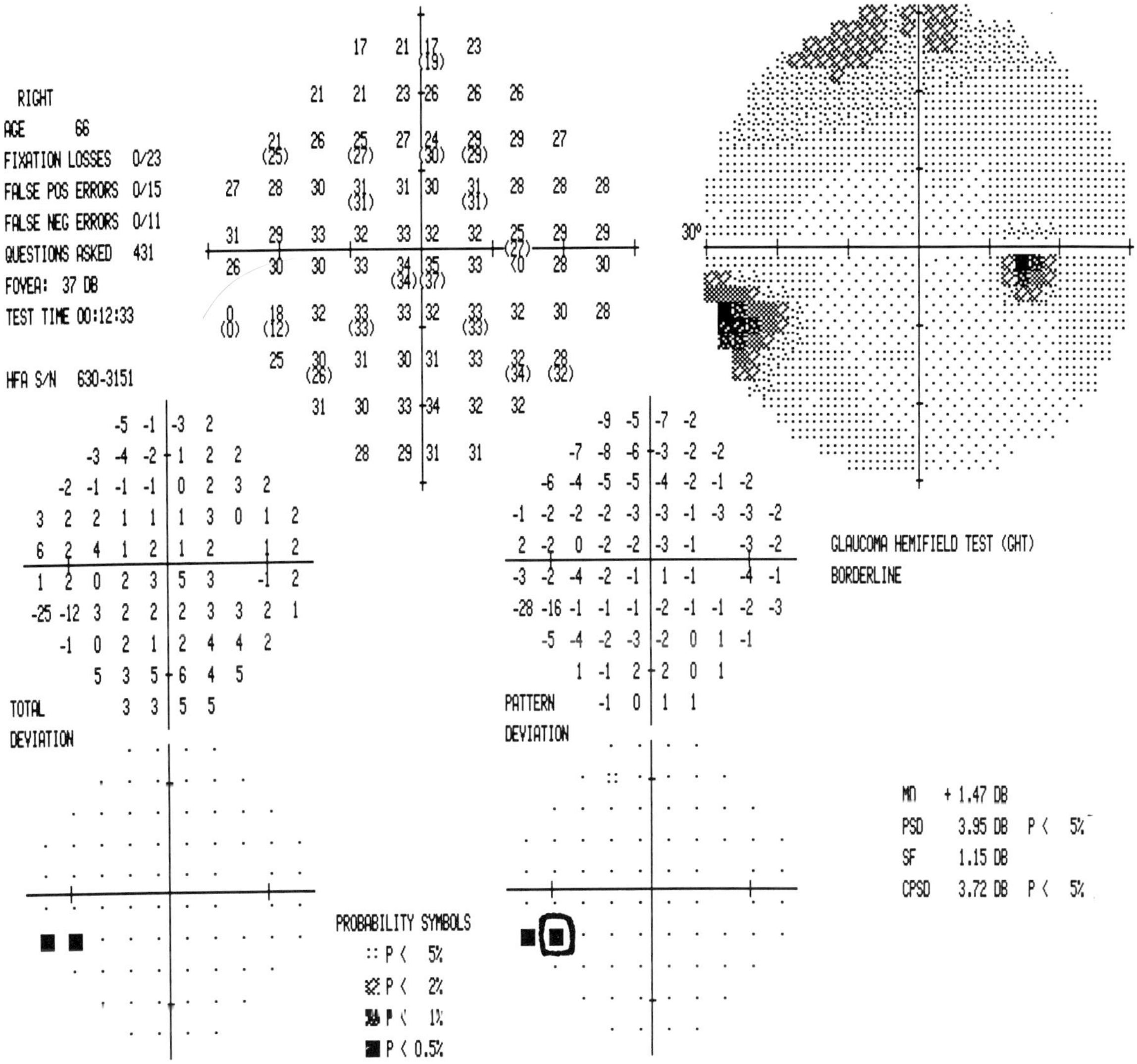

FIG. 2-38 Minimum CPSD criteria for acquired damage. Only one nonedge point in a typical location *(circled)* is depressed. The CPSD is depressed at the 5% level and the glaucoma hemifield test (GHT) is borderline

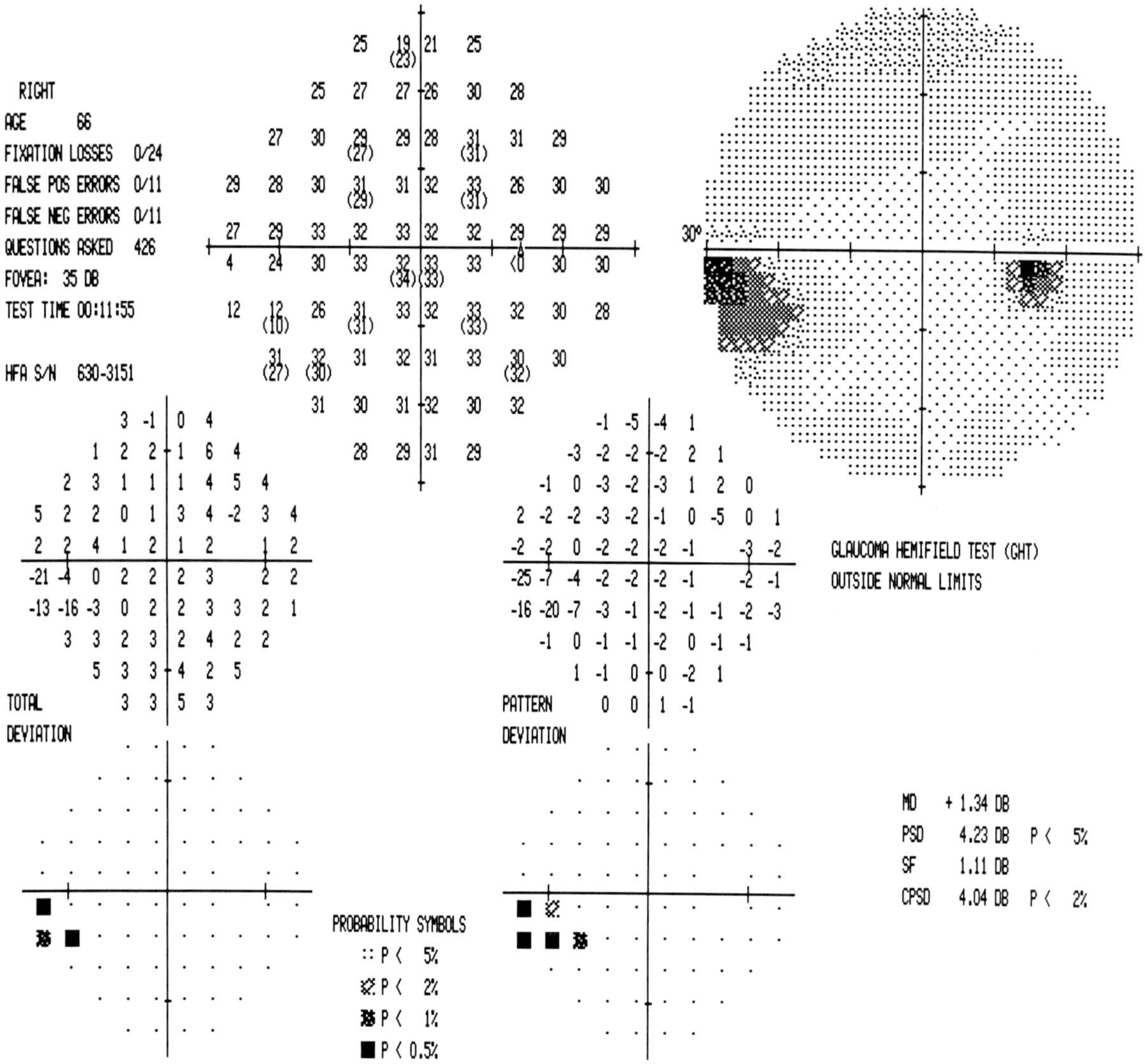

FIG. 2-39 Subsequent (3 months later) field of the patient illustrated in Fig. 2-38, which satisfies all three sets of criteria for abnormality: the glaucoma hemifield test (GHT) criterion, the pattern deviation criterion, and the CPSD criterion. The mean deviation is above normal for age.

CLASSIFICATION OF DEFECTS

It is useful at times to categorize patients by the degree of their field damage. For discussion purposes, we refer to visual field defects as early, moderate, and severe. Of course, damage is a continuum, classes are artificial, and it is possible to find fields that do not seem to be properly classified by a given set of criteria. Since we will make management recommendations based on the degree of field loss, however, it seems appropriate to define terms. In practice we usually look at a field and decide how it looks without a detailed, explicit determination of whether it "fits" into one or another category. Our general divisions are based on two criteria: overall extent of damage and proximity to fixation of damage. A small, dense, central defect weighs more heavily than does a somewhat larger but just as dense peripheral defect. Examples of fields we would classify into each group follow, in addition to some definitions. In all cases, it is assumed that the only cause of field loss is glaucoma and that the field test being interpreted is a Humphrey Central 30-2.

Early defect *(Figs. 2-40 through 2-42).* Damage should be neither extensive nor near fixation. The following three conditions should be met:

- The mean deviation index (MD) is less than −6 dB
- On the pattern deviation plot, fewer than 25% (18) of the points are depressed below the 5% level and fewer than 10 points are depressed below the 1% level
- No point in the central 5° has a sensitivity of less than 15 dB

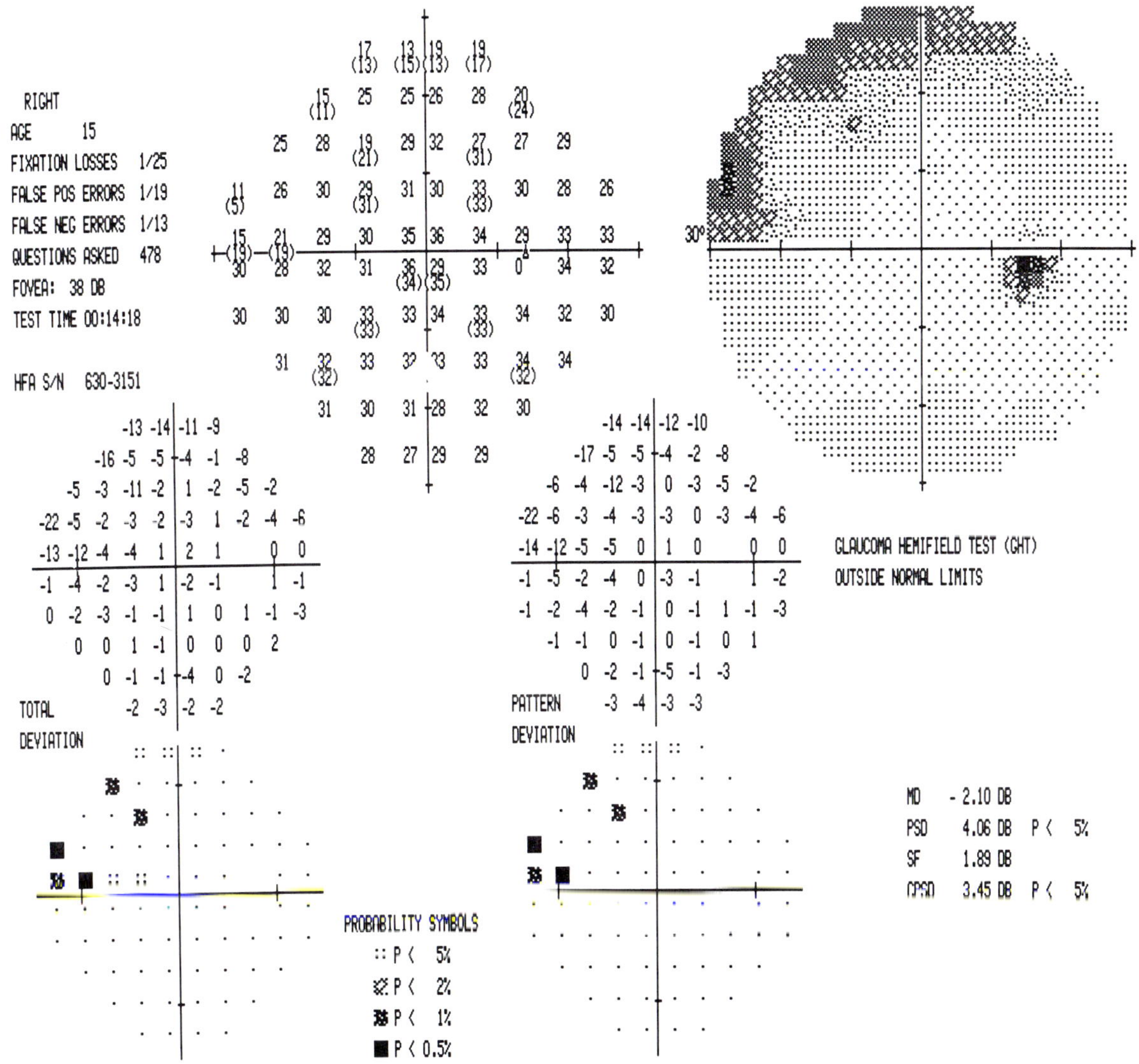

FIG. 2-40 Mild field defect. Field loss is typical for glaucoma but is neither extensive nor near fixation.

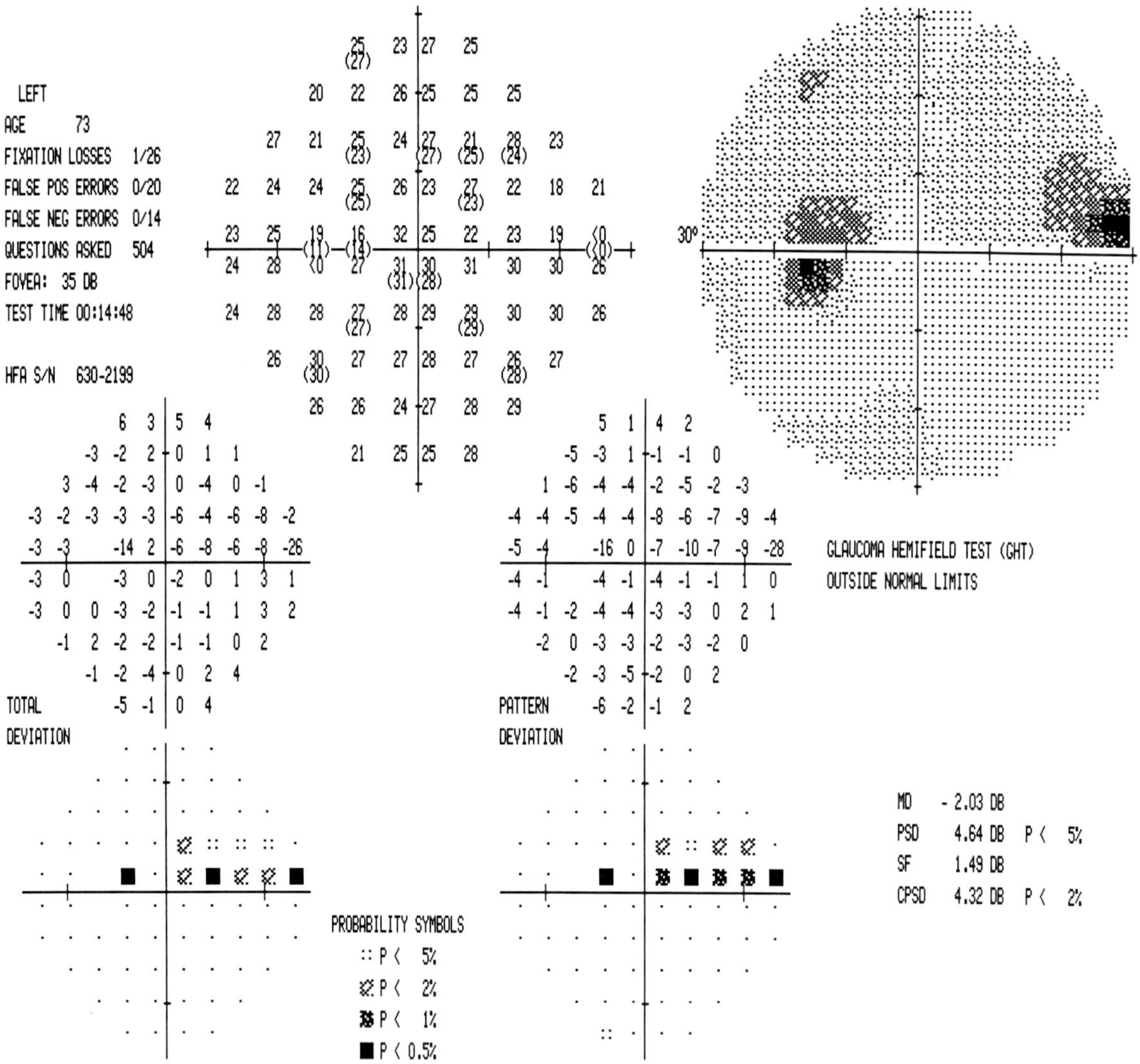

FIG. 2-41 Mild field defect. The abnormality extends to the central points, but the defect is shallow centrally and only one hemifield is involved.

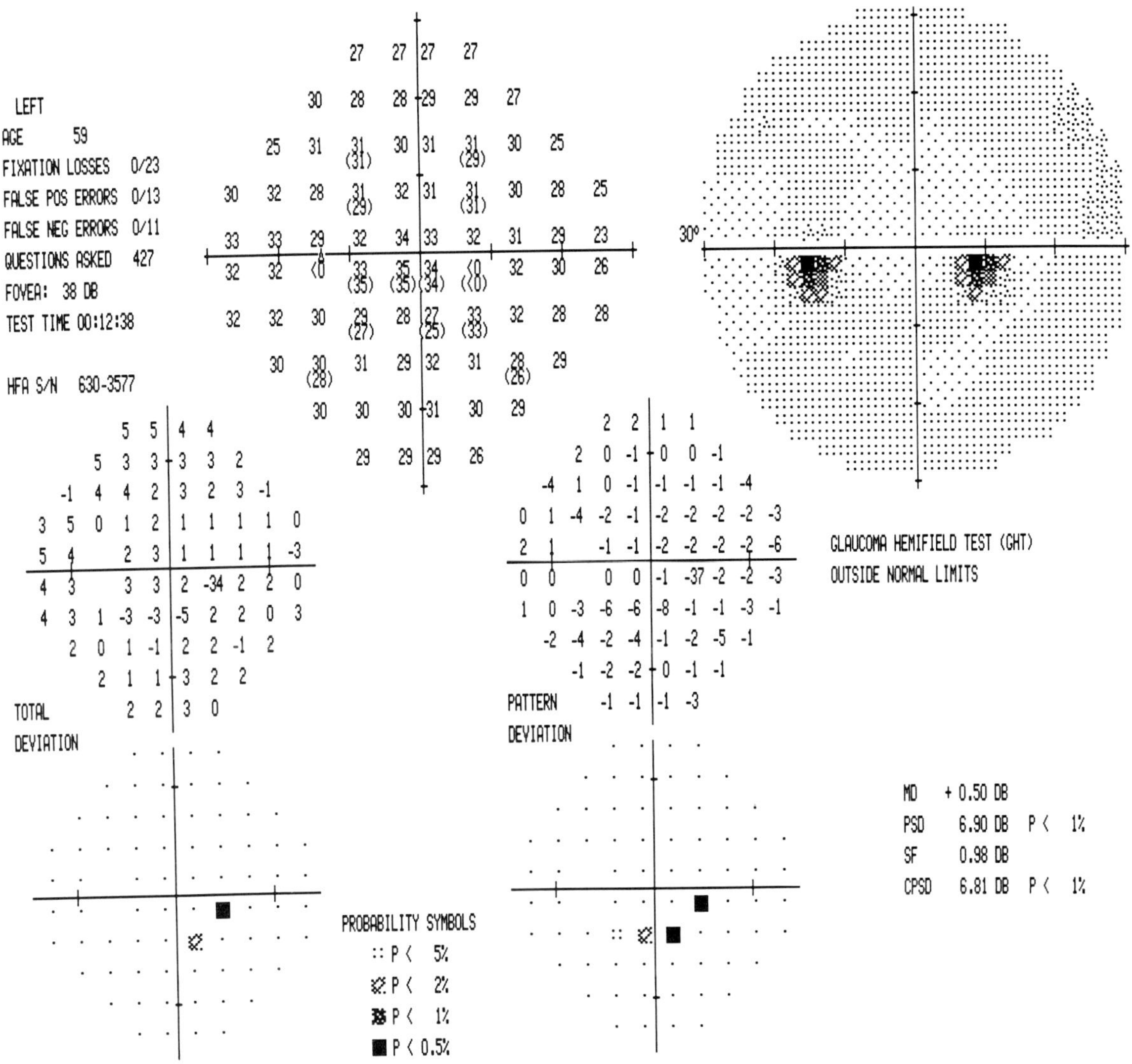

FIG. 2-42 Mild field defect. This dense localized defect falls outside the central 5°. Although it fits the criteria for a mild defect, it is more worrisome than the defects in Figs. 2-40 and 2-41.

Moderate defect *(Figs. 2-43 through 2-45).* Damage may be significant, but there should not be profound central field damage, and there should not be significant central field damage in both hemifields. The following four conditions should be met:

- The mean defect is less than −12 dB
- On the pattern deviation plot, fewer than 50% (37) of the points are depressed below the 5% level and fewer than 20 points are depressed below the 1% level
- No point in the central 5° has a sensitivity of 0 dB
- Only one hemifield may have a point with sensitivity of <15 dB within 5° of fixation

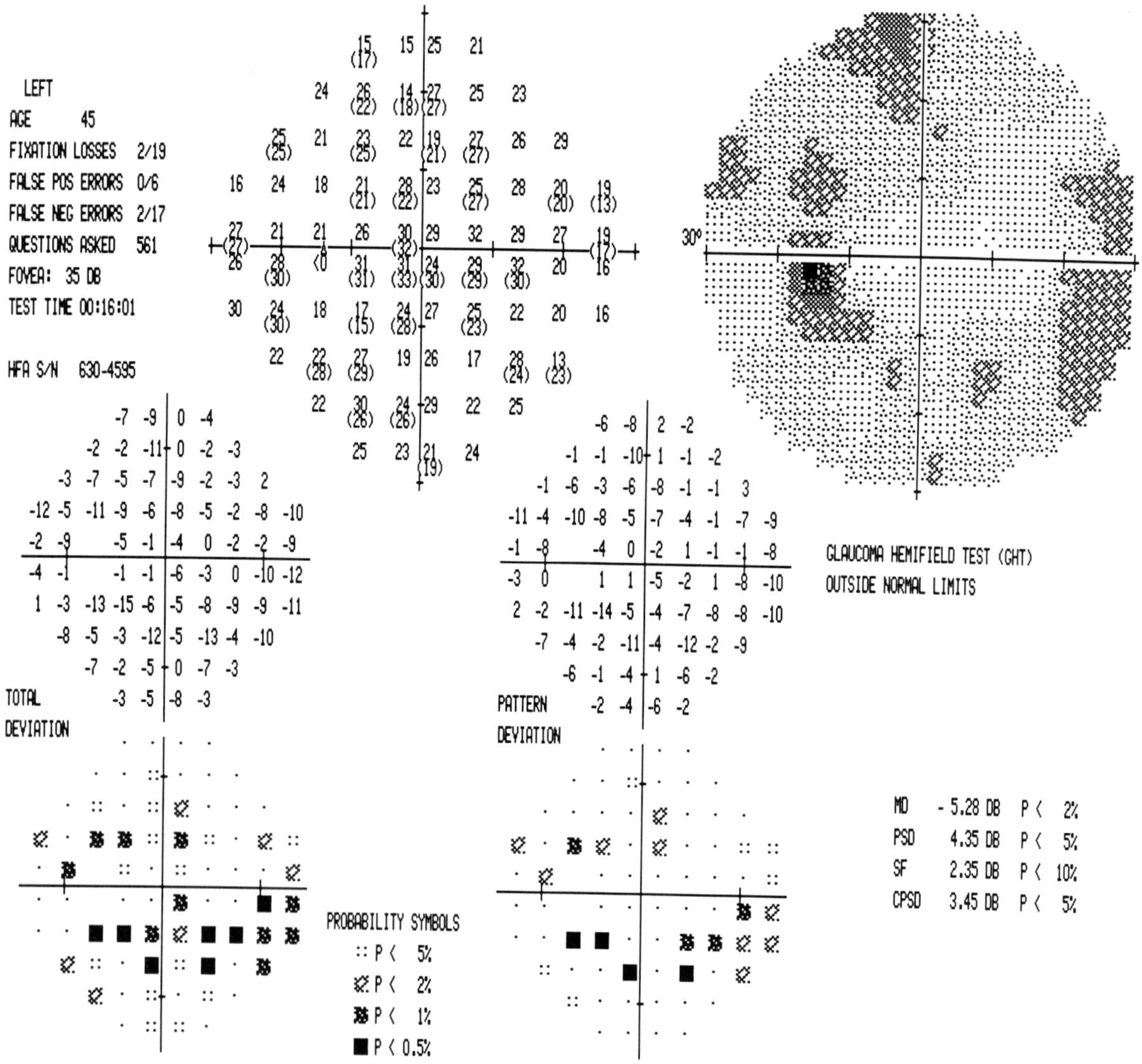

FIG. 2-43 Moderate field defect. Damage is widespread, but the central field is largely spared, and the foveal threshold and acuity are normal.

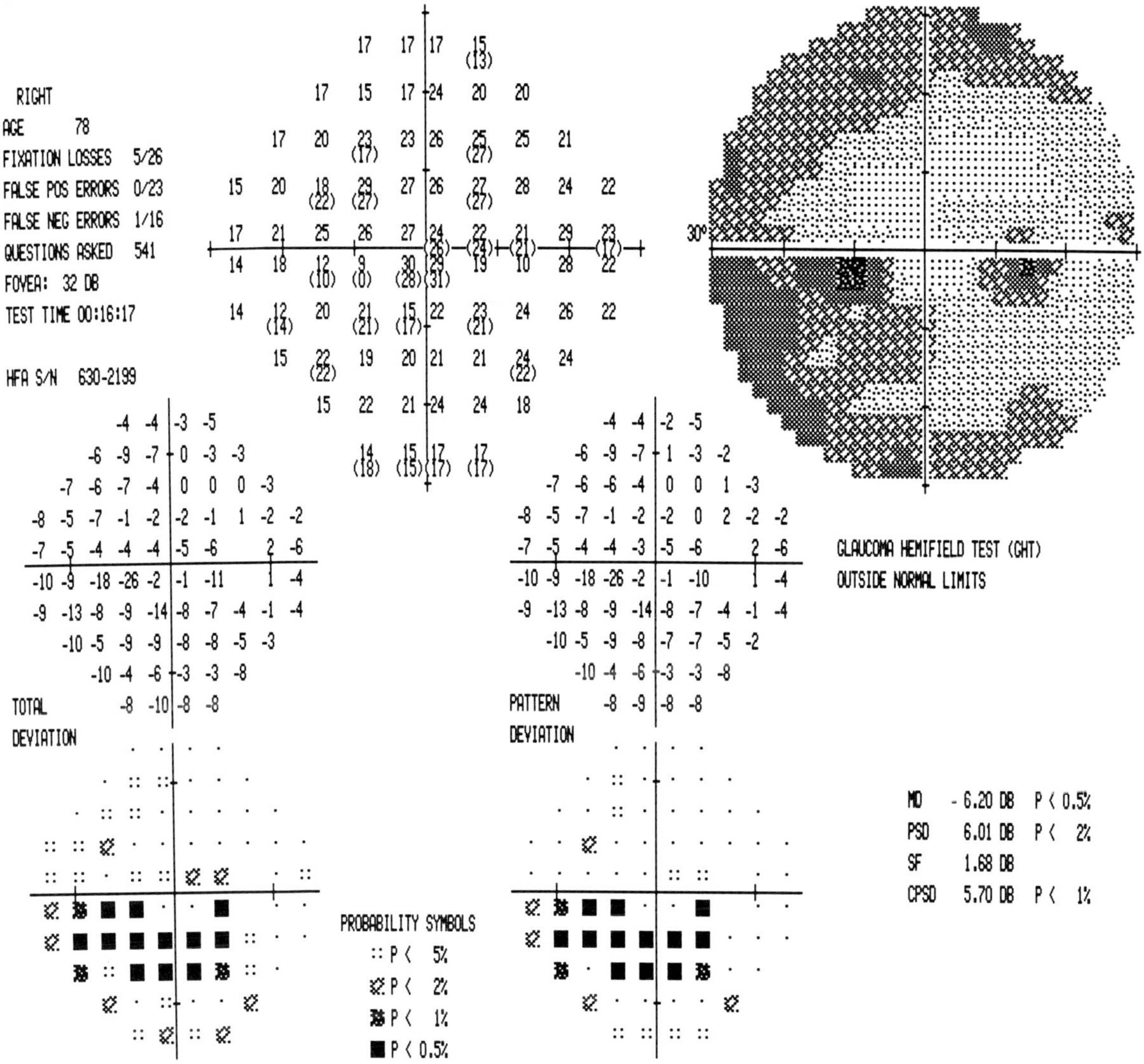

FIG. 2-44 Moderate field defect. Most of the damage is confined to the inferior hemifield, and the central points are relatively spared. (Also appears in Anderson DR: *Automated static perimetry*, St. Louis, 1991, CV Mosby.)

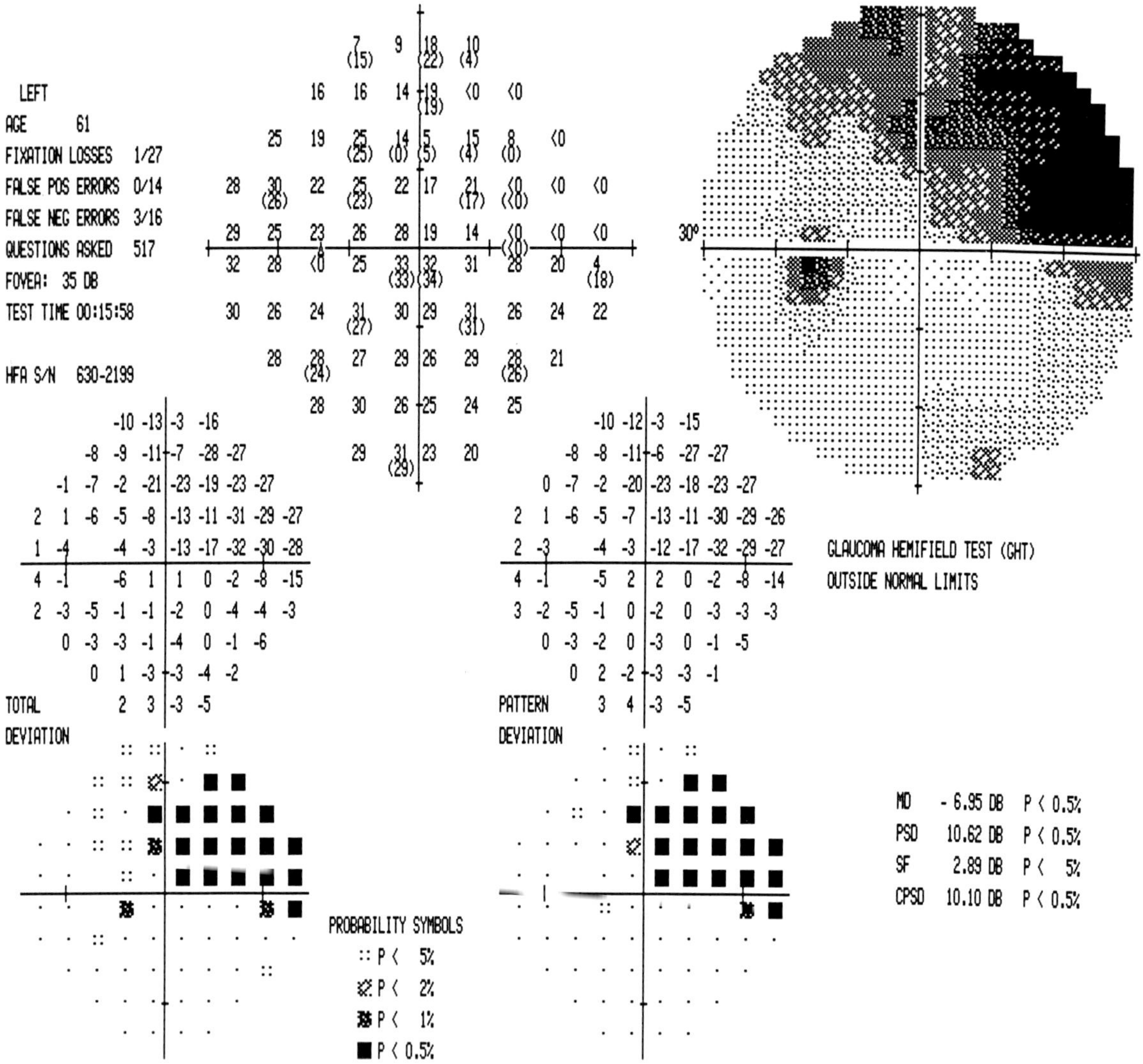

FIG. 2-45 Moderate field defect. The superior hemifield shows significant damage, but the inferior hemifield is only mildly involved.

Severe defect *(Figs. 2-46 through 2-48).* Any of the following findings indicate severe field loss:

- The mean defect is greater than −12 dB
- On the pattern deviation plot, more than 50% (37) of the points are depressed below the 5% level or more than 20 points are depressed below the 1% level
- Any point in the central 5° has a sensitivity of 0 dB
- There are points within the central 5° with sensitivity <15 dB in both hemifields

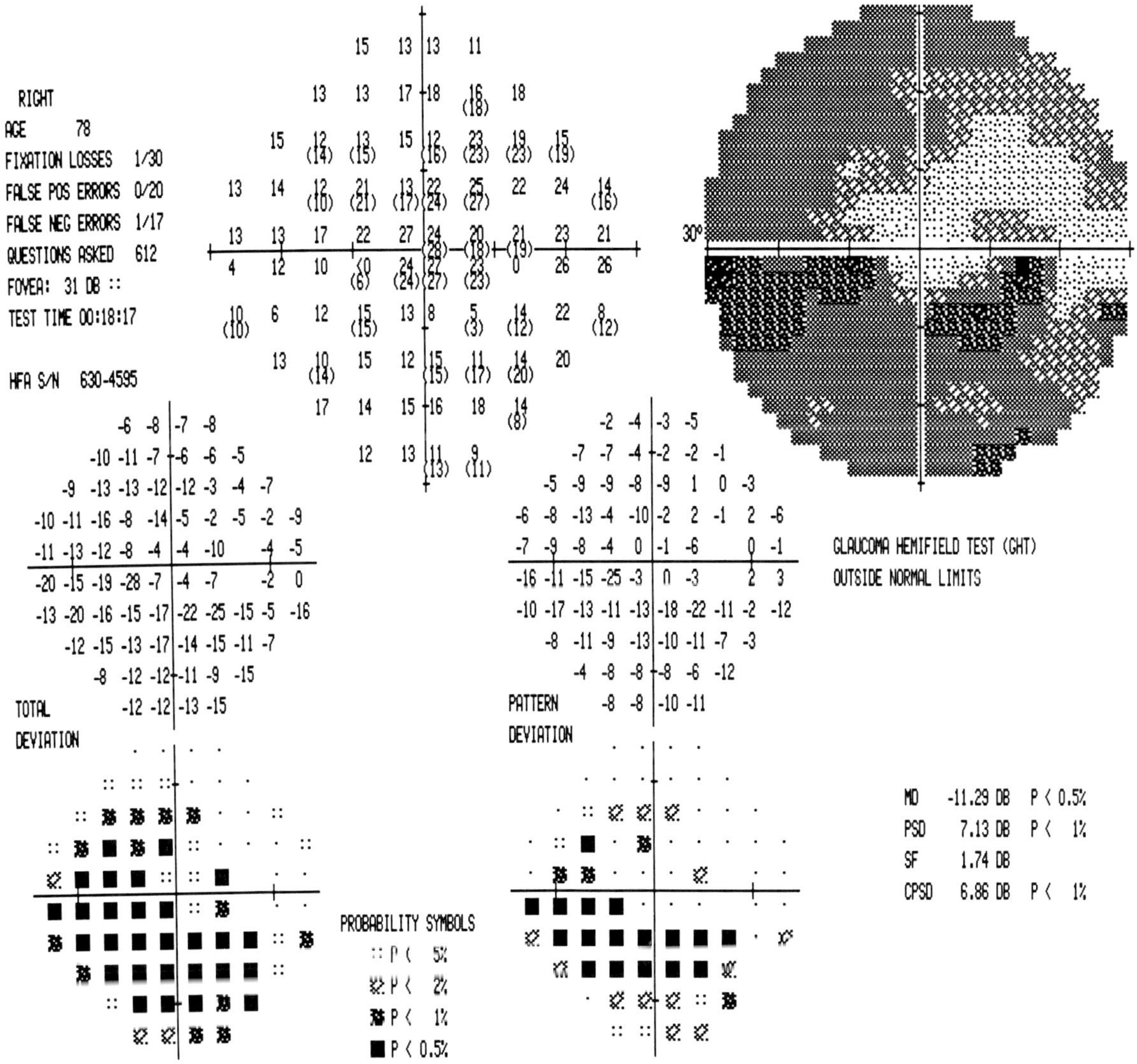

FIG. 2-46 Severe field defect. More than half the points are depressed on the pattern deviation plot, and more than 20 of these are at a 1% or 0.5% level.

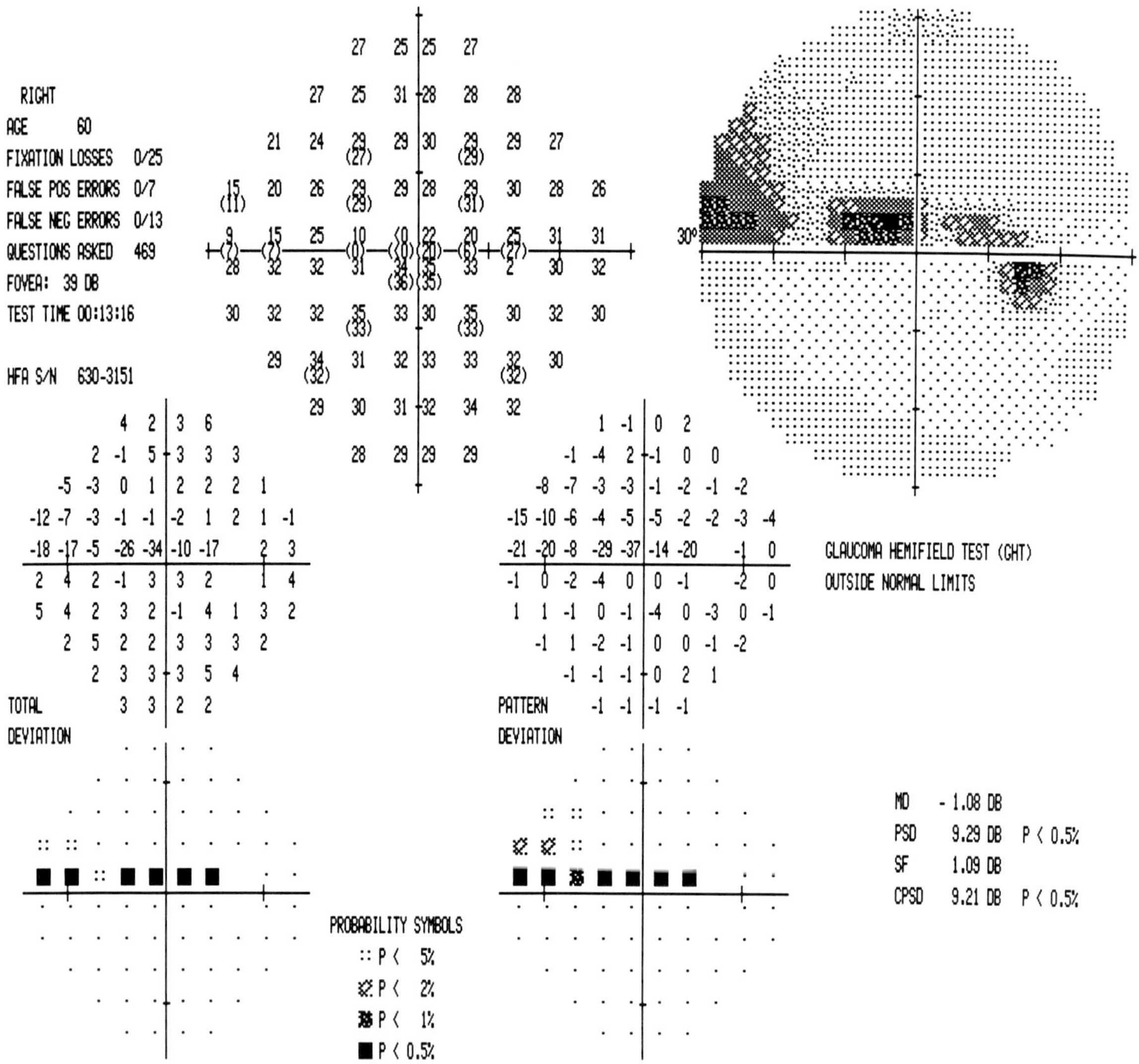

FIG. 2-47 Severe field defect. Although only a small number of points are depressed, this dense defect splits fixation.

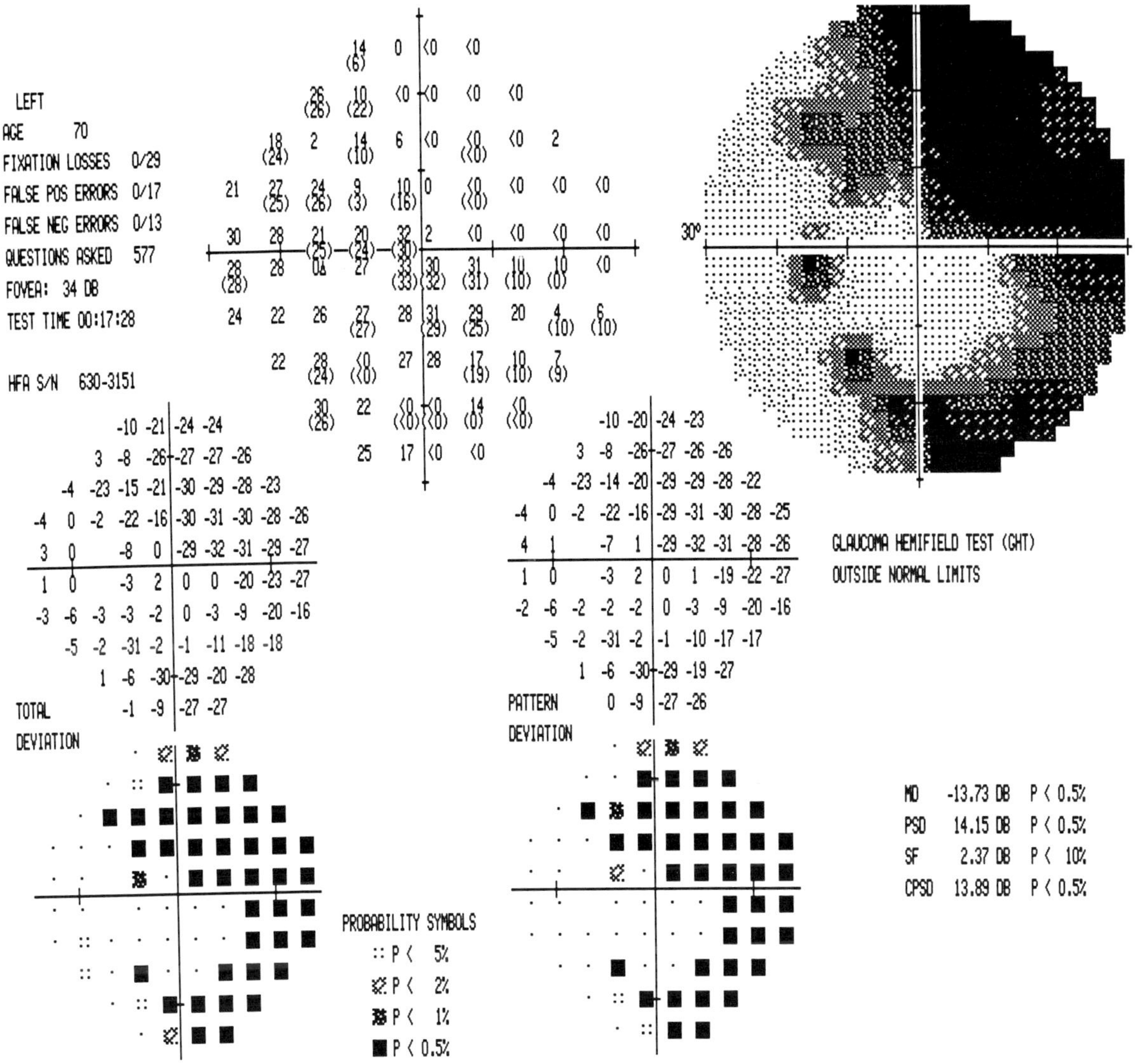

FIG. 2-48 Severe field defect.

DISTINGUISHING BETWEEN GLAUCOMA PATIENTS AND GLAUCOMA SUSPECTS

Fully manifest glaucoma consists of a clearly abnormal pressure that is not only outside the normal range (22 mm Hg or more) but also has caused recognizable characteristic glaucomatous excavation and recognizable glaucomatous visual field loss. In the setting of an elevated intraocular pressure, a diagnosis of glaucoma versus glaucoma suspect is made as shown in Chart 2-2. If a person has elevated pressure in both eyes but fully manifested glaucoma in only one eye, we classify the patient as having bilateral glaucoma.

Despite the emphasis often placed on finding the earliest possible disc or field abnormality, we do not recommend expending excess energy on trying to separate patients with early or mild glaucoma from those without manifest disease. The easy ones are easy; and the hard ones are, on initial examination, usually impossible to distinguish perfectly. Time may reveal whether the person has a physiologic variant that resembles early glaucoma, has nonprogressive or slowly progressive glaucoma, or has the early stage of glaucoma that will progress rapidly without treatment. Once a patient is even *suspected* of having glaucoma, his or her long-term course must be followed, and the care of early glaucoma is not particularly different from the initial management of the glaucoma suspect. We have, nonetheless, separated the management of fully manifest open angle glaucoma (high pressure, cupping, field loss, open angle, and no evident secondary cause) from management of glaucoma suspects with elevated pressure for several reasons:

1. We believe that most patients with fully manifest glaucoma should have their IOP lowered.
2. We believe that most glaucoma suspects should not have their pressure lowered until the nature and rapidity of their natural course is known.
3. People may be glaucoma suspects for a variety of reasons—pressure, nerve findings, field findings, etc. We prefer to keep the guidelines for

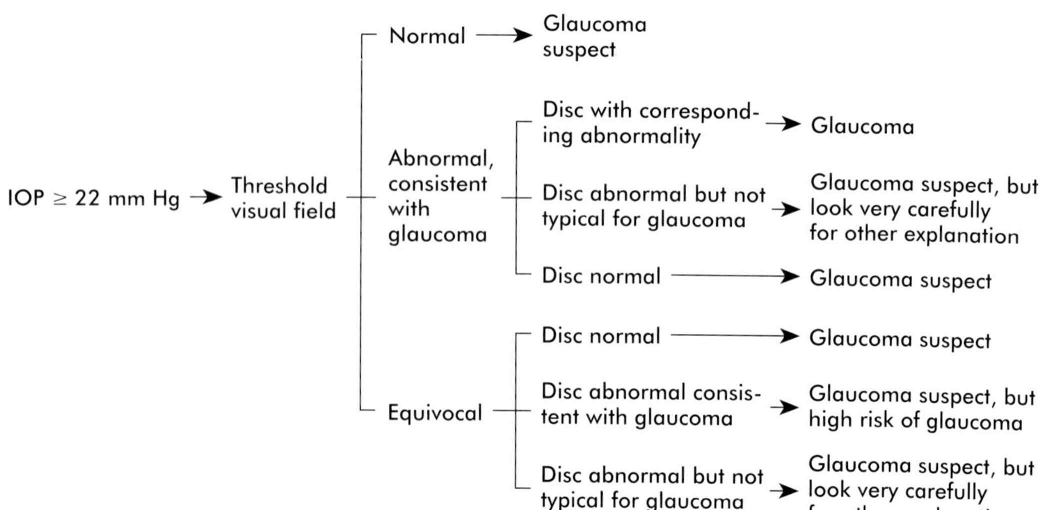

CHART 2-2 Distinguishing between glaucoma and suspected glaucoma in patients with elevated IOP.

each class of suspects separate from each other and from the guidelines for management of fully manifest open-angle glaucoma.

4. Unified management descriptions that subsume all possibilities are difficult to present comprehensibly.

There is much uncertainty involved in the care of glaucoma patients, especially early in the disease course. The fact that it is not always possible to determine who has glaucoma, even with a careful examination and a threshold visual field, is only one of the many unclear aspects of glaucoma management. We do not know at least the following about primary open-angle glaucoma: the cause, a cure, and—lacking a cure—the best available treatment to reduce disease-induced visual loss without affecting the quality of life with therapy-induced symptoms, nuisance, and undue expense. None of our treatments allow patients to see or feel better. We aim to prevent a future potential problem of uncertain magnitude and, as a result, induce various current real problems. We know that the visual function of glaucoma patients sometimes worsens greatly over the years, even if we do our best and follow the best recommendations available. The practical result is that it is rarely possible to know absolutely that all is well with a glaucoma patient. It is almost always possible, however, to develop a reasonable management plan. Our recommended treatment for primary open-angle glaucoma is described in Chapter 3.

3

Initial Treatment of Primary Open-Angle Glaucoma

Primary open-angle glaucoma (POAG) is a chronic condition. Patients who have POAG do not get better; their visual function stays the same or worsens. Treatment does not make them feel better. The physician sees no dramatic cures and receives few immediate emotional rewards. The best treatment does not always work, and some people lose vision despite the clinician's best efforts.

The picture is not uniformly grey, however. Most people with glaucoma have adequate vision for their needs throughout their lives. In addition, the management of POAG is conceptually straightforward. Attention to detail, careful follow-up, and appropriate treatment favorably affect the course of the disease. There are five basic steps to follow in managing a patient with POAG:

1. Establish a good baseline.
2. Set a reasonable goal for intraocular pressure.
3. Lower the pressure.
4. Follow up with the patient to see if the pressure goal is maintained and if the glaucomatous damage progresses.
5. Modify the pressure goal and treatment as indicated by the patient's course.

The first three steps should proceed promptly after diagnosis and together constitute the initial treatment of POAG, discussed in this chapter. The fourth and fifth steps are the chronic, ongoing steps and are discussed in Chapter 4.

The early care of patients with POAG involves frequent examinations. These multiple visits allow time for educating the patient about the irreversible nature of glaucomatous visual loss and the value of pressure reduction to avoid progressive damage. Between initial examinations, the patient may formulate new questions that require answers and may develop misconceptions that need clarification. The chronic nature of glaucoma care deserves emphasis from the start. Patient education may be the most important aspect of the chronic care of glaucoma because effective management depends not on the prescription of therapy, but on the use of therapy—consistently and for a long time. Frequent early visits convey a sense of importance about the treatment regimen.

ESTABLISHING A BASELINE

To determine whether a patient's condition is stable or is worsening over time, a precise knowledge of the patient's status at the beginning of treatment is needed. Most of the baseline data will have been gathered in the initial diagnostic evaluation, but further measurements may be needed. If possible, try to complete the baseline within the first 2 months. A good baseline includes information on the range over which IOP varies without treatment, the appearance of the angle, the status of the nerve, and the status of the visual field. Establishing such a baseline requires an initial investment of time, energy, and expense, but the investment is rewarded by making subsequent management decisions easier.

Intraocular Pressure

Pressure varies from day to day and over the course of the day, and the range within which the pressure varies is used to determine a pressure goal. If possible, obtain at least three measurements before beginning treatment. The IOP measurements should be obtained at different times of day and on two or three different days. We do not check pressures outside ordinary office hours. If the patient can obtain records of previous pressures, he or she should do so.

Angle Appearance

By definition, patients with POAG have open and unremarkable angles. The angle may shallow with time; a specific record of the initial appearance and depth of the angle should be recorded.

Disc Examination

Examination and photography of the disc is discussed in Chapter 2.

Visual Fields

The baseline visual field examination is discussed in Chapter 2. Even a patient who has fully manifest glaucoma at the time of presentation should have at least two baseline field examinations to determine the variability of repeat threshold measurements. More than two sets of fields are sometimes needed to establish a baseline free of learning effects and artifacts; rarely, establishing the visual field baseline may extend over several months. If an individual continues to improve after the second or third examination, fields should be obtained on most visits until the field levels. There is no way to make the baseline field examination easy. However, to recognize subsequent change it is necessary to invest the time, energy, and money initially.

SETTING A PRESSURE GOAL

General Considerations

Rarely, a patient may have mild glaucoma and, for example, a limited life expectancy so that the clinician elects to observe the course of the condition and intervenes only if it is more rapid than predicted. Otherwise, once the baseline is established, it is time to set a pressure goal. To determine a pressure goal, the risks and cost, including side effect cost, of treatment to lower pressure any given amount must be weighed against the risk of the pressure itself. Two useful concepts to help assess a given patient's risk of damage from elevated pressure are the estimated threshold for damage and the presence of nonpressure risk factors. In addition, the extent of damage already present determines, in part, the risk that additional damage will cause the patient noticeable visual disability and thus helps determine the importance of avoiding an increment of progression.

THRESHOLD FOR DAMAGE

Assume that each patient has some IOP level below which there will be no glaucomatous damage. (Such a safe level probably does not exist, but the rate of further damage is simply slower for successively lower pressures. It is clinically useful, however, to assume that there is some "safe" level at which the progression is acceptably slow.) This pressure is the threshold for damage for that patient. The higher his or her IOP is above the threshold, the more rapidly glaucomatous damage will progress. Once the pressure falls below threshold, additional lowering of pressure provides marginal benefit and entails unnecessary risks. We cannot determine a priori a person's threshold for damage, but the findings at the time of presentation provide clues. We assume that an asymptomatic patient with elevated IOP has had high pressure for some time, and time has shown the susceptibility of his or her disc. Thus the extent of optic nerve and visual field damage that has already occurred yields some clue to the patient's susceptibility to damage. The greater the glaucomatous damage at the time of diagnosis, the more above threshold the pressure presumably is.

NONPRESSURE RISK FACTORS

This concept was introduced in Chapter 1. Some factors other than IOP determine why an individual develops glaucomatous damage at a particular pressure. The greater the degree of damage already present at diagnosis in a person with a given IOP, the more of these other risk factors that person is presumed to possess. And the greater the unknown risk factors, the more IOP should be lowered because it is the only treatable risk factor. Conversely, a person who, despite a distinctly elevated IOP, has minimal damage probably has few additional risk factors and may not need a profoundly low IOP to prevent further damage.

EXTENT OF DAMAGE

The extent of damage is thus the major clue to the threshold for damage and for the presence of nonpressure risk factors. In addition, when setting a pressure goal, the extent of damage determines the likely effect on the patient's useful visual function if he or she has progressive damage. In an eye with extensive nerve damage and field loss, each increment of damage causes more functionally critical loss than the same increment of damage causes in a less damaged eye. Thus the greater the damage, the greater should be the attempt to lower the IOP.

Specific Numbers

With these considerations in mind, set a presure goal for each patient. We have constructed Figure 3-1 and Table 3-1 as guides (which are *arbitrary* and *imperfect*) to suggest targets based on the IOP and either the visual field or the cupping, whichever measure is of better quality in a given patient. The numbers only suggest an initial treatment goal. In a given person, the suggested goal may represent too much or too little IOP lowering. Only over time will the answer be known. Most people have findings that, following these guides, warrant lowering IOP between 20% and 40%, depending on the degree of associated damage. Thus for a patient with an average pretreatment IOP of 30 mm Hg and severe damage represented by a 0.8 cup and extensive field loss, a treatment goal would be to lower IOP 40% to 18 mm Hg or even to aim for a 50% lowering to 15 mm Hg. If the damage is mild with a 0.4 cup and minimal field damage, the goal would be 23 or 24 mm Hg, a 20% to 25% reduction. As in this example, many of the goals suggested by this chart will be higher than "normal," or conversely will be considerably less than the upper limit of normal pressure. That the "goal" does not coincide with the limit of the normal range in no way negates the importance of IOP lowering.

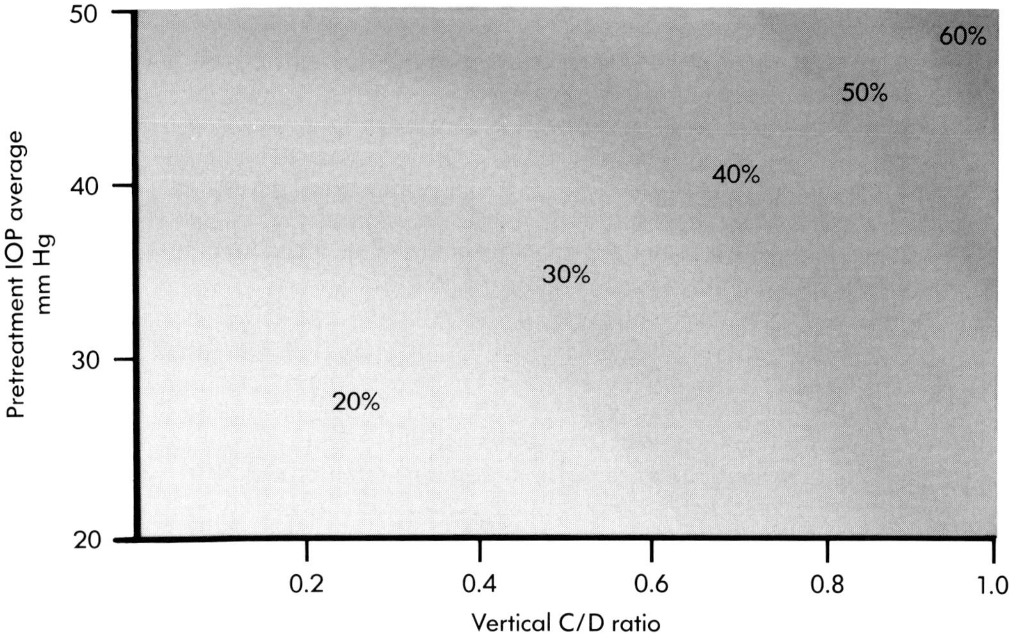

FIG. 3-1 Initial IOP goal in POAG based on disc and pressure data. The percentages refer to the decrease compared to the average pretreatment IOP.

TABLE 3-1 ***Suggested Initial Pressure Goal in POAG***

Visual field loss	Initial Average IOP (mm Hg) 50	40	30	20	
Mild	30	25	23	16	Goal (mm Hg)
Moderate	25	25	20	14	
Severe	20	20	15	10	

TREATMENT APPROACHES TO LOWER IOP

Therapeutic Options

Once a pressure goal has been determined for a patient, institute therapy to try to achieve the goal. It is currently assumed—although possibly not true—that the beneficial effect of lowering IOP is independent of how the lowering is achieved. That is, we treat glaucoma as if the nerve does not care if the pressure is 14 mm Hg because of a drop, a pill, a laser treatment, or surgery. Each treatment has different side effects, and the appropriate order in which to institute therapies is a subject of current dispute. The three major suggested courses are the following:

- Start with topical therapy. If this is ineffective, either perform laser trabeculoplasty or add carbonic anhydrase inhibitors. If the IOP remains too high, add the pills or do laser surgery, whichever has not been tried. If the pressure is still too high, filtration surgery is indicated.
- Perform laser trabeculoplasty first. If the pressure is not low enough, add topical therapy. If the pressure remains too high, add carbonic anhydrase inhibitors. If this is not sufficient, filtration surgery is indicated.
- Perform filtration surgery first. The next steps if the surgery is ineffective are generally not specified when this possibility is discussed, perhaps because it is at such variance with conventional management that discussion tends to be focused on the first step.

For each of these courses, reasonable supporting and opposing arguments exist. Some of the major points regarding each approach are summarized as follows.

MEDICINE FIRST, LASER SECOND, FILTRATION THIRD

Supporting arguments. This is the most commonly followed, traditional course. Easily tolerated topical medications lower pressure in most patients. Medications can be stopped or altered easily, and unlike either laser or filtration surgery, topical medications rarely cause acute ocular complications. The most severe systemic reactions (asthma, congestive heart failure) occur rarely; taking a good medical history usually alerts the physician to a patient's risk for such problems. If topical medicines fail to achieve the pressure goal after a short time, laser trabeculoplasty or carbonic anhydrase inhibitors often lower pressure enough. If both fail, filtration surgery can always be performed.

Drawbacks. Ocular medications are expensive and bothersome to use. Many people are unable or unwilling to use them regularly. When the patient misses a dose or takes a dose late, the pressure may rise and nerve damage may occur. All topical therapies have side effects. When people must use drops daily, their quality of life suffers, and they are constantly aware of their disease. Topical medications may promote changes in the conjunctiva that limit the success of subsequent filtering surgery.

LASER FIRST, MEDICINE SECOND, FILTRATION THIRD

Supporting arguments. Laser trabeculoplasty safely lowers the IOP in most people who have POAG. It may eliminate, reduce, or postpone the need for topical medications. After treatment, laser surgery causes no daily nuisance and requires no compliance except for routine follow-up visits. Laser exerts its effect 24 hours a day. Thus when successful, laser therapy obviates constant, day-in, day-out, attention. If laser surgery proves ineffective, then topical or systemic medications can still be used. Laser treatment has not been shown to limit the success of filtering surgery performed subsequently.

Drawbacks. Laser trabeculoplasty is often a temporary treatment that loses its effect over time. Most people treated initially with the laser require medications, and the laser provides only a fairly short reprieve. It is expensive and may cause IOP elevations that may damage the eye. In the rare event that the IOP is actually raised instead of lowered, the patient may require surgery that he or she would otherwise have avoided.

FILTERING SURGERY FIRST

Supporting arguments. After a successful procedure, the patient leads a fairly normal life and usually visits the eye doctor less frequently than do glaucoma patients treated in other ways. Successful surgery often achieves pressures lower than can be obtained with medications, and the pressure control is full time. If surgery precedes topical therapy, the success rate of surgery may be higher than reported for patients treated medically first, because eye drops cause irritation and conjunctival changes. If surgery fails, medications and lasers may then be tried. Filtering surgery costs more than other treatments initially, but over time surgery is less expensive because of fewer doctor visits and reduced medication expenses.

Drawbacks. Surgery is not always successful, and successful surgery may fail after several years, a relatively short time in relation to the patient's life. Intraocular surgery carries a risk of infrequent but immediate, severe, potentially blinding, complications. The presence of a bleb places the patient at an ongoing increased risk of endophthalmitis. Glaucoma surgery may make cataracts develop more quickly. Previously successful surgery may fail after cataract extraction. If surgery were to be done as the usual initial treatment for patients with primary open-angle glaucoma, it would place may patients who would do very well with less risky management at risk for these complications.

Suggested Approach

We subscribe in general to the topical medication first philosophy. Our general management course for POAG is as follows:

1. Topical therapy that proves free of bothersome side effects
2. Laser trabeculoplasty
3. Topical therapy with side effects that are tolerable
4. Carbonic anhydrase inhibitor therapy if well tolerated
5. Filtration surgery

We quickly determine if a patient is one who will easily achieve satisfactory pressure control with well-tolerated topical therapy. Over the last decade, we have begun to move promptly beyond topical therapy if the patient tolerates medication poorly. We are less likely than before to encourage forbearance with a regimen of multiple medications and are more ready to perform a laser treatment or to do filtering surgery than 10 years ago. However, we initially manage most newly diagnosed patients with eye drops.

PRINCIPLES OF TOPICAL THERAPY

Several general principles contribute to the goal of maximizing the therapeutic effect of each topical medication while minimizing side effects. These principles are:

1. *Start with the least offensive drug first*. This is a subjective judgment. The considerations include ocular and systemic side effects, cost, and dosage frequency.
2. *Start with a low concentration of the drug*. Systemic and ocular side effects

are usually dose dependent. If you can achieve the pressure goal in a given patient at a low dose, do so.

3. *Treat unilaterally first to assess effect.* Pressure varies during the day and from day to day, but the two eyes generally vary together. If you treat one eye initially, you will be able, at least in part, to separate drug effect from diurnal or day-to-day variation. If a drug proves effective, then begin its use in both eyes. β-Blockers have small contralateral effects, but these effects do not negate the value of uniocular trials.
4. *Encourage lid closure after drop use.* Gentle lid closure for several minutes after drop use increases the contact time between the eye drops and the cornea by removing the lacrimal pumping action of the blink. More medication enters the eye and less medication enters the systemic circulation because there is less drainage onto the nasal mucosa via the nasolacrimal duct. Nasolacrimal duct obstruction for several minutes is an alternative if the patient has difficulty controlling his or her blinking.
5. *Use as few medications as possible.* Two medications are more difficult to use regularly than one medication. Medicine that is used four times a day is less desirable than medicine that is required only once or twice a day.
6. *If more than one drop is used, allow time for each drop to be absorbed.* The cul-de-sac holds less than one drop. If a patient instills two different drops, one immediately after the other, one of two things happens. Either the second drop washes the first one out (and onto the cheek, where it is wasted, or into the lacrimal system, where it enters the systemic circulation), or the two drops mix and dilute one another. Because the amount of drug absorbed into the eye relates to its concentration, such a mix is less effective than the two drugs separated by enough time for the first to be absorbed. The ideal spacing for drops depends on a variety of variables, particularly the patient's rate of blinking. We assume that many patients reduce our time recommendations and thus suggest 10 to 15 minutes in the hope of achieving at least 10 minutes of separation.
7. *Give the patient written instructions.* It is not easy for calm, medically sophisticated people to remember medication instructions. Anxious patients often completely misunderstand or forget directions.

USUAL EFFECTS OF VARIOUS MEDICATIONS

In addition to following these general guidelines, it is useful to have a general expectation of various drug treatments when starting glaucoma treatment. Understanding the concept of outflow pressure, discussed and illustrated in the following box, is useful.

Outflow Pressure and Glaucoma Medications

Glaucoma medications either decrease the amount of aqueous humor formed or decrease the resistance to the outflow of aqueous humor. Medications do not lower pressure by a fixed amount, nor do they lower pressure by a fixed percentage. For example, a particularly effective drug that reduces aqueous humor formation by 50% will not lower the pressure by 50%, but will lower it halfway from the starting pressure toward the episcleral venous pressure. Thus if episcleral venous pressure is 10 mm Hg, a pressure of 20 mm Hg will be lowered halfway toward 10 mm Hg, resulting in a pressure of 15 mm Hg (a 25% decrease). Similarly, a pressure of 30 mm Hg will be lowered to 20 mm Hg (halfway to 10 mm Hg), a 33% lowering. A pressure of 40 mm Hg will fall 38% to 25 mm Hg, etc.

If the pressure is already lowered by one drug, both the percent and magnitude of pressure decrease from a second, equally effective drug (one that provides another 50% lowering of aqueous humor production) will be less than the first. The first drug may lower the pressure 10 mm Hg from 30 mm Hg to 20 mm Hg, whereas the second achieves only an additional 5 mm Hg decrease, from 20 mm Hg to 15 mm Hg. The following example illustrates the concept of outflow pressure.

Episcleral venous pressure is 10 mm Hg.
Drug A decreases outflow pressure by 40%.
Drug B decreases outflow pressure by 33%.

Pretreatment IOP	**40 mm Hg**	**30 mm Hg**	**20 mm Hg**
Outflow pressure	30 mm Hg	20 mm Hg	10 mm Hg
Effect of A	*12 mm Hg*	*8 mm Hg*	*4 mm Hg*
IOP after A	28 mm Hg	22 mm Hg	16 mm Hg
(New outflow pressure)	(18 mm Hg)	(12 mm Hg)	(6 mm Hg)
Effect of B	*6 mm Hg*	*4 mm Hg*	*2 mm Hg*
IOP after A and B	22 mm Hg	18 mm Hg	14 mm Hg

With the same two drugs, the patient with the initial pressure of 40 mm Hg will have a decrease of 18 mm Hg and the patient with the initial pressure of 20 mm Hg will have a decrease of 6 mm Hg. This example demonstrates two points about how much effect to expect from medication:

- The higher the initial pressure, the greater the decrease in pressure for a given medicine
- The first drug used will probably provide the greatest numerical change in pressure

A rough guide to the effect of various medications on the outflow pressure follows:*

Timolol or levobunolol	35% to 45%
Metipranolol	25% to 35%
Betaxolol	25% to 35%
Dipivefrin	25% to 35%
Pilocarpine 1%	20% to 25%
Pilocarpine 4%	25% to 35%
Echothiophate iodide 0.125%	35% to 45%
Methazolamide 50 mg b.i.d.	25% to 35%
Acetazolamide (Diamox Sequels) b.i.d.	35% to 50%

*Refer to the readings at the end of the chapter (p. 83) for more extensive data.

TREA... RE: SPECIFICS

...f the major groups of topical medications ...st commonly begin treatment with a β- ... initial therapy is a miotic, usually pilo- ...in (we do not begin treatment with any ... summarizes our standard progression

... Glaucoma Medications

β-Blockers

...antages	Disadvantages
• They have few local side effects and are used once or twice a day. • They do not affect pupil size or accommodation.	• They may precipitate or exacerbate cardiac failure, asthma, or respiratory failure. • They may decrease libido or cause impotence. • Most are expensive.

Pilocarpine/Carbachol

Advantages	Disadvantages
• They have few systemic complications. • Pilocarpine is inexpensive.	• They cause miosis and spasm of accommodation, which may blur vision and hamper long-term disc and visual field assessment. • They increase vascular permeability and may lead to posterior synechiae formation. • Over time, they may cause the anterior chamber to become shallow and may cause chronic angle closure. • The drops are used three or four times a day, and the once-daily gel causes blurry vision in the morning. • Their use may contribute to retinal breaks and retinal detachments (unproved).

Echothiophate iodide/Demecarium bromide

Advantages	Disadvantages
• They are effective in lowering the pressure, and they are used once or twice a day. • They work well in aphakic and pseudophakic individuals.	• They have all the disadvantages of pilocarpine drops, but to a greater extent. • They may cause conjunctival cicatrization and accelerate cataract formation.

Dipivefrin

Advantages	Disadvantages
• It causes few visual side effects and does not cause miosis or spasm of accommodation. • It has minimal systemic side effects.	• It causes reactive conjunctival hyperemia and results in a chronically inflamed eye, even in patients without symptoms. • It commonly causes papillary conjunctivitis and an allergic response with prolonged use. • It may cause macular edema in aphakic and pseudophakic patients.

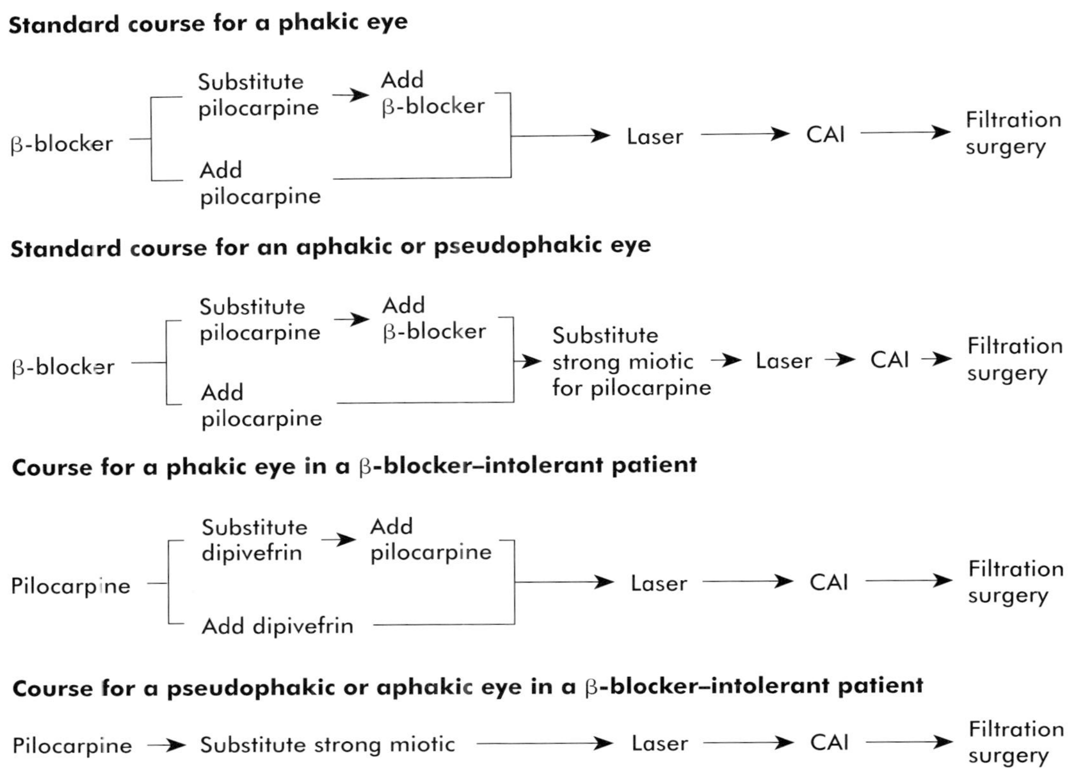

CHART 3-1 Progression of treatment in POAG. The decision to add a second medication or to substitute single medication is discussed in the text.

of treatment. Our approach to treatment beginning with each of the ordinary initial medications follows.

β-BLOCKER AS A FIRST MEDICINE

At this writing, there are four β-blockers available for ophthalmic use in the United States. The following considerations apply to the decision of which β-blocking agent to use first in a given patient: selectivity, relative pressure-lowering ability, formulation (solution vs. suspension), clinical experience, and cost.

Selectivity. Timolol, levobunolol, and metipranolol are nonselective (β_1- and β_2-) blockers; betaxolol is a cardioselective or β_1-blocker. The nonselective blockers, in addition to decreasing aqueous output, also increase airway resistance and decrease the cardiac output and the cardiac response to exercise. These drugs may precipitate asthma, respiratory failure, and congestive heart failure. The β_1 selective blocker has substantially less effect on the bronchial smooth muscle than nonselective drugs, and thus respiratory complications are much less common with betaxolol than with the others. Betaxolol does have some effect on respiratory muscle, and it has been associated with respiratory complications.

Relative pressure-lowering effect. Timolol and levobunolol in 0.5% concentration are approximately equal in effect and lower the IOP slightly more than metipranolol 0.3%. Timolol and levobunolol also are slightly more effective in lowering IOP than betaxolol.

Formulation. All the β-blockers are available in solutions. Betaxolol is also available as a suspension. Particles in the suspension remain in the cul-de-sac and thus available to enter the eye longer than does the medication in solution, and the ocular effect of betaxolol 0.25% suspension is equivalent to betaxolol 0.5% solution. This ocular equivalence results in a lower systemic dose per unit of ocular dose. Suspensions must be shaken, however, to ensure that the concentration is accurate and consistent.

Clinical experience. The longer a medication has been in use and the more people who have used it, the greater the chance that unusual effects will have surfaced. Timolol has the longest record, followed by levobunolol, betaxolol, and metipranolol.

Cost. Prices vary geographically and from pharmacy to pharmacy, depending on a variety of factors, but as Table 3-3 illustrates, the various β-blockers range widely in cost.

For a healthy patient who has no contraindications to β-blockade, we usually prescribe a nonselective β-blocker. Levobunolol and timolol are interchangeable as our first choice, and we sometimes instruct the pharmacist to dispense the less expensive drug. When cost is a significant consideration, we prescribe metipranolol.

When treating an individual who has respiratory or cardiac disease, we consult with the patient's internist or family practitioner before prescribing a β-blocker unless the patient is already taking a β-blocking agent. In this case, we assume that the internist would approve of using topical β-blockers. (In such individuals, the eye may already be partially or fully treated with a β-blocker, and topical therapy may achieve little.) If the patient is not using a systemic β-blocker and if a trial of selective β-blocker treatment is considered safe, we order betaxolol suspension. We begin therapy in one eye at a time, and the patient is cautioned to notify us promptly of any changes in his or her medical status. Before treating the second eye, we ask specifically about symptoms because bilateral treatment doubles the systemic dose.

TABLE 3-3 ***Cost of β-blockers at Different Pharmacies in the Miami Area (April 1992)***

	Pharmacies				
	1	2	3	4	5
Timoptic 0.5% 10 ml	$27.30	$33.95	$37.99	$26.49	$32.50
Betagan 0.5% 10 ml	$36.39	$38.00	$39.99	$33.39	$36.50
Betoptic 0.5% 10 ml	$35.49	$38.95	$39.99	$33.59	$36.50
Betoptic-S 0.25% 10 ml	$37.39	$39.95	$37.99	$33.00	—
Optipranolol 0.3% 10 ml	$18.19	$21.50	$29.99	—	$16.50

After choosing a β-blocker, the clinician must decide how frequently the patient should use it. Twice-a-day usage is traditional and covers occasional missed doses, but once a day may be sufficient. If once-a-day treatment is chosen, it seems reasonable to use it immediately on arising in the morning, because β-blockage has little or no effect on aqueous formation during sleep.

MIOTIC AS A FIRST DRUG

We begin treatment with pilocarpine in patients for whom a β-blocker is contraindicated or for whom cost is a major concern. (Carbachol is a reasonable alternative choice. It is slightly stronger at maximum dosage but is more likely to have aching as a side effect.) Miotics have a number of undesirable dose-related side effects. Even in low concentrations, however, pilocarpine has a significant effect on IOP in most people with POAG. We generally start with 1% pilocarpine used four times a day in one eye, but changing to 2% and then 4% is necessary in many people with brown eyes.

Patients who find pilocarpine difficult to tolerate because of miosis, accommodative spasm, or drop frequency may find the pilocarpine Ocusert to be a useful device. Because pilocarpine is delivered continuously, the Ocusert lacks the repeated bolus effect of eye drops on the pupil and ciliary muscle. Although more expensive than drops, it is much easier to use and provides full-time drug delivery for a week. We prescribe pilocarpine drops first in our patients for two reasons. First, we want to determine the pressure response to pilocarpine. In our experience, a Pilo-20 Ocusert is more or less equivalent to 1% pilocarpine, whereas a Pilo-40 approximates pilocarpine 2% to 3%. Second, patients accept the Ocusert better after a trial of topical medication. Success in using the Ocusert depends on careful instruction and supervised practice in inserting and removing the device. Sometimes there is a burst effect of transient overdose when an Ocusert is first placed in the eye. If the device is placed in the eye at bedtime, the effects of any burst are resolved by morning. The patient may also soak the Ocusert device in a glass of water for an hour before placing it in the eye to eliminate the initial excessive release. If a patient is using an Ocusert, his or her pressure should be checked both early in the week and at the end of the week to determine whether the pressure effect lasts for the full 7 days that the manufacturer recommends. Sometimes this device should be changed every 5 days or so.

We rarely use an irreversible anticholinesterase as an initial drug, even in patients who have had lens extractions. Both echothiophate iodide and demecarium bromide, known commonly as the "strong mitotics," have more side effects, such as posterior synechiae formation, conjunctival irritation, and scarring, than does pilocarpine. However, the strong mitotics are valuable; we frequently use them in individuals who have had cataract extractions if other topical medications are ineffective or intolerable. In such cases they are often effective and obviate surgery. These medications work well when used once a day.

DIPIVEFRIN AS A FIRST DRUG

We infrequently prescribe dipivefrin as an initial drug, and we never begin treatment with any of the other epinephrine compounds because of the increased systemic and topical dose effects relative to the intraocular effect. An appropriate candidate for initial dipivefrin treatment would be an individual for whom all β-blockers are contraindicated and in whom pilocarpine is so certain to be intolerable (for example a young person with a small, central posterior subcapsular cataract) that a trial seems to be a waste of time.

Evaluation and Modification of Initial Treatment

INITIAL MEDICATION EVALUATION

After instituting treatment on one eye, the next step is to determine its effectiveness in lowering the IOP. The initial treatment and the extent of the patient's disease determine the timing of follow-up. β-Blockers lower the IOP promptly, but the pressure may take some weeks to stabilize and usually does so at a higher pressure than that which immediately follows the initial dose. Thus the clinician can conclude quickly (in a day or two) that β-blockers are inadequate, but it may take a month or two to be certain that initially lowered IOP will remain adequately low to move on to chronic follow-up. Pilocarpine achieves its full effect within hours of the first dose. Dipivefrin takes a few weeks to achieve its full effect, although most of its effect occurs promptly. If we begin treatment with either a β-blocker or dipivefrin, we prefer to wait about a month for the pressure to stabilize before retesting the pressure. If we begin treatment with pilocarpine, we may recheck the patient in a week. If the patient has very high pressure and significant damage, we may check the pressure the next day. It is usually possible to quickly determine if the first drug, or indeed full medical therapy, will be *insufficient* in such cases. However, if medical therapy is initially adequate, it is impossible to tell immediately if medical therapy will be *sufficient* over the longer term without examining the patient a month or so later.

When the patient returns for assessment of medication effect, the following determinations should be made:

- Determine if the patient is both taking and tolerating the medication. Ask whether the patient understood the directions and exactly how he or she is using the medication. Ask specifically if the patient has had side effects or any significant change in medical status. Record when the patient last took his or her medicine before the examination.
- Determine if the medication is lowering the pressure at all; if not, stop it. This is much easier if treatment was started in only one eye. If the IOP in the treated eye has decreased in relation to the untreated eye, it is reasonable to assume that it is because of the medication. Particularly if the IOP fluctuates substantially, there may be little difference between

pretreatment and posttreatment pressure on a given measurement. If the medication is not lowering the pressure, discontinue it and try a different drug or treatment. It is an unnecessary nuisance, risk, and expense to use a drug that has little or no effect.

- If the medication is lowering the pressure, decide if it is lowering it enough and modify treatment accordingly. The routine steps to follow are summarized in Chart 3-2.

PRESSURE GOAL MET

If the pressure goal has been achieved, begin medication in both eyes and have the patient return for follow-up as described in Chapter 4.

PRESSURE GOAL NOT MET

There are several routine steps if the initial regimen does not achieve the desired pressure goal.

- Increase the dose or frequency of the initial medication. For example, if

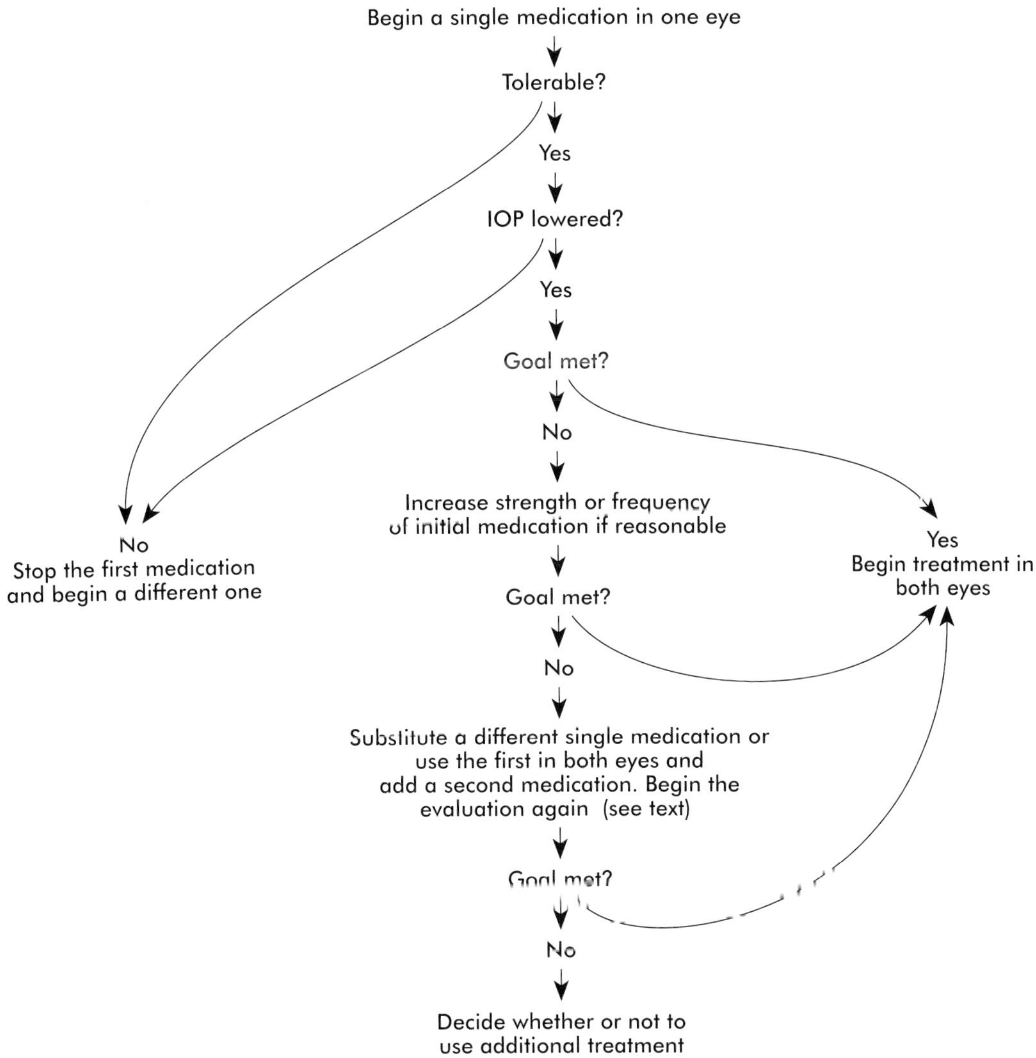

CHART 3-2 Evaluation of initial therapy.

the patient was using a β-blocker once a day, increase the frequency to twice a day. If pilocarpine was used and was well tolerated, increase the strength up to a maximum of 4%.

- When the medication is used in full dosage, decide if the pressure is close enough to the goal to accept it. Given the arbitrary nature of the pressure goals, a pressure slightly (2 or 3 mm Hg) above a patient's goal may be acceptable in a patient with mild disease. In this case, begin treatment in both eyes and move to the follow-up phase (Chapter 4). If the disease is moderate or severe, substitute or add another medication.
- Repeat the cycle after substitution or addition of medication.

MODIFICATION OF INITIAL TREATMENT

If the first medication in full dosage is effective but does not achieve a low enough pressure, the clinician must decide whether to substitute a different single medication or to add a second medication to the one already tried. This is not always a simple decision. Single-drug therapy is preferable to multiple-drug therapy, but patients usually prefer to establish their initial treatment regimen quickly. Changes that are unlikely to achieve the pressure goal are better avoided. If the desired effect is within a range for which a single drug should have a chance of achieving the pressure goal, then it is realistic to change to a different single drug.

Single-drug substitutions. If it seems reasonable to change rather than to add medication, we use the following guidelines:

- If levobunolol or timolol was insufficient alone, try pilocarpine.
- If metipranolol was not sufficient alone, try either levobunolol or timolol.
- If betaxolol was insufficient alone (presumably used because a nonselective blocker was contraindicated), try pilocarpine.
- If pilocarpine was begun because of expense rather than β-blocker contraindications and was insufficient alone, try the least expensive β-blocker in your area.
- If pilocarpine was begun because of β-blocker contraindication and was ineffective alone, try dipivefrin.
- If pilocarpine was begun in an aphakic or pseudophakic person, try one of the strong miotics.

Addition of drugs. If single-drug therapy does not achieve the individual's IOP goal, then we recommend adding drugs as follows:

- If a β-blocker was insufficient, add pilocarpine.
- If pilocarpine was insufficient, add a β-blocker (if tolerable) or dipivefrin.
- If the patient is pseudophakic or aphakic and a combination of β-blocker and pilocarpine is insufficient, try β-blocker and a strong miotic.

We rarely add dipivefrin to a regimen that already includes a β-blocker, although it may help in some cases, especially if added to the selective β-blocker betaxolol.

Evaluation for Additional Therapy: Choices

When full, well-tolerated, topical therapy lowers the pressure to some degree but does not decrease the pressure to the goal, there are two options: progress to additional treatment or observe the patient for stability. The choices for additional treatment are, in order of preference, laser trabeculoplasty, additional marginally tolerated topical therapy, carbonic anhydrase inhibitors, and filtration surgery.

LASER TRABECULOPLASTY

The technique of laser trabeculoplasty is described in standard glaucoma textbooks. We treat 180° of a patient's angle at each of two sittings separated by at least a week and usually by less than a month. If the patient's pressure remains above the pressure goal 2 months after laser trabeculoplasty, then the decision must be made whether to proceed.

TOLERATED, EVEN IF NOT WELL-TOLERATED, TOPICAL THERAPY

Most patients will not move through this step since it will already have been taken. For those patients who had bothersome but not intolerable side effects from one or more types of drops, another trial of topical therapy may be reasonable before considering carbonic anhydrase inhibitors or filtration surgery.

CARBONIC ANHYDRASE INHIBITORS

Despite their sometimes severe and rarely life-threatening complications, carbonic anhydrase inhibitors remain a useful group of drugs. We begin treatment with methazolamide 25 mg bid; if necessary, we increase the dosage to 50 mg bid or tid. If the pressure is still too high and the patient tolerates methazolamide, we change to acetazolamide 250 mg qid or to Diamox Sequels bid. Unless there is a compelling reason to avoid filtration surgery, we discontinue these medications in individuals with drowsiness, depression, renal stones, or other significant side effects.

Like other sulfonamides, carbonic anhydrase inhibitors rarely cause blood dyscrasias of varying severity, including fatal aplastic anemia. There has been some controversy about whether individuals treated with such medications should have regular complete blood counts performed. Recommendations regarding blood tests involve questions of the standard of care, the cost-benefit ratio of early detection of abnormalities, and the incidence and timing of carbonic anhydrase inhibitor associated dyscrasias. It is currently not known how frequently—if ever—early recognition of a carbonic anhydrase inhibitor-related blood dyscrasia and prompt drug withdrawal improves the ultimate outcome of the condition. In the absence of better information, it seems reasonable either to perform or to forgo blood tests. In either case, however, the patient should be advised to report systemic symptoms. (Refer to the second group of reading at the end of the chapter.)

FILTRATION SURGERY

Filtration surgery is well described in standard surgical texts. We usually perform a trabeculectomy and currently use both antiproliferative adjunctive therapy and selective suture lysis when aiming for a very low pressure. For patients for whom these are impractical, for example because of poor cooperation, we may perform full-thickness surgery.

Evaluation for Additional Therapy: Algorithm

Chart 3-3 outlines our approach to the patient in whom initial topical treatment fails to achieve the pressure goal. This algorithm deals with the newly diagnosed patient with POAG, and assumes the following definitions of disease stage:

- Mild disease: *Both* a C/D ratio of ≤0.4 and no more than mild field loss
- Moderate disease: *Both* a C/D ratio of <0.8 and no more than moderate field loss
- Severe disease: *Either* a C/D ratio of ≥0.8 or severe field loss

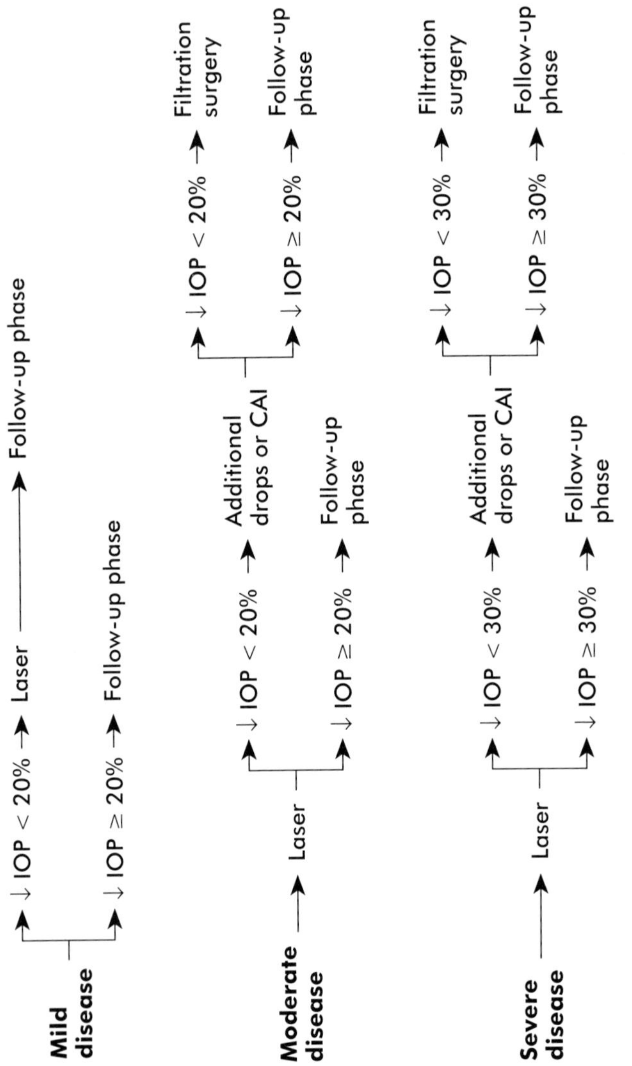

CHART 3-3 Course when goal is not met with readily tolerated topical therapy.

MILD DISEASE

- If the pressure is at least 20% lower than the baseline, regardless of whether the goal is met, proceed to chronic follow-up.
- If the pressure is not lowered at least 20%, proceed with laser treatment. Even if the laser treatment does not achieve a 20% decrease in pressure, proceed with chronic follow-up to determine the pace of damage.

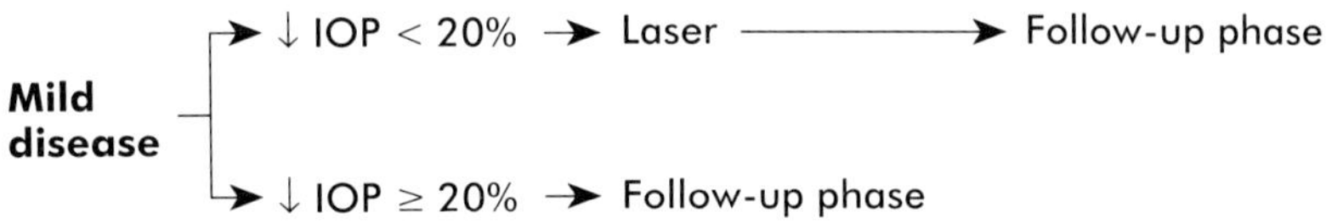

MODERATE DISEASE

- Proceed with laser trabeculoplasty.
- If the pressure is at least 20% lower than the baseline after laser treatment, regardless of whether the goal is met, follow the patient's course.
- If the pressure is not lowered at least 20%, add additional topical therapy or carbonic anhydrase inhibitors. If they are tolerated and achieve at least a 20% decrease in pressure, proceed with chronic follow-up.
- If the pressure cannot be lowered at least 20%, perform filtration surgery in one eye. If the surgery achieves the pressure goal without causing side effects that decrease the vision, perform surgery in the other eye. If the surgery either fails to lower the pressure or has visually significant side effects, follow the patient's course carefully to determine the pace of disease before operating on the other eye.

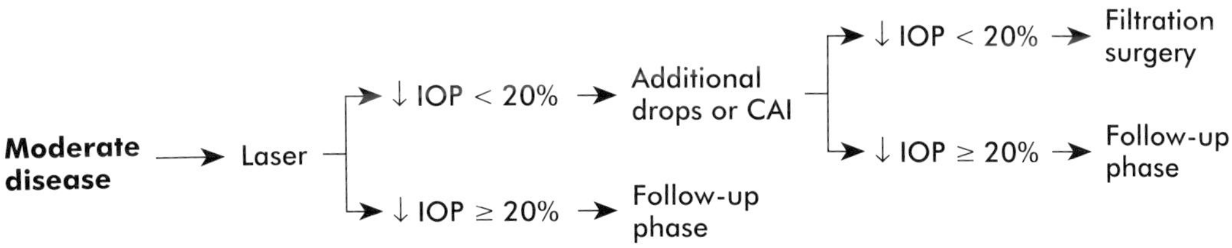

SEVERE DISEASE

- Proceed with laser trabeculoplasty.
- If the pressure is at least 30% lower than the baseline after laser treatment, regardless of whether the goal is met, observe the patient.
- If the pressure is not lowered at least 30% by laser treatment, try additional topical therapy or carbonic anhydrase inhibitors. If they are well tolerated and lower the pressure at least 30%, continue them and follow the patient's course.

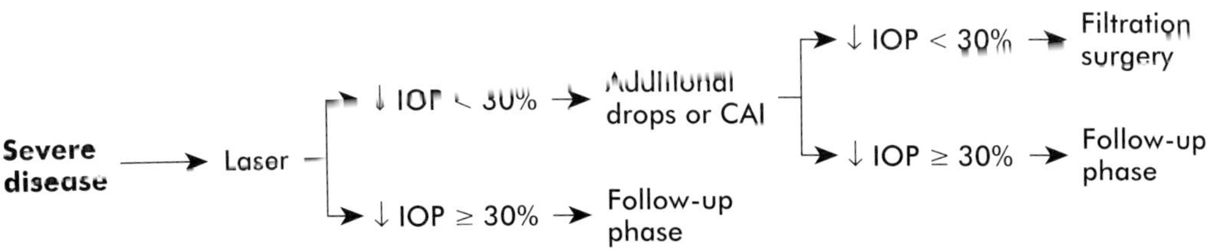

- If additional medication and laser treatment do not lower the pressure at least 30%, proceed with filtration surgery in one eye. If the surgery is successful in lowering the IOP without significant complications, perform surgery in the other eye. If the surgery is not successful, follow the patient's course carefully to determine the pace of disease before operating on the other eye.

TREATING TO LOWER THE PRESSURE: SOME VARIATIONS

Our recommended management of POAG presumes that clinicians can follow-up with their patients over time and modify their goals and treatment as indicated by their courses. In some situations, however, it is difficult or impossible to assess further progression. The most common such clinical settings are as follows:

- The patient who cannot do reliable fields
- The patient whose fundus cannot be seen well
- The patient with far-advanced glaucoma on initial observation

The Patient Who Cannot Do Reliable Fields

If a patient cannot, despite education, perform reliable visual fields, then determine if the patient can perform any reliable fields. Suprathreshold testing is not as good as threshold testing, but if reliable it is better than nothing. In patients who cannot give good field information the disc examination assumes greater importance. The greater the nerve damage, the more difficult it is to recognize a small change, and thus the more difficult it is to recognize progressive damage. In patients with less than 80% cupping, lower the IOP by the routine guidelines in Figure 3-1. In those whose cupping equals or exceeds 80%, follow the guidelines below for advanced glaucoma.

The Patient Whose Fundus Cannot Be Seen Well

In a patient whose fundus cannot be seen well because of miosis, cataract, or other media opacity, the visual field and pressure will be the key points to follow. In this case, use the pressure guides related to visual fields in Table 3-1. The visual field constriction that usually accompanies small pupils and cataracts may cause you to set a low pressure goal, but in this situation it is reasonable.

The Patient With Far-Advanced Glaucoma On Initial Observation

Even if both the disc and field can be evaluated, the more severe an individual's glaucomatous damage already is at the time of diagnosis, the more difficult it is to recognize further change in either disc or field. In addition, the more advanced a patient's glaucoma is, the greater the chance that damage will progress, and that a small additional amount of damage will cause symptomatically important worsening, such as loss of central fixation. If the disc and field are so badly damaged that further incremental damage will be difficult to recognize, we suggest the following *arbitrary* general guide:

1. Set a goal of 50% lowering of pressure or an IOP ≤15 mm Hg, whichever is less.
2. If the pressure can be decreased to this level, follow the patient's course carefully, as described in Chapter 4.
3. If this strict pressure goal cannot be achieved with medical or laser therapy, and if the patient has two seeing eyes, do filtering surgery on one of the eyes with a goal of ≤12 mm Hg.

4. If the pressure goal cannot be achieved with medical or laser therapy, and if the patient has only one seeing eye, do surgery if the pressure is either 20% above the pressure goal or is less than 30% below the baseline pressures.

After completing the initial steps of management, glaucoma care moves into the chronic follow-up phase, described in Chapter 4.

BIBLIOGRAPHY

* Few studies of the IOP response to medication present data on outflow pressure. However, it is often possible to calculate the approximate value using the mean untreated and treated pressures. The data in the outflow pressure table (p. 71) are derived from the following studies:

Berson FG, Cohen HB, Foerster RJ, Lass JH, Novack GD, Duzman E: Levobunolol compared with timolol for the long-term control of elevated intraocular pressure, *Arch Ophthalmol* 103:379, 1985.

Berson FG, Epstein DL: Separate and combined effects of timolol maleate and acetazolamide in open-angle glaucoma, *Am J Ophthalmol* 92:788, 1981.

Berson FG, Epstein DL, Grant WM, Hutchinson BT, Dobbs PC: Acetazolamide dosage forms in the treatment of glaucoma, *Arch Ophthalmol* 98:1051, 1980.

Dahlen K, Epstein DL, Grant WM, Hutchinson BT, Prien EL, Krall JM: A repeated dose-response study of methazolamide in glaucoma, *Arch Ophthalmol* 96:2214, 1978.

Drance SM, Nash PA: The dose response of human intraocular pressure to pilocarpine, *Can J Ophthalmol* 6:9, 1971.

Harris LS: Dose-response analysis of echotiopate iodide, *Arch Ophthalmol* 86:502, 1971.

Kaback MB, Podos SM, Harbin TS, Mandell A, Becker B: The effects of dipivalyl epinephrine on the eye, *Am J Ophthalmol* 81:768, 1976.

Kass MA, Mandell AI, Goldbert I, Paine M, Becker B: Dipivefrin and epinephrine treatment of elevated intraocular pressure, *Arch Ophthalmol* 97:1865, 1979.

Kohn AN, Moss AP, Hargett NA, Ritch R, Smith H, Podos SM: Clinical comparison of dipivalyl epinephrine and epinephrine in the treatment of glaucoma, *Am J Ophthalmol* 87:196, 1979.

Long DA, Johns GE, Mullen RS, et al: Levobunolol and betaxolol. A double-masked controlled comparison of efficacy and safety in patients with elevated intraocular pressure. *Ophthalmology* 95:735, 1988.

Mertz M: Results of a 6 weeks' multicenter double-blind trial. Metipranolol versus timolol. In Merte H-J, editor: *Metipranolol. Pharmacology of beta-blocking agents and use of metipranolol in ophthalmology.* First Metipranolol Symposium, Berlin 1983. New York, 1983, Springer-Verlag.

Mills KB, Wright G: A blind randomised crossover trial comparing metipranolol 0.3% with timolol 0.25% in open-angle glaucoma: a pilot study, *Br J Ophthalmol* 70:39, 1986.

Pratt-Johnson JA, Drance SM, Innes R: Comparison between pilocarpine and echothiophate for chronic simple glaucoma, *Arch Ophthalmol* 81:485, 1976.

Serle JB, Lustgarten JS, Podos SM: A clinical trial of metipranolol, a noncardioselective beta-adrenergic antagonist, in ocular hypertension, *Am J Ophthalmol* 112:302, 1991.

Stewart RH, Kimbrough RL, Ward RL: Betaxolol vs timolol. A six-month double-blind comparison, *Arch Ophthalmol* 104:46, 1986.

Soll DB: Evaluation of timolol in chronic open-angle glaucoma. Once a day vs twice a day, *Archiv Ophthalmol* 98:2178, 1980.

Stone RA, Zimmerman TJ, Shin DH, Becker B, Kass MA: Low-dose methazolamide and intraocular pressure, *Am J Ophthalmol* 83:674, 1977.

Weinreb RN, Caldwell DR, Goode SM, et al: A double-masked three-month comparison between 0.25% betaxolol suspension and 0.5% betaxolol ophthalmic solution, *Am J Ophthalmol* 110:189, 1990.

Zimmerman TJ, Kass MA, Yablonski ME, Becker B: Timolol maleate. Efficacy and safety, *Arch Ophthalmol* 97:656, 1979.

The following references present the major points of view regarding blood tests and carbonic anhydrase inhibitors.

Fraunfelder FT, Meyer SM, Bagby GC, Dreis MW: Hematologic reactions to carbonic anhydrase inhibitors, *Am J Ophthalmol* 100:79, 1985.

Johnson T, Kass MA: Hematologic reactions to carbonic anhydrase inhibitors, *Am J Ophthalmol* 101:128, 1986 (letter).

Keisu M, Wiholm B-E, Ost A, Mortimer O: Acetazolamide-associated aplastic anaemia, *J Intern Med* 228:627, 1990.

Mogk LG, Cyrlin MN: Blood dyscrasias and carbonic anhydrase inhibitors, *Ophthalmology* 95:768, 1988.

Werblin TP, Pollack IP, Liss RA: Aplastic anemia and agranulocytosis in patients using methazolamide for glaucoma, *JAMA* 241:2817, 1979.

Zimran A, Beutler E: Can this risk of acetazolamide-induced aplastic anemia be decreased by periodic monitoring of blood cell counts? *Am J Ophthalmol* 104:654, 1987 (editorial).

4

Follow-Up of Primary Open-Angle Glaucoma

Establishing a baseline, setting an initial pressure goal, and achieving the initial pressure goal with treatment usually take a few months. The fourth and fifth steps in the management of primary open-angle glaucoma, following up on the patient's course and modifying treatment as indicated, continue for the patient's lifetime (see box below).

PATIENT FOLLOW-UP

The underlying purpose of examining a patient with POAG on a regular basis is to improve the chance of preserving vision. The more prosaic reasons include monitoring the effects—both desired and undesired—of therapy, maintaining the patient's motivation to care for his or her disease, determining if the pressure goal continues to be met, recognizing progressive damage, and modifying the pressure goal and management if needed to achieve optimal visual preservation. Three major questions arise in relation to follow-up:

- How frequently should the patient be examined?
- What should be tested at follow-up examinations?
- How is it determined whether the patient's condition is stable or is worsening?

Frequency of Examinations

Specific follow-up examples appear in the following sections. In general, we see patients frequently in the first 2 or 3 years of their (recognized) disease, when we are uncertain of the pace of their condition and when they need to be reminded of the importance of continuous treatment. We examine patients with severe disease more frequently than those who have mild disease. We gradually

Chronic Glaucoma Management Steps

1. Establish a good baseline.
2. Set a reasonable goal for IOP.
3. Lower the pressure.
4. Continue to observe the patient to determine whether the pressure goal is met and if the glaucomatous damage progresses.
5. Modify the pressure goal and treatment as indicated by the patient's course.

lengthen the interval between examinations in patients whose conditions prove stable for 2 or 3 years.

These guidelines may translate into weekly to monthly visits early in a patient's course, while the baseline is being established, a goal is being set, and treatment is instituted to reach the goal. Then the interval lengthens gradually to once or twice a year provided the patient's course remains stable. If the pressure becomes uncontrolled or if damage progresses, we evaluate the patient and modify management as necessary. We revert to more frequent visits and again slowly reduce the visit frequency.

Content of Follow-Up Examinations

HISTORY

Always take an interval history, particularly regarding possible side effects of medicine and changes in general health. Ask the patient to describe the schedule he or she is using for the treatment regimen; it may not correspond to the schedule prescribed.

VISION

Always check the visual acuity.

IOP

Check the IOP in both eyes and record the time of measurement and time of last medication. Although patients do not always take every dose of their medication, most people do use their medicine before visiting the doctor. Thus an IOP measurement at or below the patient's goal cannot ensure that the pressure is always low, but an IOP above the target generally indicates that the prescribed regimen does not achieve the pressure goal.

GONIOSCOPY

Gonioscopy should be performed at least yearly because the lens grows. Examine the patient with a gonioprism soon after adding a miotic to the treatment regimen because miotics may narrow the angle in direct relation to their strength.

FUNDUS EXAMINATION

Look for hemorrhages on the disc at every visit. Except in individuals with very small pupils or significant cataracts, a direct ophthalmoscope provides an adequate view of the nerve to recognize blood. Dilate the patient's pupils at least once a year to compare the optic nerve to the baseline and to examine the fundus. If the patient is using miotics, dilate the pupil every 6 months to decrease posterior synechiae formation. (If the patient does not otherwise need to be examined, it may be reasonable to prescribe dilating drops for the patient to use at home.) When the pupil is dilated, examine the disc with a lens that provides a magnified binocular view. As noted before, we prefer either a Hruby lens or a contact lens over the 78D and 90D noncontact indirect fundus lens because the direct lenses provide a better stereoscopic image. Use a slit beam to delineate the contour of the cup. Examine the macula and the retinal periphery; glaucoma patients are susceptible to other eye conditions.

VISUAL FIELDS

By the time most patients move into the follow-up phase of their care, they should have their field baseline established (Chapter 2). If a patient has significant variability or improves over the first four or five fields, obtaining the field baseline may extend into what is ordinarily the follow-up period. In such people, obtain a visual field test on most or all visits until a good, stable baseline is obtained.

Frequent fields early in the course of follow-up give a sense of the patient's variability and provide the opportunity to recognize unexpected rapid progression. If a series of several fields is stable over approximately 2 years, it is reasonable to extend the interval between field examinations, because the years of stability establish that if the patient is progressing at the selected pressure goal, such progression is not rapid. If the pressure rises or a disc hemorrhage is noted on a visit when the patient does not have a field examination, we promptly repeat the test to help interpret the pressure or disc change.

Threshold visual field examinations require extensive time. This makes them difficult for patients to perform and expensive to administer. Shorter visual field test algorithms are being studied, and some are emerging as available optional programs on the computerized perimeter (Fig. 4-1). It is not yet clear which of the faster tests compromise the physician's ability to reliably detect a change from baseline and which tests remain adequately accurate. If shorter, faster tests are shown to be adequate, we will use them. In the meantime, we use full threshold programs for patient follow-up.

VISUAL FIELDS AND MIOTIC DROPS

Miotic drops decrease the measured sensitivity on visual field tests. This effect confounds the comparison of fields obtained while the patient is using miotics to a baseline obtained before miotic use. It is possible to dilate patients' eyes for their visual fields, but this maneuver involves ocular manipulation before the field examination and lengthens the examination. In addition, dilation may raise the IOP. Since recognizing *change* is the key element in follow-up, it is possible to simply obtain a baseline on miotics and continue to test the field with the pupils constricted. However, if the overall sensitivity of the field is markedly diminished, it becomes difficult to recognize small changes (Fig. 4-2). We recommend the following compromise:

- Obtain an ordinary set of baseline fields
- Shortly after beginning miotic use, perform another field examination. If it is markedly worse than the initial baseline, dilate the pupil and repeat the field. If the dilated field approximates the baseline, henceforth dilate the patient's eyes for field examination.
- If the field examination during miotic treatment is only slightly worse than the baseline and the dilated field is not substantially better than the field when miotics are used, or if the field obtained during miotic use is almost the same as the baseline, measure a second field during miotic use at the patient's next visit and use these two fields as a new baseline.
- If the field obtained during miotic use appears in the future to have worsened, obtain a field with the patient's pupils dilated as the second (confirmatory) field examination. If it does not confirm worsening, use dilated fields thereafter for patient follow-up.

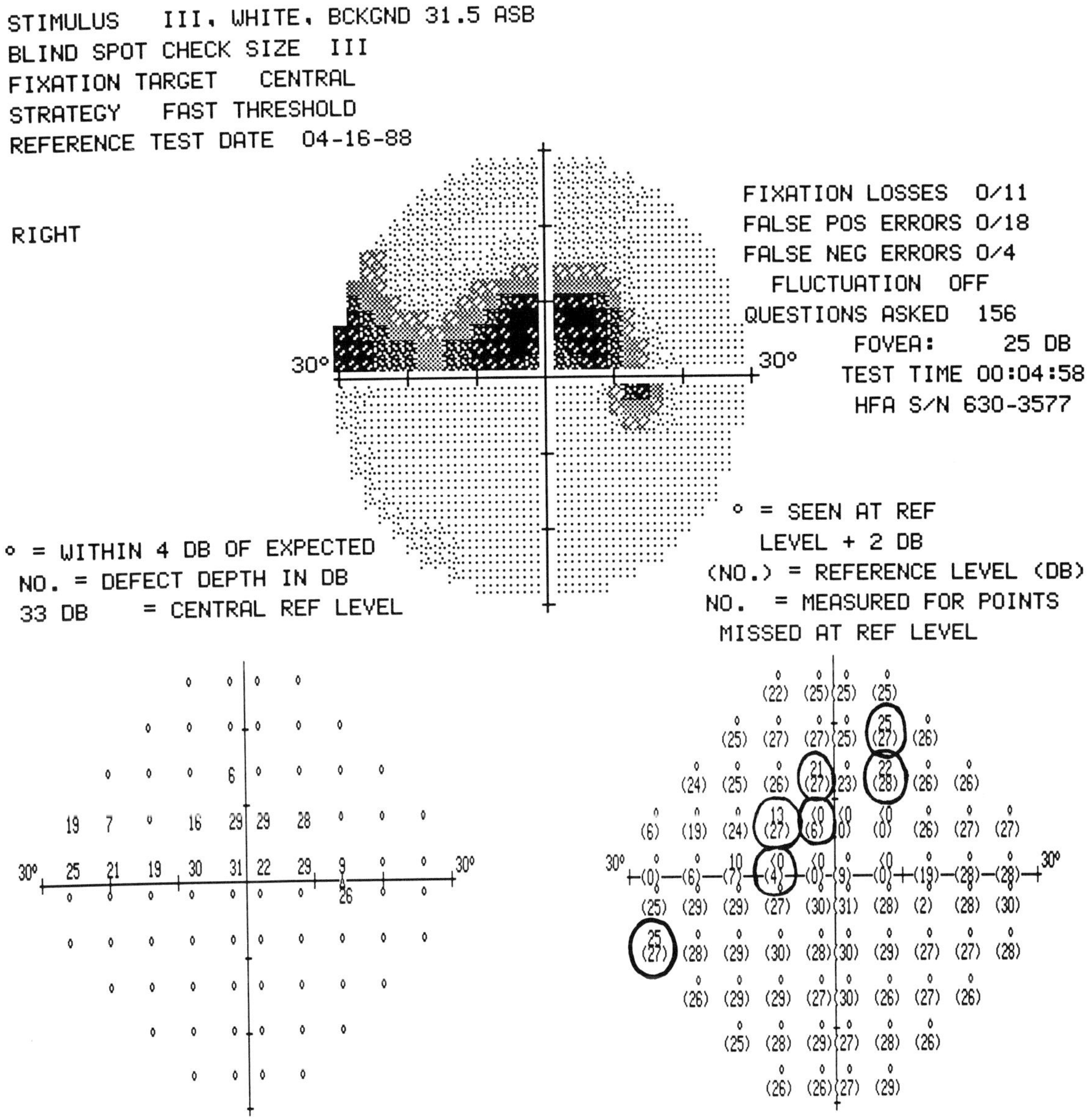

FIG. 4-1 Fast threshold. The grey scale and defect plot are the same as for a Master field. The lower right plot shows the results of testing each point with a stimulus 2 dB above the Master field value (presented in parentheses). If the stimulus was seen it is recorded as a o, if not seen, the threshold is determined and appears above the Master value. The *circled points* have lower threshold values than the Master field.

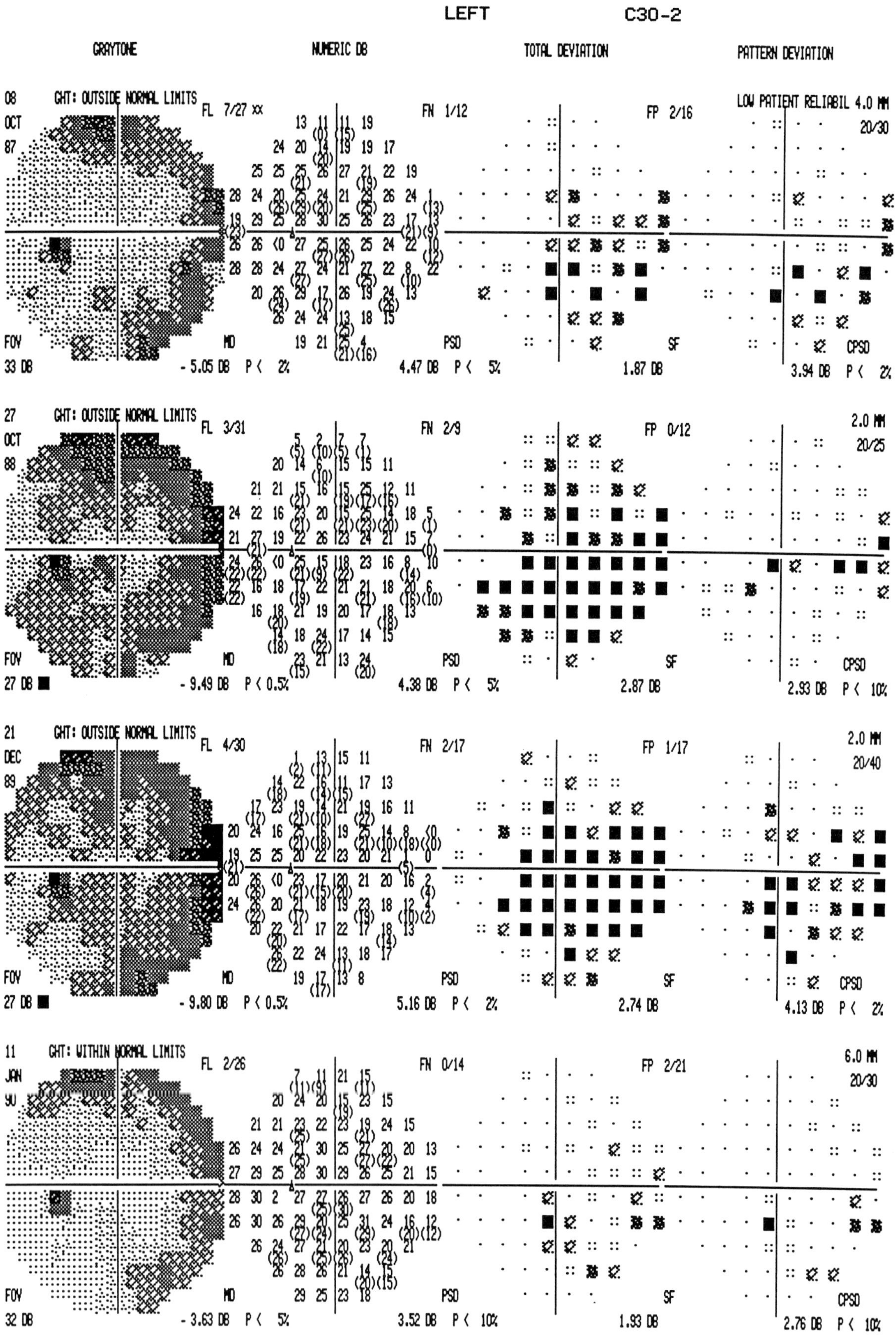

FIG. 4-2 Effect of miosis on the visual field. Between the first and second field examination, pilocarpine 2% was begun. Before examination 4, the pupil was dilated, and the field results returned to the initial level.

Follow-Up Planning Examples

The following hypothetical patient examples illustrate our recommendations for initial follow-up plans. How we decide whether the patient's condition is stable is discussed later; these examples outline our rationale about the frequency and nature of follow-up visits. Note that the frequency schedule and content of visits relate to the severity of the disease, to length of patient follow-up, and to the use of miotic drops. On all visits when the patient does not have his or her pupils dilated, examine the nerve with a direct ophthalmoscope to detect any hemorrhages.

CASE AB—EASILY CONTROLLED MILD GLAUCOMA

A 60-year-old asymptomatic woman is first seen with an IOP of 32 mm Hg. Her cup/disc ratio is 0.5, and her discs have neural rim tissue of good color without notches or hemorrhages. Baseline examinations completed over the course of 2 months include two static visual fields that show mild field loss, pressure measurements that, before any treatment, average 30 mm Hg (range, 27 to 33 mm Hg), and excellent-quality optic nerve photographs. The initial goal is a 30% lowering of pressure, or a pressure that varies between about 19 and 23 mm Hg on treatment. Treatment with a β-blocker in one eye results in a pressure of 21 mm Hg in the treated eye and 30 mm Hg in the untreated eye after 1 month. Treatment in both eyes is recommended.

- When should this patient be reexamined?
- What should be tested on follow-up?

A patient who has only early visual field loss despite a pressure in the high 20s to low 30s probably has a fairly high threshold for damage and probably has few nonpressure risk factors. Visual field and optic nerve changes may develop over time, but initially the focus is on whether the pressure remains below the target pressure and whether the patient tolerates the medication. It is reasonable to examine this person in a month or so and again 2 months later to check the pressure. If it remains low, reexamine the patient again in 3 months (6 months into follow-up) to monitor the pressure and repeat the visual field. If the patient's field is stable and the pressure remains within the goal, see the patient again in 3 months to test the pressure. In another 3 months (now 12 months into follow-up), perform another visual field examination, check the pressure, repeat gonioscopy, and dilate the patient's pupils to examine the disc and the rest of the fundus. Compare the discs to the photographs. If the field remains stable after two examinations 6 months apart for another year, and if the pressure remains within the target range, then continue to check the pressure every 6 months but increase the interval of field examinations to every year for 3 or 4 more years. Perform gonioscopy and dilate the pupils yearly; compare the discs to the baseline photographs. If the patient's condition is still stable after 5 years of follow-up, it is reasonable to examine the patient fully every 12 months. Alternatively, an office visit might be planned every 6 to 9 months to ensure that the pressure goal is maintained, with field examinations every other visit. Table 4-1 summarizes the recommended routine baseline studies and follow-up schedules for individuals with mild disease. Table 4-2 indicates the additional recommendations for patients using miotics.

TABLE 4-1 *Follow-up of Mild Glaucoma*

Baseline	• At least three IOP measurements at different times of day • At least two threshold visual field examinations • Gonioscopy • Disc photographs	Obtain within 2 months
Initial treatment	• Pressure checks and medication adjustments at 1- to 4-week intervals until treatment regimen is established	Complete within 2 months if possible
Follow-up		

	Months									Years 3 and after		Alternate after 5 years
	1	3	6	9	12	15	18	21	24	Every 6 months	Every year	Every year
IOP	X	X	X	X	X		X		X	X	X	X
Visual field			X		X		X		X		X	X
Gonioscopy					X				X		X	X
Undilated disc examination	X	X	X	X			X			X		
Dilated disc and fundus examination					X				X		X	X
Disc photos	Repeat only if the patient's condition is suspected of worsening.											

TABLE 4-2 *Follow-up of Mild Glaucoma in a Patient Who Uses Miotic Drops*

Baseline	• At least three IOP measurements at different times of day • At least two threshold visual field examinations • Gonioscopy • Disc photographs	Obtain within 2 months
Initial treatment	• Pressure checks and medication adjustments at 1- to 4-week intervals until treatment regimen is established	Complete within 2 months if possible

Follow-up

	Months									Years 3 and after		(Alternate) after 5 years
	1	3	6	9	12	15	18	21	24	Every 6 months	Every year	Every year
IOP	X	X	X	X	X		X		X	X	X	X
Visual field	X (Baseline with miotic)	X			X		X		X		X	X
Gonioscopy	X (Miotic)				X				X		X	
Undilated disc examination	X	X		X								
Dilated disc and fundus examination			X		X		X		X	X	X	X*
	(Because of miotic use, the pupil is dilated every 6 months)											
Disc photos	Repeat only if the patient's condition is suspected of worsening.											

*If the patient is seen only once a year, he or she may use dilating drops at home to avoid posterior synechiae formation.

CASE CD—PROBABLY CONTROLLED MODERATE GLAUCOMA

A 59-year-old man has untreated pressures that average 28 mm Hg (range, 24 to 32 mm Hg). His cup-disc ratio is 0.7 with a notch inferotemporally in both optic nerves and with corresponding superonasal visual field defects that are consistent on two sets of baseline fields. A goal of decreasing pressure by 30% gives a target pressure of 20 mm Hg. The patient has severe asthma, and his internist believes that β-blocker use is contraindicated. Treatment of one eye with pilocarpine 1% results in pressures of 22 mm Hg in the treated eye and 31 mm Hg in the untreated eye after a 2-week trial. Pilocarpine 2% produces intolerable symptoms after 1 day, and the patient is advised to use pilocarpine 1% for both eyes and dipivefrin in one eye. One month later the pressure is 18 mm Hg in the eye with both drugs and 22 mm Hg in the eye with only pilocarpine. He is advised to use both medications in both eyes.

- When should this patient be re-examined?
- What should be tested on follow-up?

This patient has significant disease, but he has responded nicely to medication. His threshold for damage is probably lower than that of patient AB, but he is unlikely to show measurable optic nerve or visual field changes after only a few months. The purpose of the initial follow-up examination is to ensure that the pressure remains low. However, with the addition of a miotic, his visual field test will change and the status of his angle may alter. Therefore the field test and gonioscopy should be repeated soon after determining that, at least initially, he will use a miotic. Schedule a follow-up visual field, pressure check, and gonioscopy a month or so after beginning bilateral treatment with the two drugs. This time course allows for stabilization of the effect of the dipivefrin. Arrange a second baseline field examination during miotic use and a follow-up pressure check in another 2 months. Recheck the visual field, pressure, gonioscopy, and the fundus (dilated) in another 3 months (now 6 months into follow-up). Check the pressure in 3 months; 3 months later (now 12 months into follow-up), repeat the field examination, pressure check, gonioscopy, and dilated funduscopy. If the patient's condition remains stable, perform a visual field examination, monitor the pressure, and dilate the pupils every 6 months for another 2 years or so and examine the angle every year. If the field and pressure remain satisfactory, the visual field examination and gonioscopy could be done yearly and the pressure tested every 6 months. Table 4-3 summarizes the follow-up schedule for patients with moderate glaucoma; Table 4-4 includes the additional examinations for a person using a miotic drop.

TABLE 4-3 *Follow-up of Moderate Glaucoma*

Baseline	• At least three IOP measurements at different times of day • At least two threshold visual field examinations • Gonioscopy • Disc photographs	Obtain within 2 months
Initial treatment	• Pressure checks and medication adjustments at 1-4-week intervals until treatment regimen is established	Complete within 2 months if possible

Follow-up

	Months					Years 2 through 4		Years 5 and after	
	1	3	6	9	12	Every 6 months	Every year	Every 6 months	Every year
IOP	X	X	X	X	X	X	X	X	X
Visual field			X		X	X	X		X
Gonioscopy					X		X		X
Undilated disc examination	X	X	X	X		X		X	
Dilated disc and fundus examination					X		X		X
Disc photos	Repeat only if the patient's condition is suspected of worsening.								

TABLE 4-4 *Follow-up of Moderate Glaucoma in a Patient Who Uses Miotic Drops*

Baseline	• At least three IOP measurements at different times of day • At least two threshold visual field examinations • Gonioscopy • Disc photographs	Obtain within 2 months
Initial treatment	• Pressure checks and medication adjustments at 1- to 4-week intervals until treatment regimen is established	Complete within 2 months if possible

Follow-up

	Months					Years 2 through 4		Years 5 and after	
	1	**3**	**6**	**9**	**12**	**Every 6 months**	**Every year**	**Every 6 months**	**Every year**
IOP	X	X	X	X	X	X	X	X	X
Visual field	X (Baseline on miotic)	X	X		X	X	X		X
Gonioscopy	X (Miotic)				X		X		X
Undilated disc examination	X	X		X					
Dilated disc and fundus examination			X		X	X	X	X	X
Disc photos	Repeat only if the patient's condition is suspected of worsening.								

CASE EF—MARGINALLY CONTROLLED SEVERE GLAUCOMA

A 64-year-old man with pressures without treatment averaging 26 mm Hg (range, 23 to 29 mm Hg), has a cup/disc ratio of 0.8 with significant visual field loss. Baseline fields are of good quality given the extent of damage, but there is a moderate amount of variation, particularly in the damaged areas. The target pressure is 16 mm Hg. After he uses a β-blocker in one eye for 2 weeks, the pressure measures 19 mm Hg in the treated eye and 27 mm Hg in the untreated eye. Treatment is begun in both eyes, and 1 month later the pressure is 19 mm Hg in each eye. With the addition of pilocarpine to one eye, the pressure decreases in 2 weeks to 16 mm Hg in the eye treated with both drops and is 20 mm Hg in the eye only on a β-blocker. He is advised to use pilocarpine and β-blocker in both eyes.

- When should this patient be reexamined?
- What should be tested on follow-up?

This patient has severe disease and a pressure goal that has been barely attained. He probably has more nonpressure risk factors than the other two patients and thus has a lower threshold for damage. It will be difficult to recognize additional small increments of visual field loss in this patient because of the inherent variability of damaged fields. Examine this patient in about a month to check the visual field and angle during miotic use and to check the pressure. If the pressure is still controlled, recheck the pressure and obtain a second baseline field examination during miotic use in another 2 months; check the IOP and dilate the pupils for fundoscopy in 2 more months (5 months into follow-up). Repeat the pressure measurement and visual field test in 2 more months and the pressure determination in another 2 months (9 months into follow-up). Thereafter, check the pressure and field every 3 months for perhaps a total of 24 months and dilate the pupils on alternate visits because of miotic use. Repeat gonioscopy once a year. If the fields and pressures remain stable, the frequency of visits and fields may be decreased to every 6 months for another 2 to 3 years. If the patient's condition is stable for 5 years, continue to examine the patient every 6 months, but check the field on every other visit (i.e., once a year) as long as the pressure remains in the range in which the field had been stable. Tables 4-5 and 4-6 outline follow-up courses for patients with severe disease treated without or with miotic drops.

TABLE 4-5 *Follow-up of Severe Glaucoma*

Baseline

- At least three IOP measurements at different times of day
- At least two threshold visual field examinations
- Gonioscopy
- Disc photographs

Obtain within 2 months

Initial treatment

- Pressure checks and medication adjustments at 1- to 4-week intervals until treatment regimen is established

Complete within 2 months if possible

Follow-up

	Months										Years 3 through 5		Years 6 and after	
	1	3	5	7	9	12	15	18	21	24	Every 6 months	Every year	Every 6 months	Every year
IOP	X	X	X	X	X	X	X	X	X	X	X	X	X	X
Visual field		X		X		X	X	X	X	X	X	X		X
Gonioscopy						X				X		X		X
Undilated disc examination	X	X		X	X		X	X	X		X		X	
Dilated disc and fundus examination			X			X				X		X		X
Disc photos	Repeat only if the patient's condition is suspected of worsening.													

TABLE 4-6 *Follow-up of Severe Glaucoma in a Patient Who Uses Miotic Drops*

Baseline

- At least three ICP measurements at different times of day
- At least two threshold visual field examinations
- Gonioscopy
- Disc photographs

Obtain within 2 months

Initial treatment

- Pressure checks and medication adjustments at 1- to 4-week intervals until treatment regimen is established

Complete within 2 months if possible

Follow-up

	Months										Years 3 through 5		Years 6 and after	
	1	3	5	7	9	12	15	18	21	24	Every 6 months	Every year	Every 6 months	Every year
IOP	X	X	X	X	X	X	X	X	X	X	X	X	X	X
Visual field	X (Baseline on miotic)	X		X		X	X	X	X	X	X	X		X
Gonioscopy	X (Miotic)					X				X		X		X
Undilated disc examination	X	X		X	X		X		X					
Dilated disc and fundus examination			X			X		X		X	X	X	X	X
Disc photos	Repeat only if the patient's condition is suspected of worsening.													

Recognition of Progressive Damage

Glaucoma rarely causes symptoms until it is very advanced, therefore only in severe cases will the patient be able to tell the clinician that his or her vision is decreasing. Similarly, the visual acuity rarely alerts the clinician to deterioration because it does not decrease appreciably until glaucoma is profoundly advanced, although use of miotics, especially in conjunction with cataract, may dim the vision or decrease the measured acuity.

The pressure, the appearance of the nerve, and the visual field are the three determinations on which to rely in deciding if a patient's condition is worsening or remaining stable over time. The management of progressive damage is discussed beginning on page 116.

PRESSURE AS A GUIDE

Early in the course of glaucoma, the pressure offers mainly negative information. Regardless of how low the IOP is on a follow-up examination, a patient may undergo further damage either because of a low threshold for damage or because of variable compliance. But if the pressure measures consistently at a level known or reasonably presumed to be above the threshold, this information is useful. If the pressure rises into the range of the baseline IOP, assume that the eye is probably undergoing further damage. Any therapeutic decision based on pressure alone should be made only after pressure measurements on at least two occasions. Do not act on a single pressure reading that is out of line with the usual for the patient.

OPTIC NERVE AS A GUIDE

Cupping. The appearance of the optic nerve helps most in the chronic follow-up of patients with early to moderate glaucoma. Consider the role of the nerve photographs in the following hypothetical patient.

Case GH. In 1991 a 65-year-old patient is first seen by a clinician. The patient brings her records from the past 10 years of glaucoma care. There are 14 pages of photocopied records; the pretreatment pressures in 1981 were 25 and 27 mm Hg. With therapy the pressures have varied between 17 and 23 mm Hg, with most readings approximately 19 mm Hg. In 1981 the patient's nerves were described as "0.5." The clinician has copies of eight sets of kinetic fields done on Goldmann-type perimeters in four different offices, and the fields show variably plotted Bjerrum's defects. Two fields done on a Fieldmaster perimeter, one field done on an Octopus perimeter, and three fields done on a Humphrey perimeter show comparable abnormalities. The last three fields look as if they might be worsening, but the patient reports that over the past 4 years a cataract has been developing. Her vision, which was 20/20 in 1981, is now 20/50. However, her pupils dilate nicely and a clinician can obtain a good view of the nerves. She has a cup/disc ratio of 0.5 horizontally and 0.7 vertically with a notch inferotemporally in each eye. It is not known whether her condition is currently stable. Then she shows the clinician photographs taken in 1981. If the photographs look like the nerves in 1991, the clinician can be confident that the patient's condition is either stable or progressing so slowly that it cannot be determined over a decade. If the nerves in 1991 appear clearly worse than the photographs, the pressure should average less than 19 mm Hg.

Real patients like the hypothetical patient GH do exist; in such patients baseline photographs and follow-up nerve examinations are sometimes critical.

Patients who have early or moderate disease usually show convincing changes in their fields before clear changes in the nerves are evident. However, not all examiners can perform good field tests, and media opacities may develop that affect the field but do not preclude examination of the nerve. Photographs of the nerves are of little value when there is very advanced cupping.

Disc hemorrhages. The observation of a splinter hemorrhage along the disc margin on a routine disc examination may mean that a patient's condition is unstable. If a disc hemorrhage is noted on a visit that did not include a visual field examination, a visual field examination should be scheduled within the next 1 to 3 months, depending on the severity of the patient's disease. If the field shows worsening in the area corresponding to the hemorrhage, this constitutes evidence of glaucomatous progression, since the two findings support one another. If the field shows no change, another field examination should be scheduled in 3 to 6 months, depending on the severity of the disease.

VISUAL FIELD AS A GUIDE

The visual field examination usually serves as the major guide as to whether a patient's condition is stable. The ability to recognize marginal progression depends on the quality of the baseline fields as well as on the degree of initial visual field loss. The more damaged a portion of the field, the more it varies both on repeat measure (short-term fluctuation) and from day to day (long-term fluctuation), and thus the more difficult it is to recognize additional deterioration. Therefore on follow-up examinations, it should be determined whether the field shows change beyond this variation and, if it does, whether the change is related to progressive glaucomatous damage.

The only clear standard for diagnosing progressive glaucomatous damage on automated static threshold perimetry is that a change should be confirmed on a repeat examination, especially if the field change is the only sign that indicates worsening. (If the field change is confirmed by another finding, for example, a corresponding disc hemorrhage, a distinctly uncontrolled pressure, or a cup that has clearly enlarged, it may be better to repeat the field as a new baseline after taking the next appropriate management step.) Confirmation of a field change is important because whatever reasonable criteria are used to recognize marginal progression, a patient whose condition is stable will meet the criteria occasionally because of the variability in field testing. Aggressive treatment in a patient whose disease is stable is unwarranted if the clinician happens to test the field on a day when the patient's visual sensitivity was decreased by something other than progressive glaucoma.

Visual fields may deteriorate in one or more of four main ways:

- A new defect may develop in a previously normal area.
- A preexisting defect may deepen.
- A preexisting defect may expand.
- The entire field may develop decreased sensitivity.

The two fundamental interpretive approaches to the detection of progressive worsening are first, to compare each individual follow-up field, as it is obtained, to the baseline fields and second, to study the entire series of fields since diagnosis and to see if there is any feature that shows a steady decline beyond any field-to-field variability. A statistical program facilitates each approach, but both may be done without one. The following discussion deals with the use of the Statpac 2 program.

Comparison of an individual field to the field baseline. Merging the two or three fields selected as a baseline into a Master file simplifies this approach. Each subsequent field can be compared to that Master and the differences, both positive (follow-up better than Master) and negative (follow-up worse than Master) can be printed out (Figs. 4-3 through 4-7). If this method of following fields is used, each follow-up field should be compared to the Master file of the baseline fields, not to intermediate fields, to avoid missing gradual worsening. There are

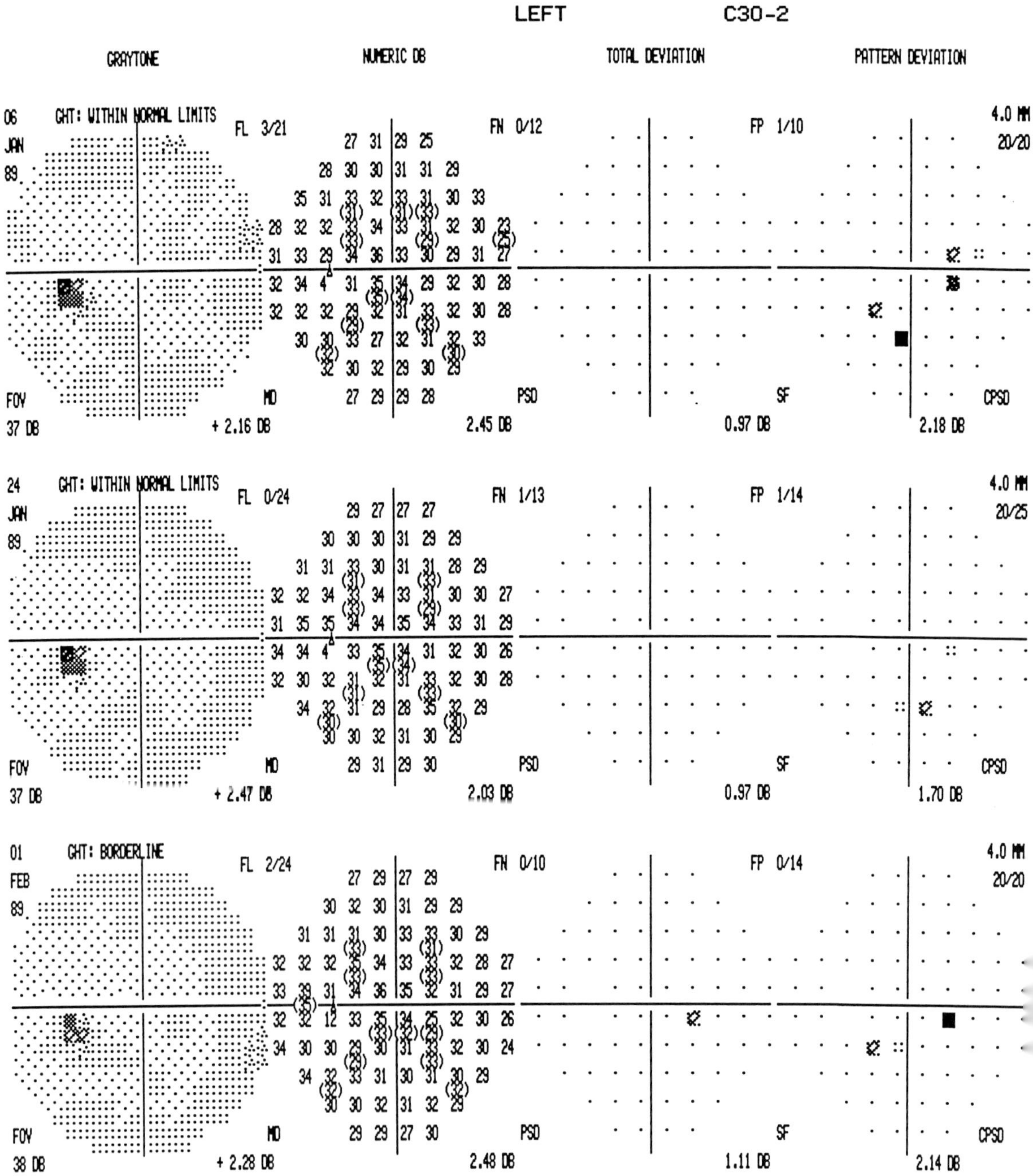

FIG. 4-3 Creation of a Master file. The three fields shown were chosen to be combined into the Master file shown in Fig. 4-4.

no criteria that have been validated or have come into common usage for what constitutes meaningful change. The following seem reasonable:

- For a new defect in a previously normal area (normal refers to points which, on the Master field, are within 4 dB of expected on the defect depth plot): Either a cluster of three or more nonedge points, each of which declines ≥5 dB compared to baseline on two consecutive fields; or a single nonedge point that declines ≥10 dB compared to baseline on two consecutive fields. See Figures 4-3 through 4-7 for an illustration of this finding.
- For deepening of a preexisting defect: A cluster of three nonedge points, each of which declines ≥10 dB compared to baseline on two consecutive fields. The confirming points may differ if they are part of a contiguous cluster (Figs. 4-8 and 4-9).

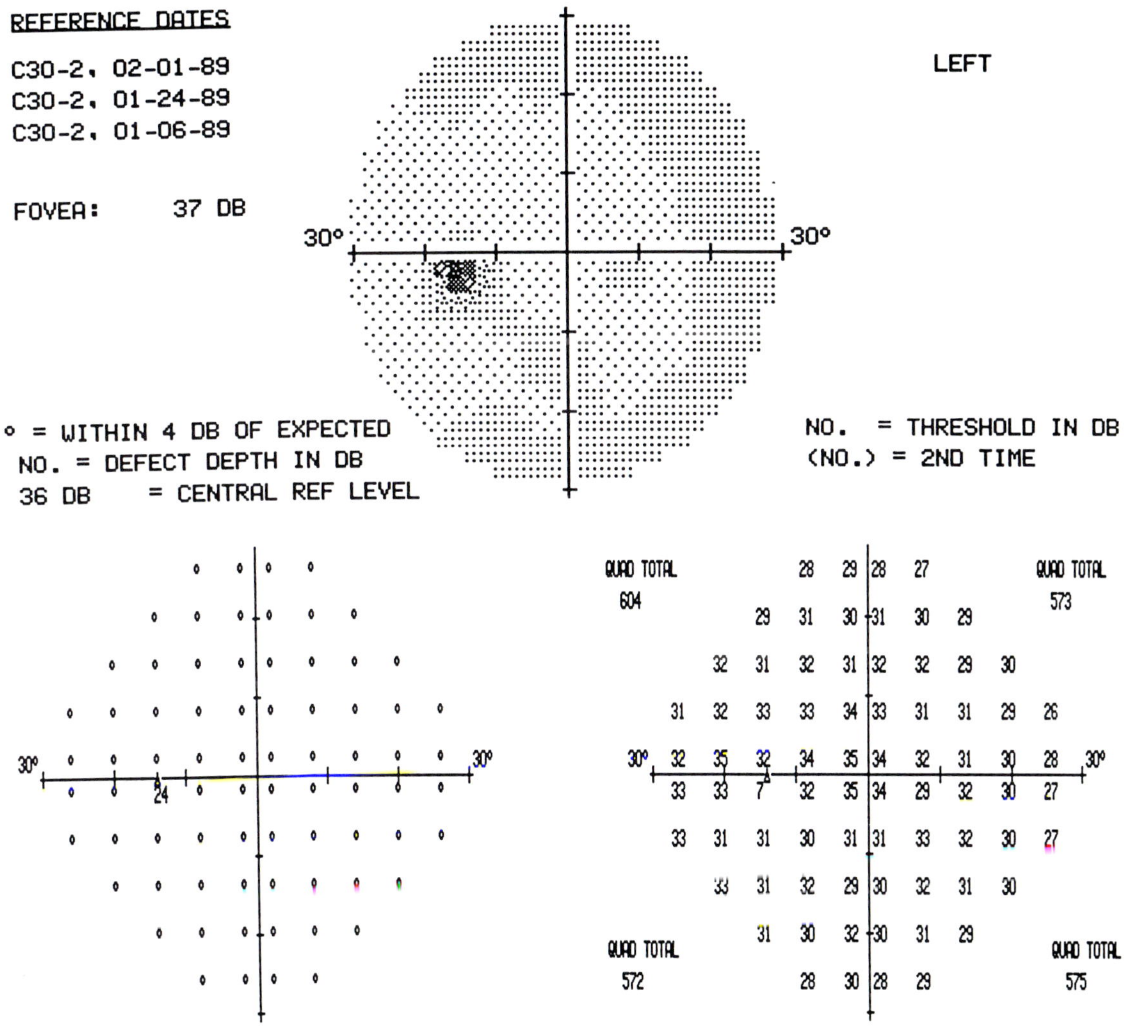

FIG. 4-4 Master file of the three fields shown in Fig. 4-3.

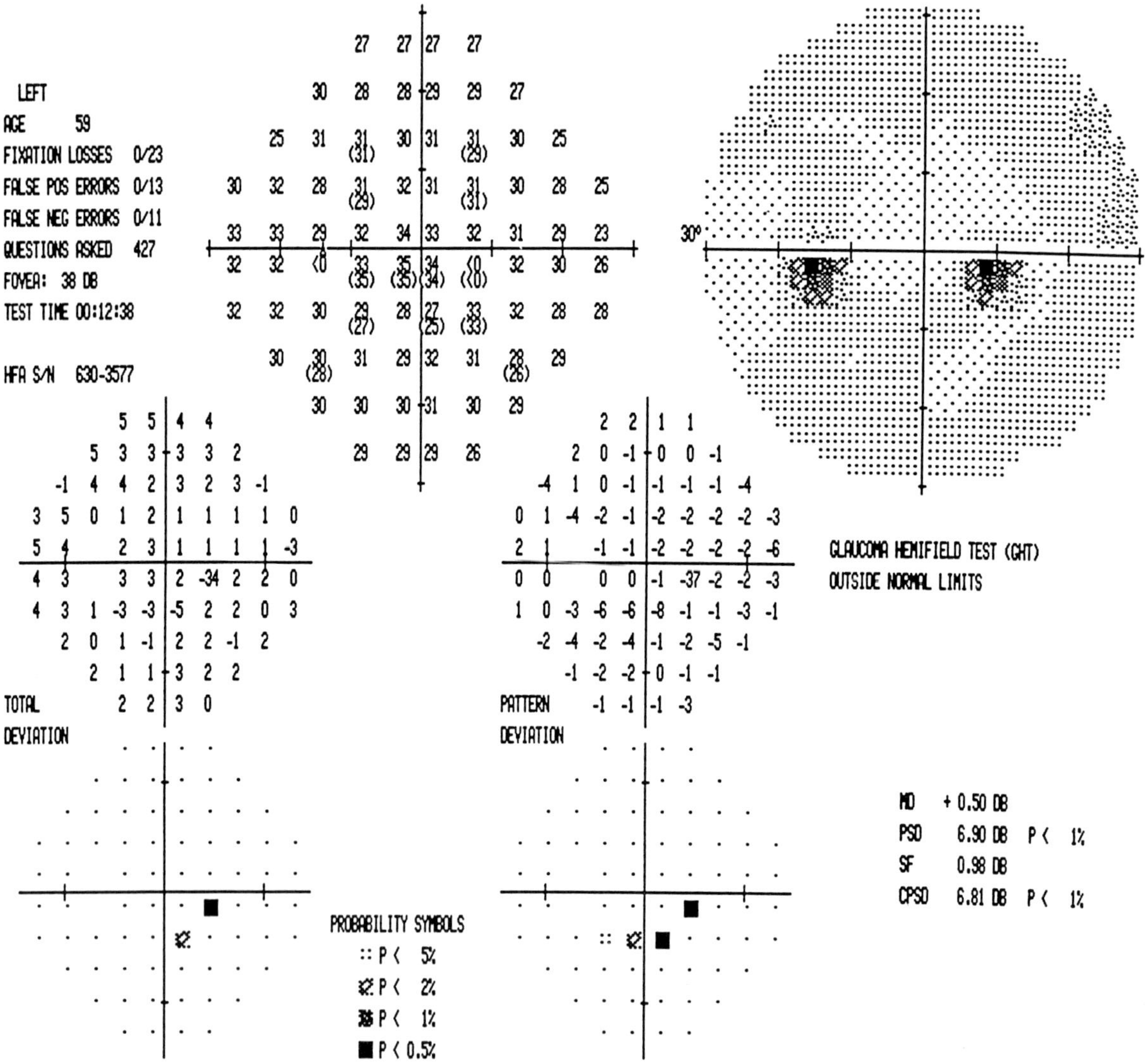

FIG. 4-5 Follow-up field obtained 15 months after the Master field (Fig. 4-4) was completed. A comparison program was run.

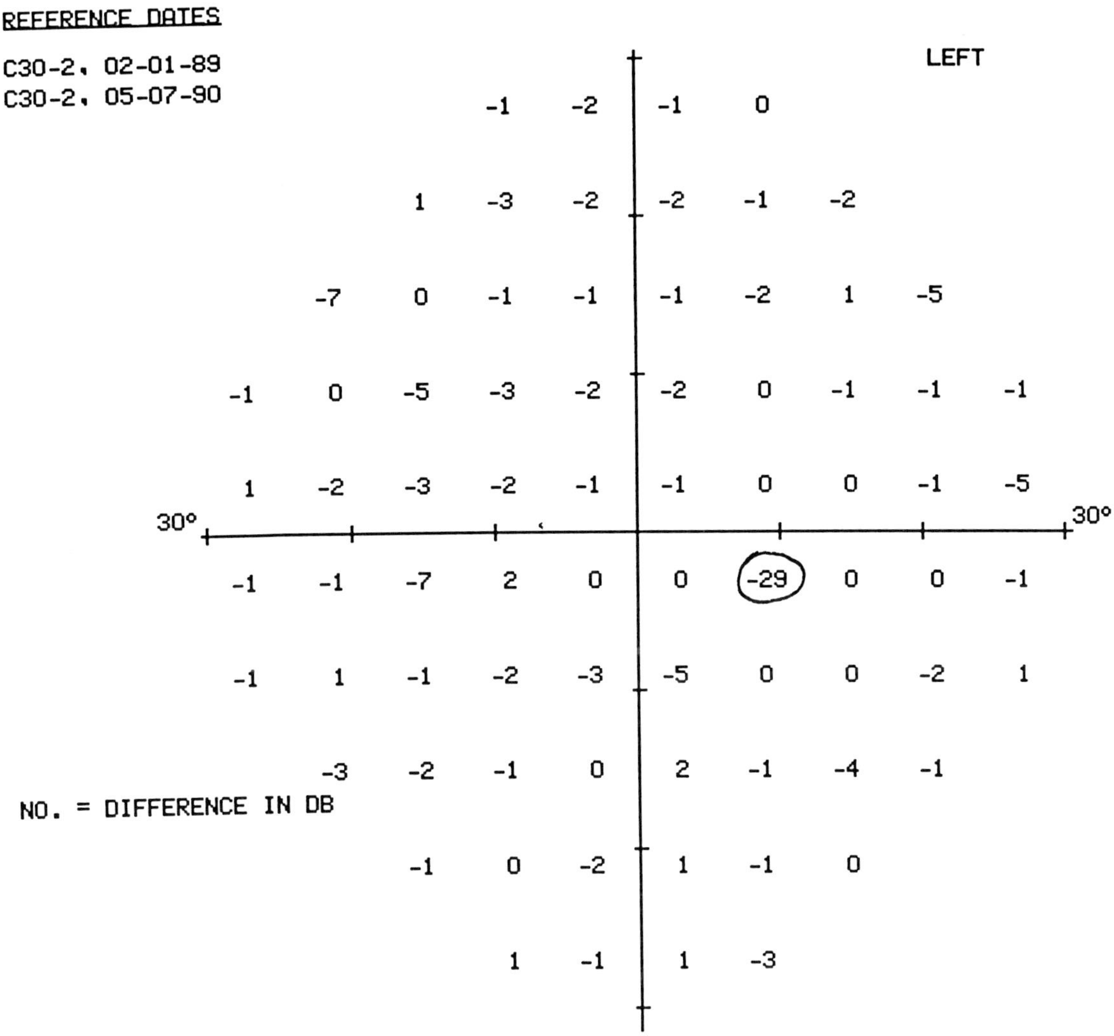

FIG. 4-6 Comparison of follow-up field in Fig. 4-5 to the Master of Fig. 4-4. Positive numbers indicate higher values on the follow-up field, negative numbers show a lower result. There is a dense localized defect *(circled)*. The field was repeated with the result shown in Fig. 4-7.

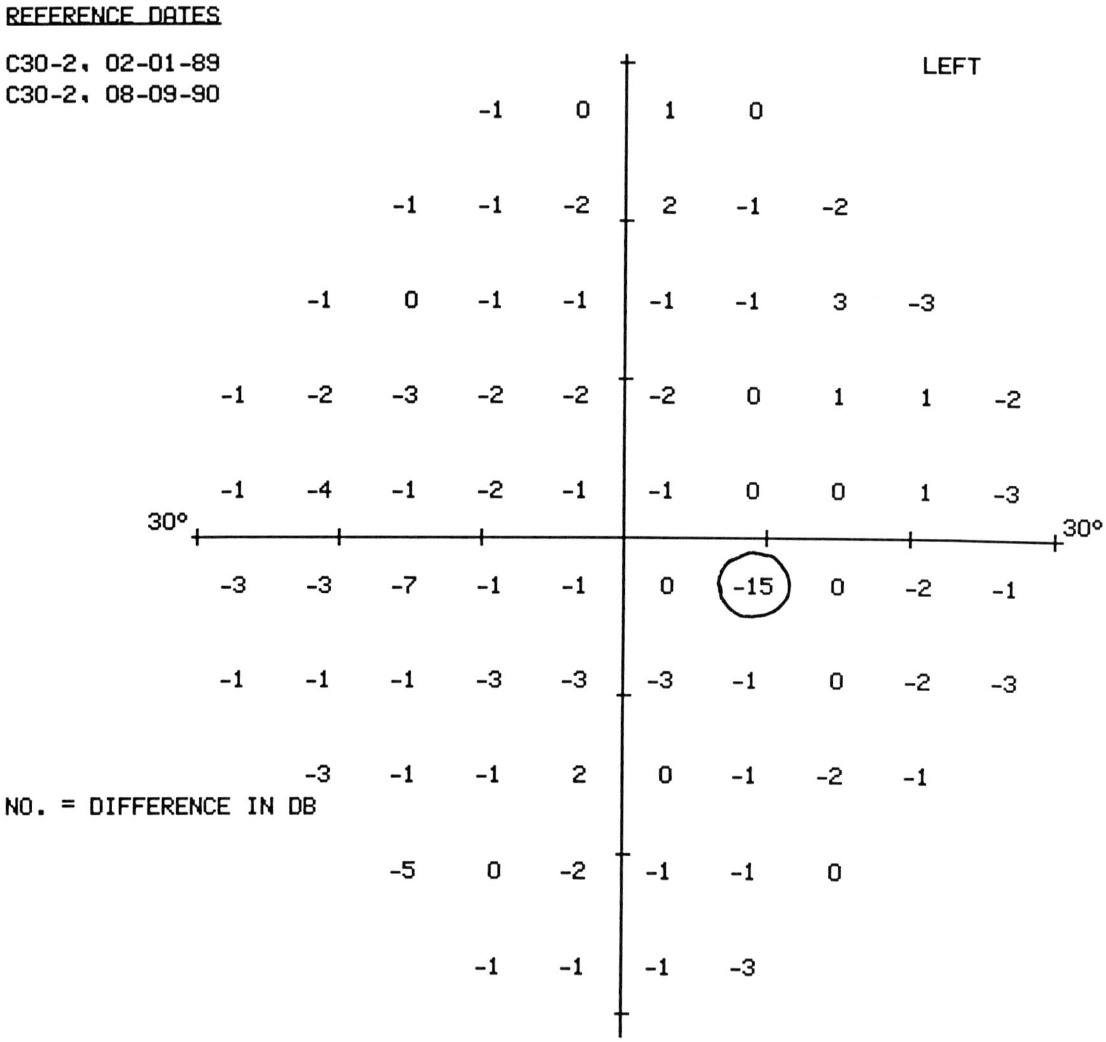

FIG. 4-7 Repeat comparison program on the patient's subsequent field confirms the defect *(circled)*.

- For expansion of a preexisting scotoma: At least two previously normal points within the central 15° or three additional previously normal points outside 15°, each of which declines ≥10 dB on two consecutive fields (Figs. 4-8 and 4-9).
- For generalized depression: This determination is best made on inspection of a series of fields, but in comparison of the recent field to baseline would be represented by a decline of all points by 3 dB on two occasions.

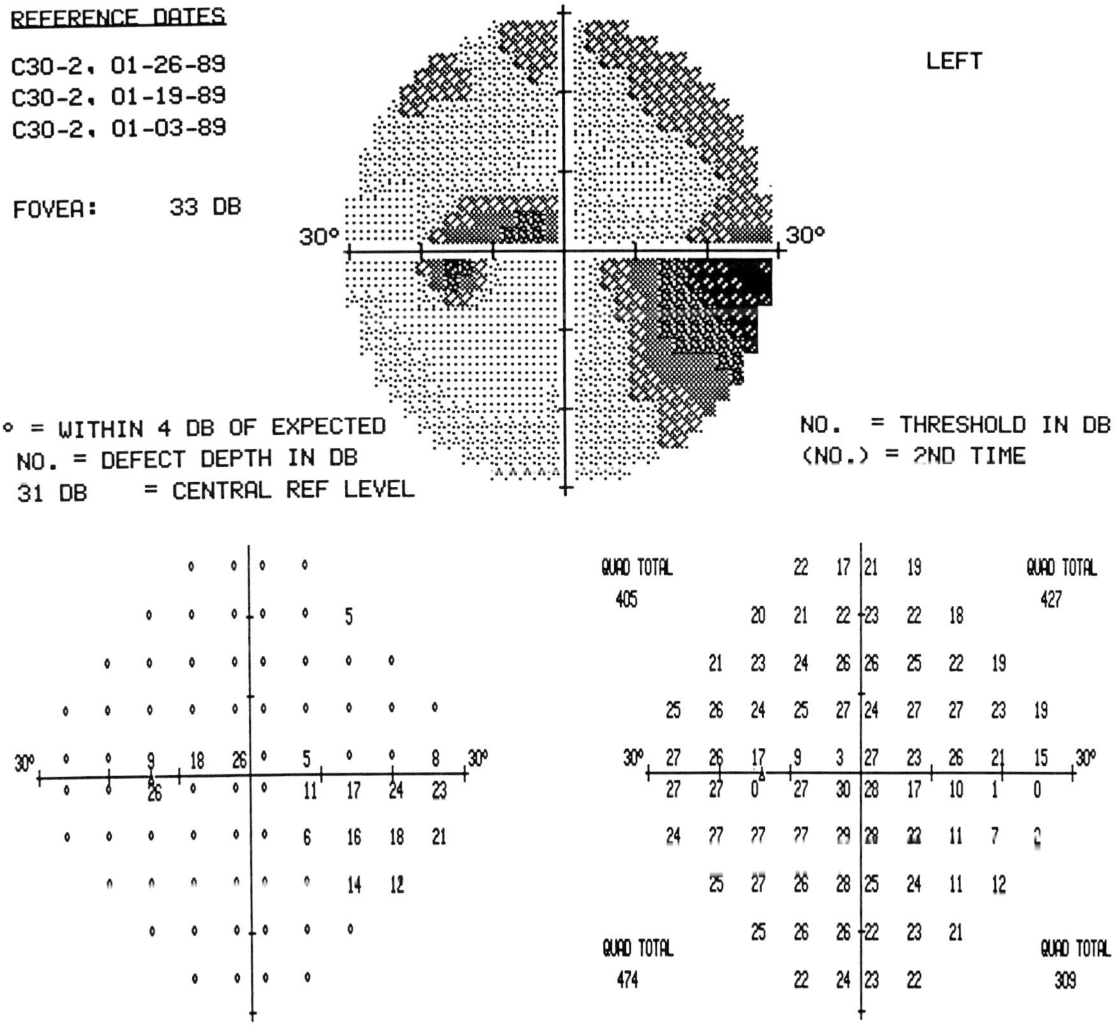

FIG. 4-8 Master file of a patient with severe field loss.

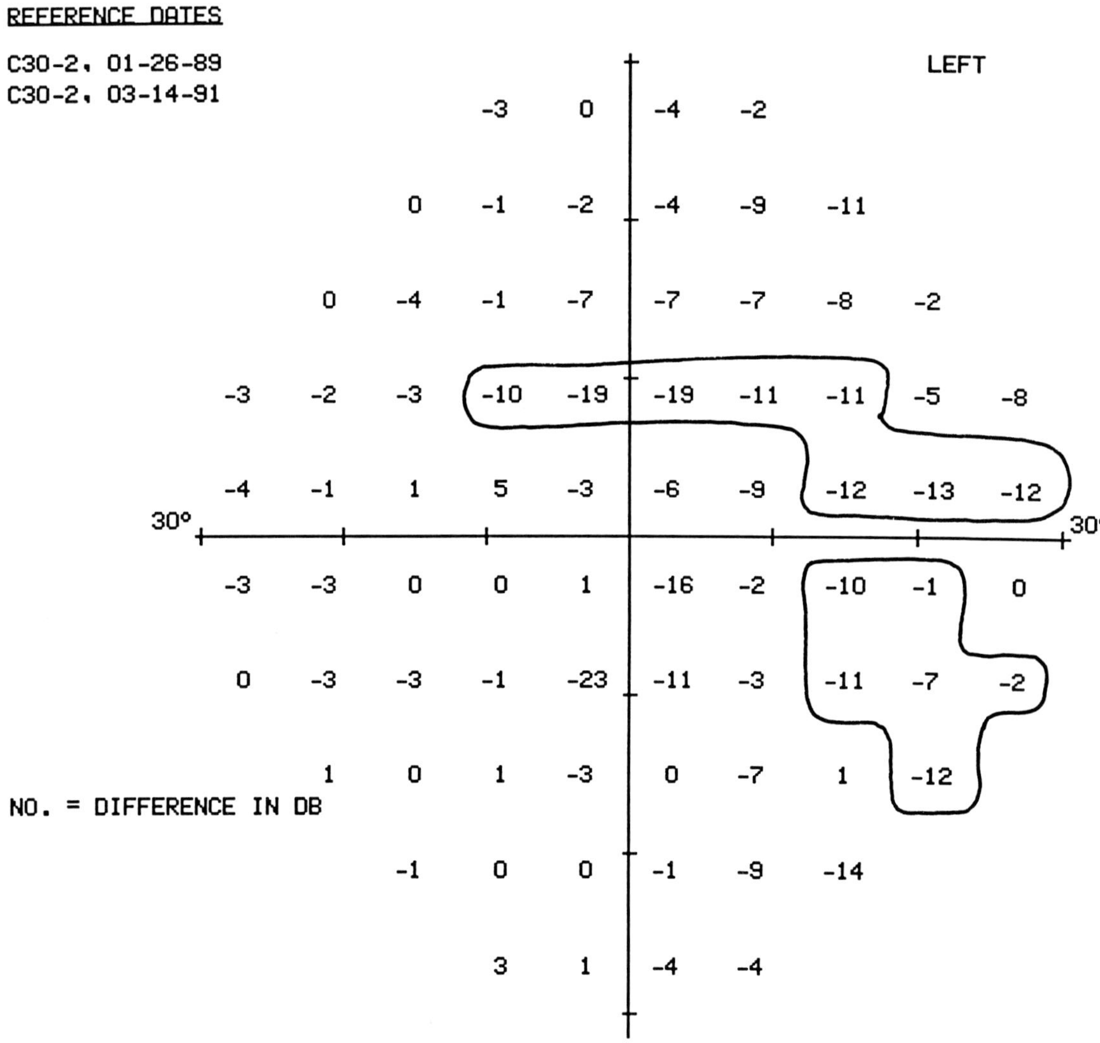

FIG. 4-9 Deepening and expansion of a scotoma. Comparison of the Master file of Fig. 4-8 to a follow-up field, shows in the superior hemifield expansion of a scotoma to involve eight *(circled)* additional points, which were previously within 4 dB of expected value. In addition, the inferior nasal scotoma has deepened. Only two nonedge points decreased by ≥10 dB, but the circled points all decreased to 0 dB, and the edge point is supported as real by the rest of the field. Repeat testing confirmed these findings.

A second way to compare individual fields to baseline fields is with the Glaucoma Change Probability program. This program analyzes a series of fields and determines the point-by-point probability that any difference between a follow-up field and the baseline examinations occurred by chance. The calculations are based on empiric data from glaucoma patients. Figures 4-10 and 4-11 illustrate the printout of a patient in whom a new defect developed. The following criteria seem reasonable for defining progression:

- For a new defect in a previously normal area: A cluster of three or more nonedge points, each of which is depressed compared to baseline at a $p < 5\%$ level on two consecutive fields (Figs. 4-10 and 4-11).

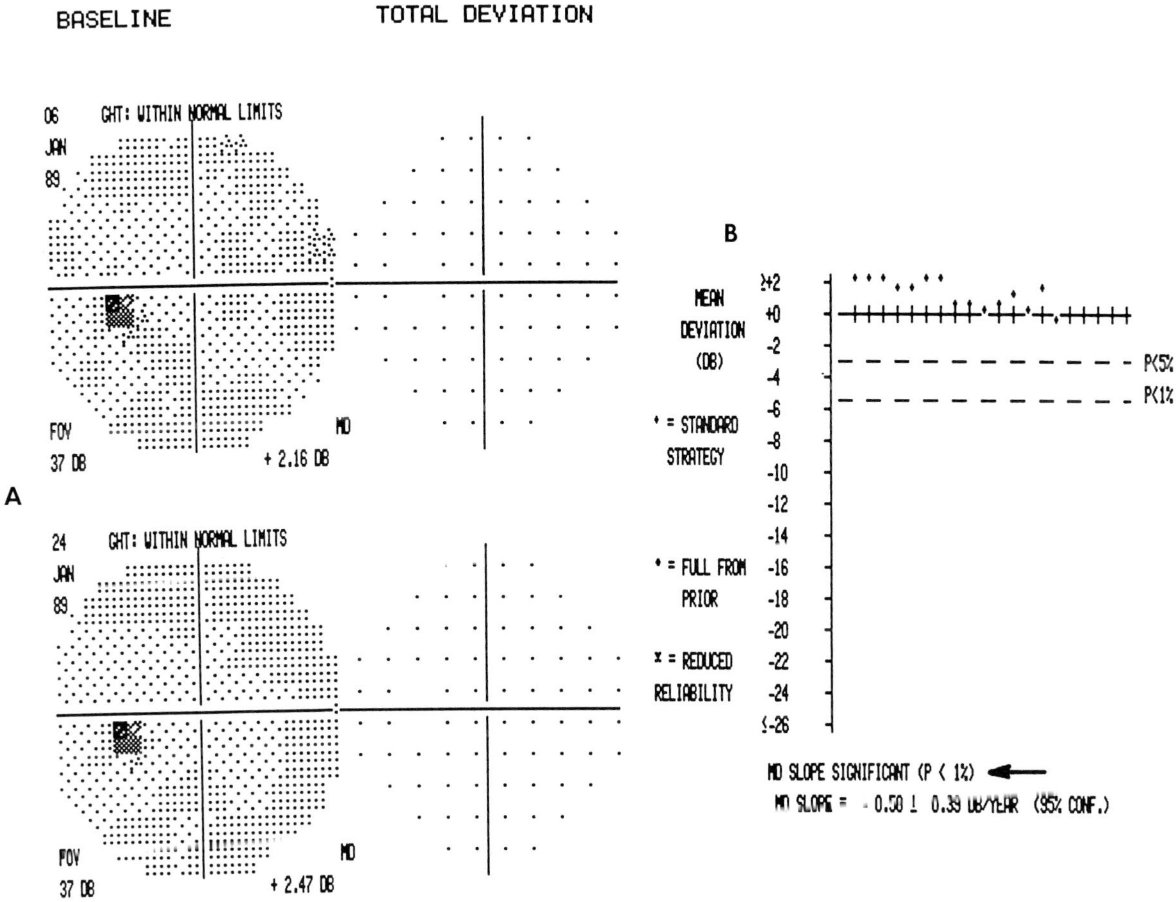

FIG. 4-10 Glaucoma change probability. **A,** Baseline fields. If two fields are chosen for the program, the first is the baseline and the second the follow-up. If three or more fields are chosen, the first two are the baseline. If five or more fields are chosen and the first field is significantly depressed relative to the others (indicating a learning effect), the second and third field are used as a baseline and a message appears on the printout. **B,** Mean deviation plot. If five or more fields are chosen, the program calculates the probability that a change occurred by chance *(arrow)*.

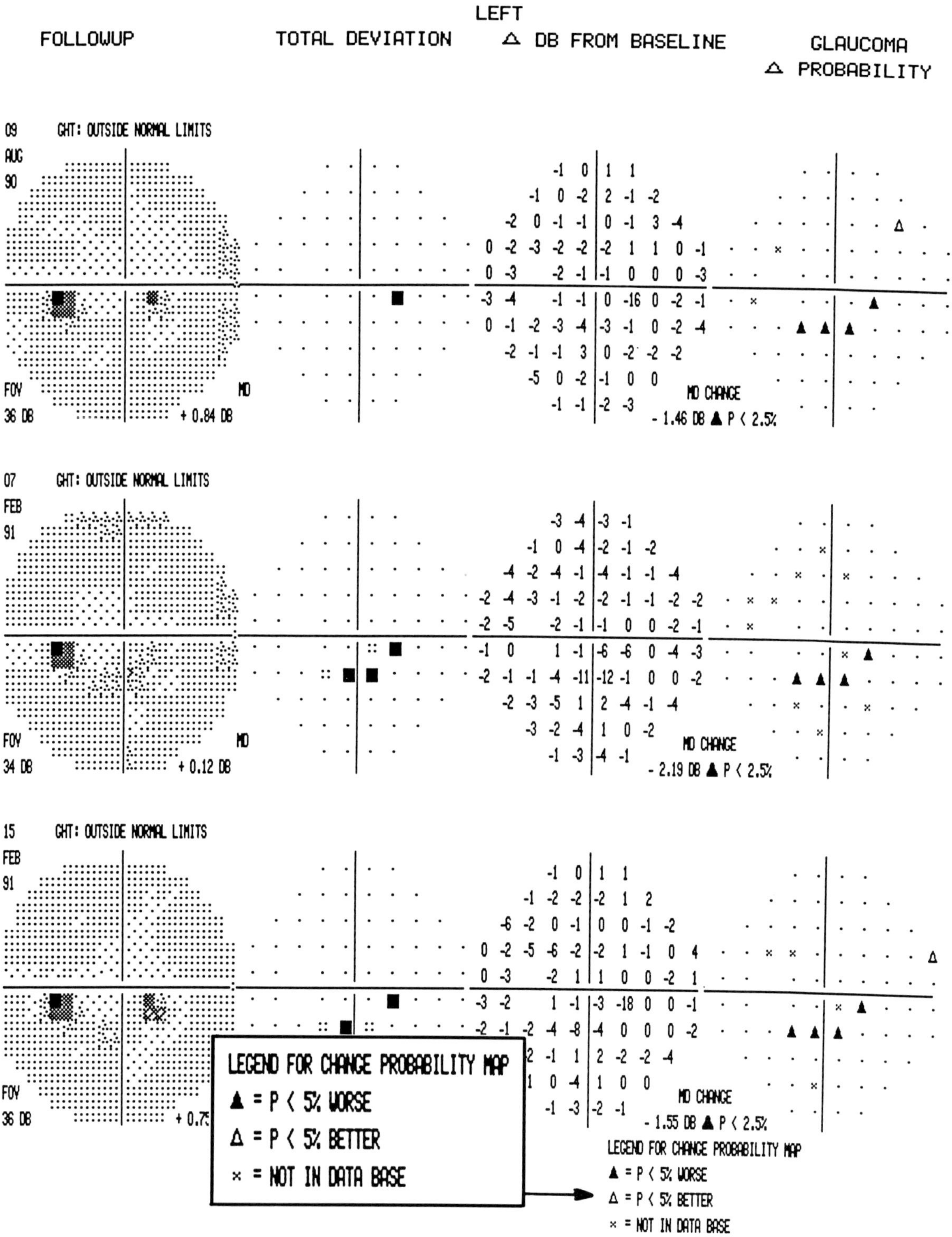

FIG. 4-11 Glaucoma change probability, follow-up fields. For each point, the program calculates the probability that a change occurred by chance. The *x* symbol for *not in data base* appears at points with sensitivities not included in the program's empiric data base. This patient's follow-up fields demonstrate a new scotoma that is present on three consecutive fields.

- For deepening of a preexisting defect: A cluster of three nonedge points or three points that are part of the same scotoma, each of which worsens at least 5 dB and each of which is depressed compared to baseline at a $p < 5\%$ level on two consecutive fields. The confirming points may differ if they are a part of a contiguous cluster or if they are separated by points that were so depressed on the baseline that they were not in the data base (Figs. 4-12 and 4-13).
- For expansion of a preexisting defect: At least two previously normal points within the central 15° or three previously normal points outside 15° that are depressed at a $p < 5\%$ level compared to baseline on two consecutive fields.
- For generalized depression: A decline in the mean deviation that is significant at the 1% level and is not explained by media opacity or pupil size (Fig. 4-10).

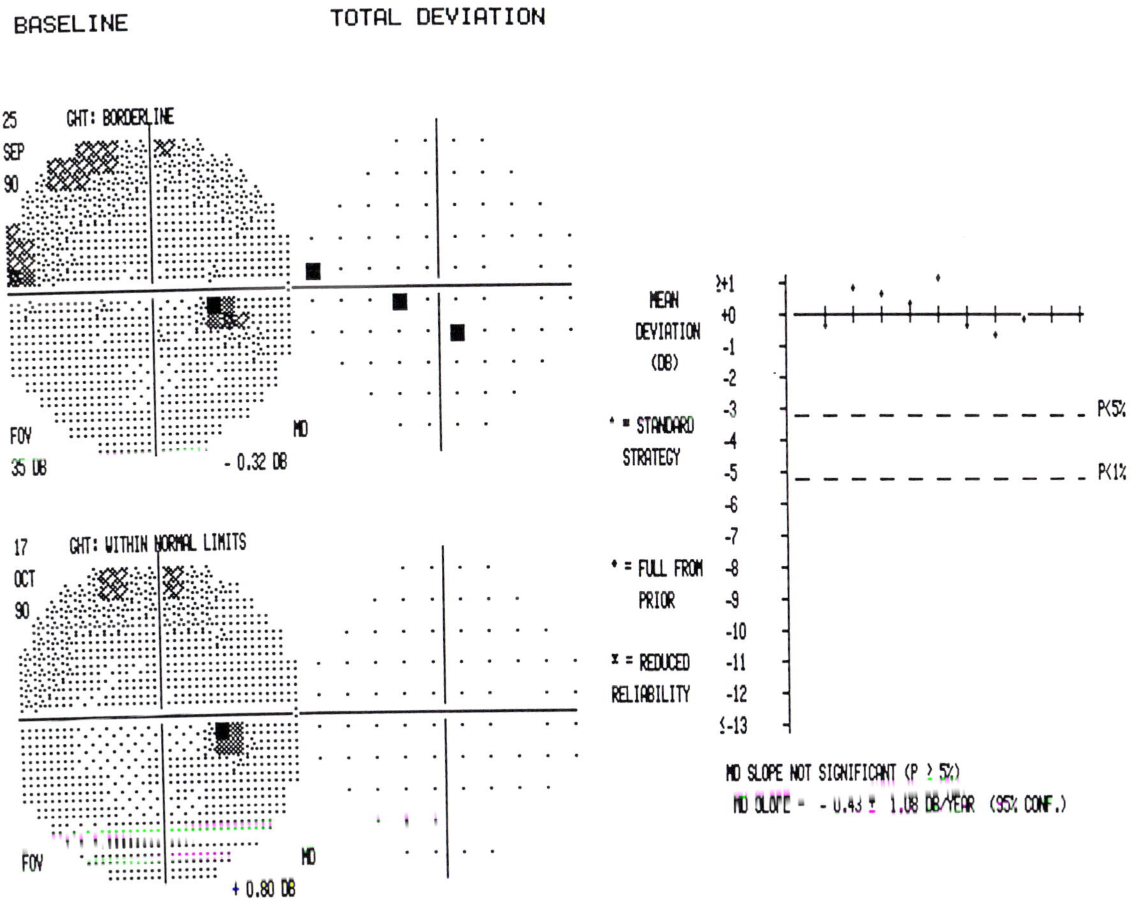

FIG. 4-12 Deepening and expansion of a preexisting scotoma, baseline fields. A single nonedge point is depressed at a $p < 5\%$ level relative to normal on one test. Follow-up is shown in Fig. 4-13.

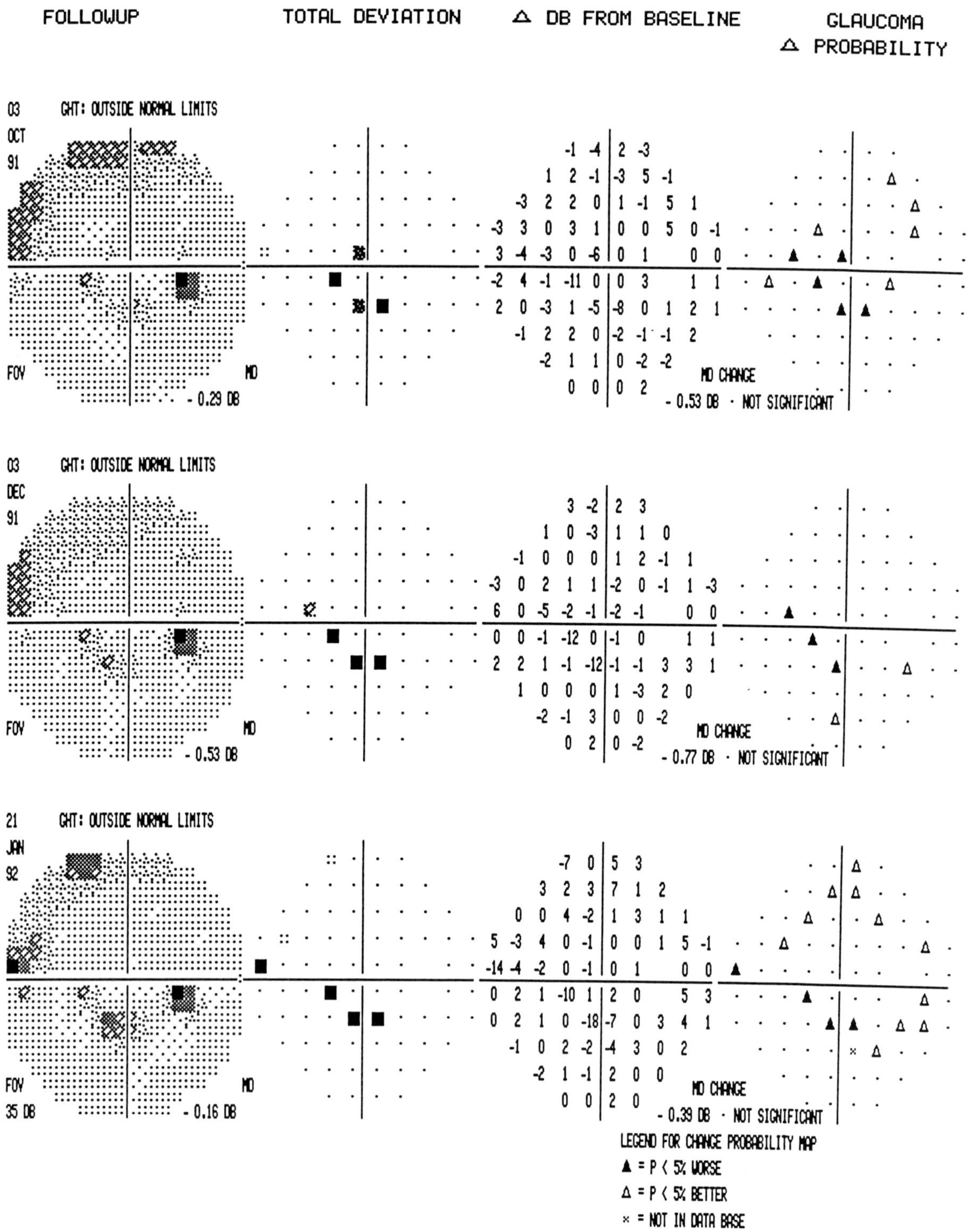

FIG. 4-13 Deepening and expansion of a preexisting scotoma, follow-up fields. The initially abnormal point has declined and the scotoma extends to involve additional points in a typical location.

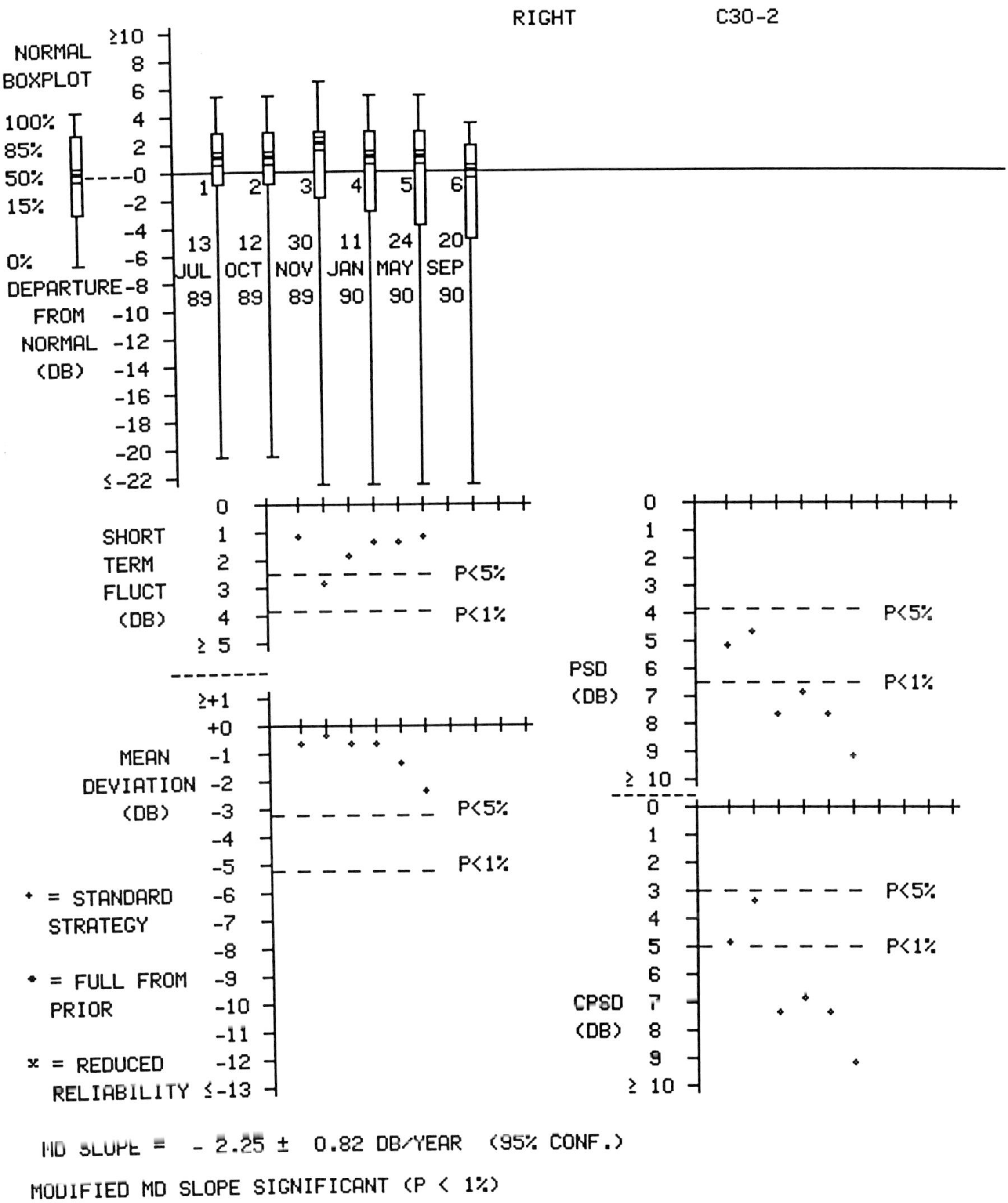

FIG. 4-14 Change analysis program showing progression of glaucomatous damage (discussed in text).

Examination of the entire series of fields. Figs. 4-14 and 4-15 show a change analysis and overview printout of a series of fields obtained over 14 months. Each part of the printout provides support for the diagnosis of worsening damage. The boxplot lengthens downward, indicating an increasing number of depressed points. The short-term fluctuation remains stable, decreasing the suspicion that changes are spurious. The mean deviation gradually but steadily declines. The pattern standard deviation (PSD) and corrected pattern standard deviation (CPSD) increase, indicating an increase in the irregularity of the visual field. Of these indices, the decline in the PSD or CPSD is the most impressive

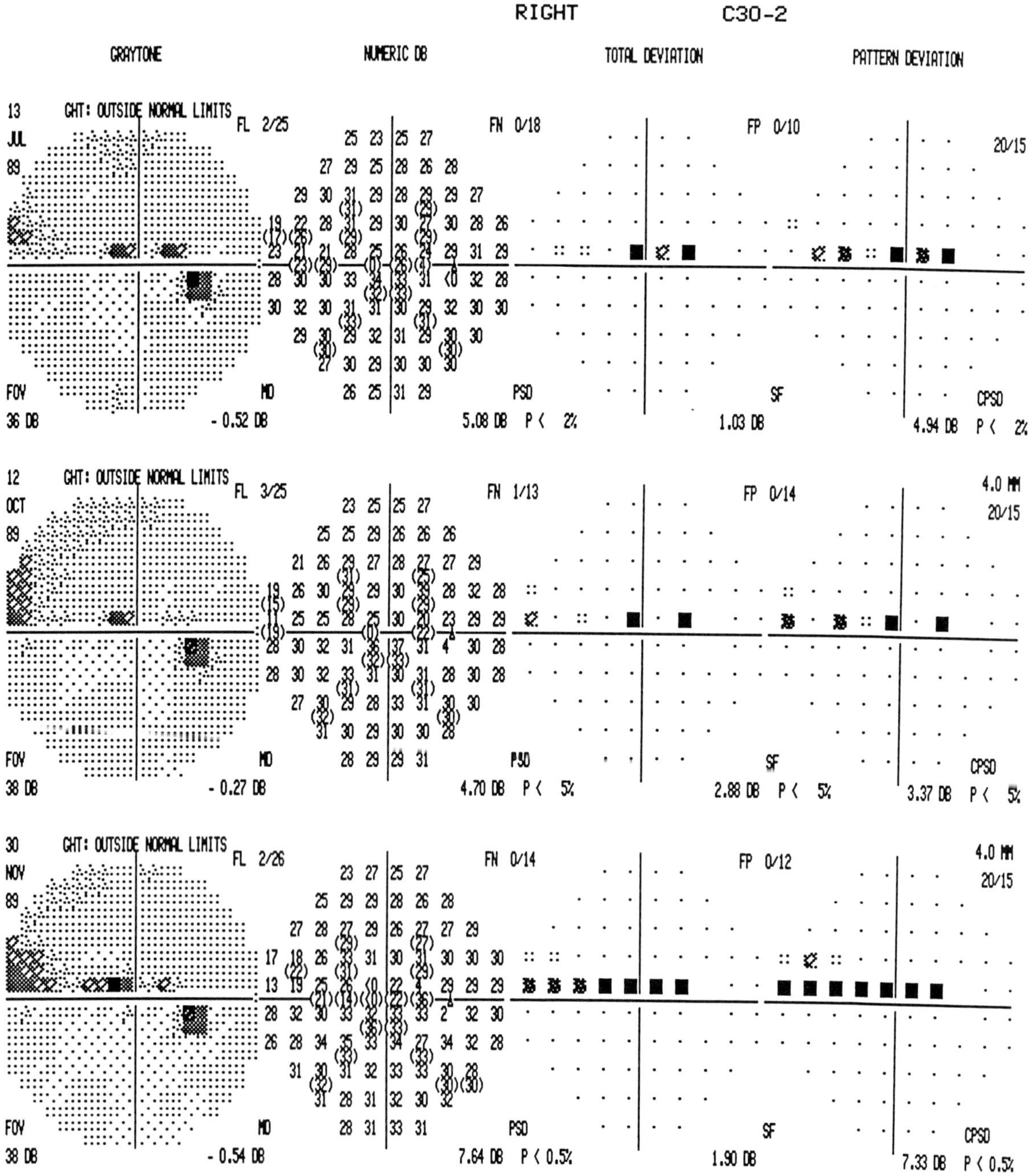

FIG. 4-15 Overview corresponding to Fig. 4-14.

declines. The pattern standard deviation (PSD) and corrected pattern standard deviation (CPSD) increase, indicating an increase in the irregularity of the visual field. Of these indices, the decline in the PSD or CPSD is the most impressive because it indicates that the decline is not generalized but is greater in some areas than in others. (However, if the PSD or CPSD is very abnormal initially, it may not be helpful in follow-up). A minimum criterion for progression in a

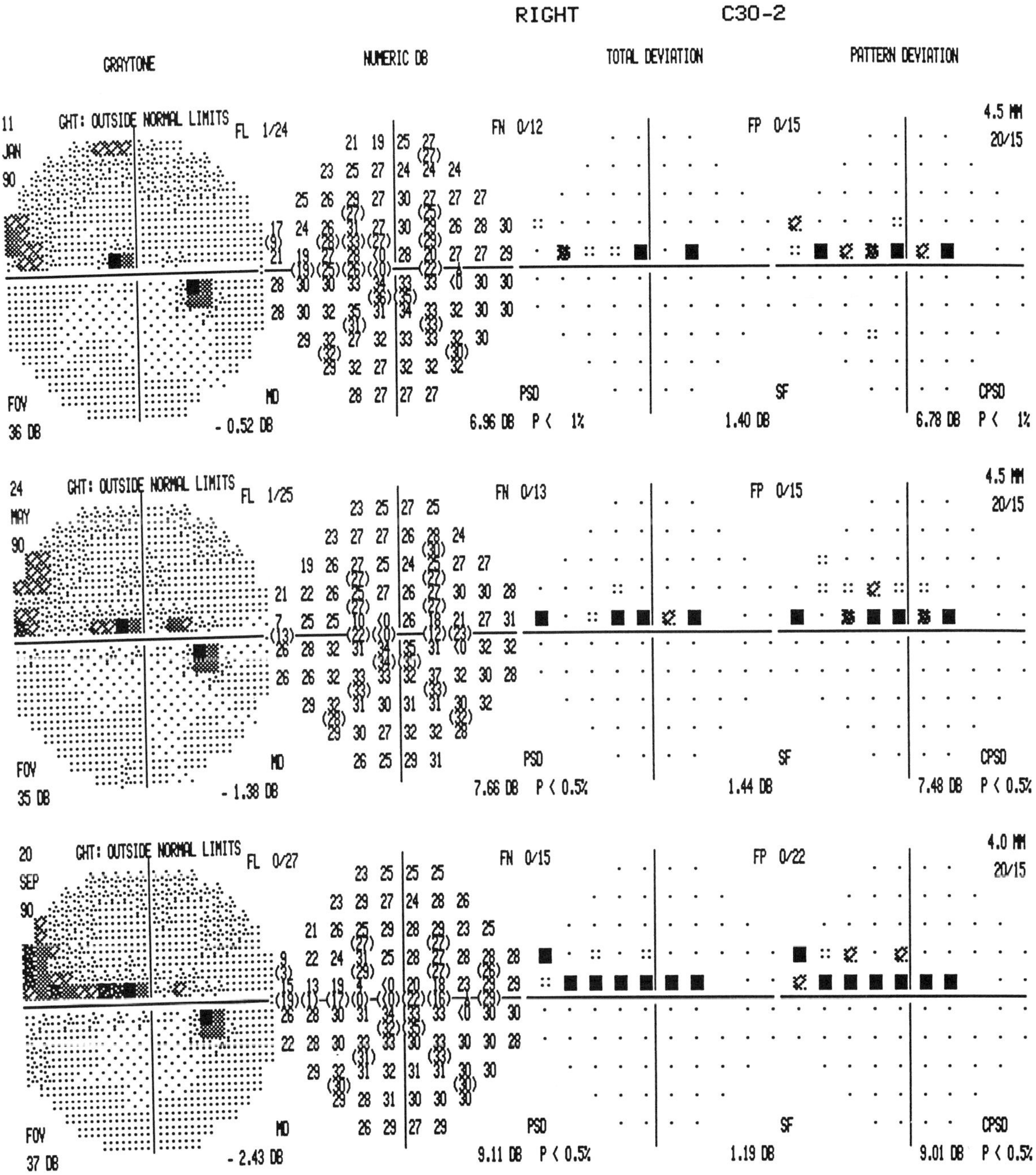

FIG. 4-15, cont'd Overview corresponding to Fig. 4-14.

series of fields is either a decline in the mean deviation that is significant at a 1% level and is not explained by media opacity or pupil size, or a CPSD that declines more or less steadily on at least five fields. Detailed examination of the overview printout Fig. 4-15 shows that the point-by-point criteria for progression are also met. (See box below.)

The limitations of statistical programs and visual fields. Statistical programs provide probabilities, but they do not practice medicine. They do not determine if a change is a transient physiologic one or a permanent pathologic change. They do not determine if a change is related to glaucoma or to a vascular accident, tumor, or stroke. The field needs to be interpreted in light of the entire clinical picture.

Summary of Criteria for Field Progression

FOR A NEW DEFECT IN A PREVIOUSLY NORMAL AREA

- A cluster of three or more nonedge points, each of which declines ≥5 dB compared to baseline on two consecutive fields.

or

- A single nonedge point that declines ≥10 bB compared to baseline on two consecutive fields.

or

- A cluster of three or more nonedge points, each of which declines at a $p < 5\%$ level compared to baseline on two consecutive fields.

FOR DEEPENING OF A PREEXISTING DEFECT

- A cluster of three nonedge points, each of which declines ≥10 dB compared to baseline on two consecutive fields. The confirming points may differ if they are part of a contiguous cluster.

or

- A cluster of three nonedge points or three points that are part of the same scotoma, each of which worsens at least 5 dB and is depressed compared to baseline at a $p < 5\%$ level on two consecutive fields. The confirming points may differ if they are part of a contiguous cluster or are separated by points not in the data base.

FOR EXPANSION OF A PREEXISTING SCOTOMA INTO CONTIGUOUS POINTS

- At least two previously normal points within the central 15° or three additional previously normal points outside 15°, each of which declines ≥10 dB each on two consecutive fields.

or

- At least two previously normal points within the central 15° or three previously normal points outside 15°, each of which is depressed at a $p < 5\%$ level compared to baseline on two consecutive fields.

FOR GENERALIZED DEPRESSION

- A decline in the mean deviation that is significant at the $p < 1\%$ level and is not explained by media opacity or pupil size.

or

- A CPSD that shows an obvious trend based on at least five consecutive fields.

or

- A decline of ≥3 dB at all points on two consecutive fields that is not explained by media opacity or pupil size.

MODIFYING PRESSURE GOALS

If a person with glaucoma tolerates his or her treatment, if the pressure stays at or below the goal, and if the nerve and visual fields remain stable, we do not modify the treatment or ponder whether the pressure goal is too low. It is time to reassess the patient's management when the patient develops intolerance to medication, when the pressure rises beyond the goals, or when the nerve or field shows progression.

If, after a period of stability, medication intolerance develops or if the pressure rises higher than the goal, it may be appropriate to modify the pressure goal upward unless a slight change in therapy reestablishes the target pressure. The longer the patient had been followed up without progression before developing medication intolerance or exceeding the pressure goal, the more confident the clinician can be that the pressure maintained during that interval was indeed low enough, and that a somewhat higher IOP *might* be adequate. In general, if the patient's condition has been stable for at least a year, we are willing to reset the pressure goal up to 4 mm Hg higher in a patient with early to moderate disease and up to 2 mm Hg above the initial goal in a patient with severe disease.

If the goal is reset upward, then the patient should be followed up closely for a time to determine stability. A patient with mild disease should have a visual field test every 6 months for 1 year; a patient with moderate disease every 6 months for 2 years, and a patient with severe disease every 3 months for a year and then every 6 months for another year.

If the glaucomatous damage progresses, the pressure goal should usually be revised downward. Reassess the risk/benefit ratio of more aggressive treatment given the patient's duration and degree of disease before pursuing aggressive treatment. A patient with mild disease who is 70 years old and whose condition worsens slightly over a decade may be at less visual risk from IOP than he or she would be from filtration surgery for example.

MODIFYING TREATMENT

Medication Intolerance

A common circumstance that requires a change in management is the development of intolerance to medication that was originally tolerated. Sometimes an alternate medication or laser trabeculoplasty achieves the pressure goal easily. However, if the pressure rises above the target pressure, the goal should be reevaluated as described above. The sequence for additional treatment follows the guides in Chapter 4.

LOCAL INTOLERANCE

Drops may cause contact dermatitis of the eyelids and an associated conjunctival allergic reaction, with itching as a prominent symptom. Chronic reactive hyperemia or follicular conjunctivitis on a nonallergic basis may also occur, as may a pemphigold type of conjunctival shrinkage. Whatever the basis, if symptomatic cutaneous or conjunctival reaction develops, then discontinue the medication. Sometimes a preservative-free formulation of the medication can be used, but it is usually more expeditious to use some other therapy. If the conjunctival reaction could have represented viral or bacterial conjunctivitis, try the medication again in one eye for a few days after the inflammation resolves.

β-BLOCKER INTOLERANCE

If either respiratory or cardiac disease develops that could be related to β-blockade, discontinue the β-blocker while determining if the drug is indeed contributing to the problem. Tolerated β-blocker treatment does not usually become intolerable *suddenly* in the absence of another process. Thus a patient who notes a sudden change in symptomatology should have a prompt evaluation by his or her general medical physician.

Individuals who become intolerant to betaxolol cannot use any other β-blocker. Those who develop respiratory intolerance to a nonselective β-blocker may tolerate betaxolol. Do not use betaxolol in patients who develop cardiac failure with nonselective blockers.

MIOTIC INTOLERANCE

Intolerance to previously tolerated miotics most commonly appears when a cataract develops. Because of the usual order of drop use, most such patients will either be using a β-blocker or will be intolerant of them. If the pressure goal is not achieved with drops, we recommend laser trabeculoplasty and carbonic anhydrase inhibitors as outlined in Chapter 3. If the pressure cannot be controlled with these measures but had been well controlled with miotics, a plain cataract extraction, rather than a filtering operation, suffices. If the disease is moderate or severe, cataract extraction may be combined with a filtration procedure.

CARBONIC ANHYDRASE INHIBITOR INTOLERANCE

Use of carbonic anhydrase inhibitors is rare unless patients both have significant disease and fail to achieve control on other treatment. Symptomatic side effects usually occur when the medication is first started. However, lethargy and depression may be insidious, either not recognized at first or not attributed to the drug until some later time. Late intolerance may also arise because the patient grows tired of the side effects of the pills. Either way, relative intolerance of carbonic anhydrase inhibitors usually involves choosing to live with side effects, having a higher than desired pressure, or having glaucoma surgery. A reasonable course in a patient with relative intolerance is to stop the carbonic anhydrase inhibitor, perform filtering surgery in one eye, and observe the other eye. If the operated eye does well, surgery on the second eye can be done. If the surgery does not go well on the first eye, either because of poor pressure control or visually significant side effects, and if the unoperated eye worsens, the clinician and the patient may elect to use the carbonic anhydrase inhibitors and tolerate the side effects rather than do surgery on the second eye.

Pressure Increase

Pressure increase includes a variety of situations, most of which fall into one of three groups: a sudden marked increase in IOP compared to previous readings, a mild change in pressure that results in pressure above the goal, or a gradual increase in IOP over several visits regardless of whether the pressure goal is passed. *In each case, examine the eye for some obvious cause such as inflammation and perform gonioscopy to rule out the development of angle closure.* If angle closure is found, it is usually secondary to pupillary block and iridectomy is the appropriate treatment. If no obvious cause is found, then the likely explanations and management depend on the circumstances of presentation.

SUDDEN DRAMATIC INCREASE IN PRESSURE

Patients with POAG rarely have rapid changes in their conditions. If a pressure reading is distinctly elevated compared to previous readings, the three most common explanations (other than angle closure) in our experience are that the patient failed to use his or her medication, that the patient has pseudoexfoliative glaucoma that was not previously detected, or that the patient is under unusual major stress (a child using drugs has been jailed, a spouse has died, a bitter divorce has gone to court, etc.). The latter cause (stress) is one that we have noted frequently enough to accept as a valid reason for escape from pressure control.

If the patient missed a dose of medication but his or her condition is otherwise stable and the patient denies frequent noncompliance, recheck the pressure after the person uses his or her medication. If the examination reveals pseudoexfoliative material and a second IOP determination confirms the pressure rise, proceed with additional treatment following the guidelines for POAG. Patients in this situation usually require laser treatment or filtration surgery if the pressure is to be kept at or below the target set. If the patient is undergoing unusual stress and the examination does not reveal any other explanation, then the patient should return soon and the pressure should be rechecked. If the pressure is so high or the eye is so damaged that it requires prompt treatment, proceed with additional treatment as described in Chapter 3. Otherwise, it is often acceptable to allow the stress and the pressure to subside rather than to modify the patient's regimen. Sometimes the pressure rises suddenly and no explanation is found. In such cases, progress with additional treatment as described in Chapter 3.

MILD CHANGE IN PRESSURE THAT INCREASES PRESSURE ABOVE THE GOAL

Consider, for example, a pressure rise, compared to previous IOP, of 5 mm Hg that increases the pressure 2 mm Hg above the goal in a person without progressive nerve or field damage. If the higher IOP is still below the initial untreated pressure and if the patient's condition has been stable for at least a year, it may be appropriate to modify the pressure goal as previously discussed.

If the patient has not been followed up long enough to determine stability, we recommend rechecking the pressure on a different day before changing the treatment course. For patients with mild disease, recheck the pressure within 2 months. For patients with moderate disease, recheck within 1 month, and recheck patients with severe disease within 2 weeks. If the pressure remains elevated beyond the target pressure on repeat pressure checking, proceed as described in Chapter 3.

GRADUAL RISE IN PRESSURE OVER TIME

If gonioscopy with compression fails to show chronic angle closure, then the usual explanation for this finding is that either the medications are gradually losing their effectiveness or that the underlying pathologic resistance to aqueous humor outflow is rising. Provided the pressure remains below the goal and the field remains stable, observe the patient without changing treatment. If the pressure rises above the target pressure, reevaluate the goal as described above. Then, if indicated, proceed with additional treatment as described in Chapter 3.

Worsening Visual Fields or Disc

Most patients who show worsening of their fields or whose nerves appear to have deteriorated compared to their baseline photos fit into one of three general classes: rapid worsening despite achievement and maintenance of the pressure goal, rapid worsening associated with failure to achieve the desired pressure goal, and gradual worsening with or without achievement of the pressure goal.

Unless the worsening is part of a generally uncontrolled situation, a repeat field test or repeat photos should confirm the worsening before management is changed.

RAPID WORSENING DESPITE ACHIEVEMENT AND MAINTENANCE OF THE PRESSURE GOAL

Probable causes. Glaucoma may progress rapidly, but unless the pressure is substantially above the threshold for damage, it usually progresses in small steps. When a patient's condition is worsening rapidly despite achievement of the desired pressure, there are four major possibilities to consider:

- The patient has a very low threshold for damage because of many non-pressure risk factors.
- The patient does not take his or her medicine between visits.
- The pressure fluctuates widely, and thus for part of the time, the pressure goal has not been achieved.
- **Something other than or in addition to glaucoma is causing the field loss.**

Although the explanation often is that the patient is not using medication properly, the possibility that additional visual loss is not related to glaucoma demands the most immediate attention. The list of urgent concerns includes—but is not limited to—tumor, anterior ischemic optic neuropathy, retinal vascular occlusion, and giant cell arteritis. If the patient has had a clearly stable course for a period of time and then shows clear deterioration, a nonglaucomatous cause must be suspected. Late deterioration can occur if the patient's general health declines and the optic nerve becomes more susceptible to pressure, but such rapid change occurs rarely.

Diagnostic approach

- Reexamine the patient. Take a careful history. This should include questions about medication compliance. Not everyone will admit to failure to use medications, but some patients will. Ask about any other symptoms that the patient may have that would coincide with either vascular events or mass lesions. Check the acuity and note if it is falling. In some people it is appropriate to use an Amsler grid and do confrontation fields to look for central scotomas. Repeat gonioscopy to check for previously missed angle closure that could be raising the pressure intermittently. Look carefully at the nerve and determine if it is consistent with the visual field changes. In particular, look for shunt vessels and pallor out of proportion with cupping that suggests nonglaucomatous optic atrophy. Examine the rest of the fundus for conditions such as vascular narrowing consistent with branch arterial occlusion.
- Study the visual field change carefully and determine if it is unusual for glaucoma. Is there a central scotoma or a homonymous defect that might be more consistent with a pathologic condition in the orbit or brain? Did a major field defect, such as a total hemifield loss or a dense fiber bundle defect, appear from one field to the next, such as might occur in a person with acute anterior ischemic optic neuropathy? If the field is atypical in any manner, proceed further. This may involve orbital echography and neuroradiologic studies. Consultation with a neurologist or neuroophthalmologist is particularly helpful in planning an appropriate diagnostic approach in this situation.
- Check the pressure at different times of the day, especially if the patient had wide pressure fluctuations before treatment.

- If all findings seem consistent with primary open-angle glaucoma, then assume that the worsening is pressure related.

Therapeutic approach. Treat any nonglaucomatous conditions identified. If the worsening is determined to be glaucomatous, reset a pressure goal 30% lower than the initial goal. When this situation arises we have generally elected to perform filtering surgery, at least in one eye, because filtration surgery is the best means to achieve a consistently very low pressure. The risks of surgery to a person whose field is deteriorating rapidly have generally seemed reasonable.

RAPID WORSENING ASSOCIATED WITH FAILURE TO ACHIEVE THE DESIRED PRESSURE GOAL

Some patients will have higher than desired pressures during follow-up. The initial pressure goal is only an estimate, and if easy measures reduce the pressure to a level near the goal, we may accept a higher than desired pressure for a while and evaluate the rate of further damage. Generally the decision to accept a pressure above the target is made when the next treatment option is either carbonic anhydrase inhibitors or filtering surgery. Of course, these patients' conditions can worsen from causes other than glaucoma, and we recommend that the fields and patient be examined carefully to confirm that any change is glaucomatous in nature. However, it is not surprising if progressive field loss develops in a patient with inadequately lowered IOP.

When a patient's condition is rapidly worsening because of glaucoma, it seems best to perform filtration surgery to achieve prompt definitive pressure control. It is usually futile to encourage compliance or try to change medications when the situation is clearly uncontrolled.

GRADUAL WORSENING REGARDLESS OF WHETHER THE PRESSURE GOAL HAS BEEN ACHIEVED

Over the years, many patients with glaucoma lose some of their visual field. Some will have "well-controlled" pressures, and some will have less than the desired pressure lowering. Worsening of the visual field usually signals that there should be a change in management. How drastic the change in pressure goal and management should be does not depend on the fact that progression occurred, but on how serious the damage was initially and the *rate* of progression on the treatment used to date.

The steps in this situation are similar to those involved in instituting treatment.

Diagnostic steps

- Determine the rate of change. The pace at which the condition is worsening helps in deciding how aggressive treatment should be to obtain an even lower pressure. If a 79-year-old person had only mild or moderate field loss initially and has had a mild enlargement of a scotoma over the past 10 years, it is reasonable not to change management unless the damage is accelerated. The same change in a 45-year-old patient almost always warrants more aggressive treatment.
- Try to determine if the patient is compliant with treatment. If poor compliance is established, it may be best to try a treatment, such as laser or filtration surgery, that does not require chronic medication use.

Therapeutic steps

- Reset the pressure goal. The degree of initial damage and rate of further change help to determine how much lower to aim in pressure control.

For example, clear-cut change may be noted over 3 years or 15 years, and the two situations are treated differently. The more rapid the change, the greater should be the additional lowering. When resetting a pressure goal, we recommend trying to achieve about a 25% further reduction (15% for slow (>5 years) progression, 35% for rapid (<2 years) progression) compared to the average pressures for the patient during the period of change.

- Treat to achieve the new pressure goal. If the rate of progression is a serious threat in a given patient, consider laser trabeculoplasty or filtering surgery if additional medical therapy does not have a prompt dramatic effect. These procedures may reduce spikes of pressure and eliminate pressure rises related to periodic nonuse of medications.
- Reestablish a baseline. The two fields that showed progression may serve as a baseline. However, if you add a miotic or if you perform surgery, it is best to obtain new fields promptly. In most cases, the clinician should take new nerve photographs. In the future, this new baseline will be used for comparison, and all the provisos about the ability to determine change apply to the new baseline.
- Start a new follow-up schedule.

Cataract Development

As long as the patient sees well enough for his or her needs and you are able, by either fundus or field examination, to follow-up with the patient adequately, there is no need to encourage cataract surgery. When the patient cannot see adequately or the cataract precludes adequate follow-up, a combined cataract extraction/intraocular lens implant/trabeculectomy may be indicated.

If a patient who has a cataract that is not yet dense enough to remove requires filtering surgery, we perform only a filtering operation.

FOLLOWING UP ON TREATMENT VARIATIONS

In Chapter 3 we outlined our initial approach to three groups of patients who did not fit easily into the routine management scheme for POAG: those who cannot do reliable fields, those whose fundus cannot be seen, and those with advanced disease when first seen. For each group, follow-up care presents the expected difficulties.

The Patient Who Cannot Do Reliable Fields

The obvious problem in following individuals who cannot perform reliable fields is that it usually takes a large increment of damage to be recognizable. The greater the degree of initial damage, the greater a problem this presents. The difficulty in following the rate of change in these patients highlights the value of field examination. As with patients with routine POAG, the frequency of follow-up depends on the degree of damage and the success with which the pressure is lowered. In general, if the nerve has only mild damage and is easily examined, it is possible to recognize mild to moderate progression if the patient has good 2× stereo baseline photographs. Once it is known that the deterioration is not rapid, follow-up may be similar to patients who can perform reliable fields. In more advanced cases, successive nerve evaluation is less valuable, and stricter pressure control monitored more frequently will be necessary. Sometimes a patient with serious visual loss can accurately describe visual fluctuations and can report meaningfully that his or her vision is or is not generally stable. In such cases, a subjective sense of deteriorating vision (especially dimming) may be the prime guide to more aggressive therapy.

Using the hypothetical patients from earlier in this chapter, we suggest the following as examples of follow-up schedules. On every visit the clinician should examine the optic disc, particularly to detect disc hemorrhages; gonioscopy should be performed yearly.

CASE AB—EASILY CONTROLLED EARLY GLAUCOMA

A 60-year-old asymptomatic woman is first seen with an IOP of 32 mm Hg, cup/disc ratio of 0.5 with rim tissue of good color without notches or hemorrhages. Baseline examinations include pressure measurements averaging 30 mm Hg (range, 27 to 33 mm Hg) and excellent-quality optic nerve photographs. Despite education and multiple attempts, the patient cannot perform reliable visual fields. The initial goal is a 30% lowering, or a pressure range between about 19 and 23 mm Hg. Treatment with a β-blocker in one eye results in a pressure of 21 mm Hg in the treated eye and 30 mm Hg in the untreated eye after 1 month. Treatment is begun in both eyes.

- When should this patient be reexamined?
- What should be tested on follow-up?

Over time, it will be important to determine if the optic nerve is developing progressive cupping, but initially the focus is on the pressure. Once the initial pressure goal is achieved, it is reasonable to examine this patient in a month or so to check the pressure. If it remains low, reexamine the patient again in 2 or 3 months and examine the optic nerve. If the nerve is stable and the pressure remains within the goal, see the patient again in 3 months (6 months into follow-up) to check the pressure and dilate the patient's pupils for fundoscopy. In another 3 months, check the pressure, and 3 months thereafter (now 12 months into follow-up), test the pressure, repeat gonioscopy, and dilate the patient's pupils to examine the disc and fundus. Check the pressure and nerve every 6 months for 2 years and perform gonioscopy yearly. If the patient's condition appears to be stable after 3 years, repeat the optic nerve photographs and compare them to the initial photographs. If they show stability, and if the pressure remains within the target range, then decrease the interval of pressure and nerve examinations to every 9 months for 2 or 3 more years. Repeat the photographs and, if they show stability, check the pressure, perform gonioscopy, and examine the nerve at least yearly. Obtain photographs every 2 years and always compare the current photographs to the *initial* photographs. If the pressure rises above the goal, manage it by the routine guides for POAG (Table 4-7).

- What should be done if this patient's condition worsens?

If on any of the repeat examinations, the condition of the nerves is worse, then reset the pressure goal at least 20% lower than the initial goal and treat the patient for moderate disease. If at least an additional 20% pressure decrease cannot be achieved medically, proceed with laser and filtering surgery.

CASE CD—PROBABLY CONTROLLED MODERATE GLAUCOMA

A 59-year-old man has untreated pressures that average 28 mm Hg (range, 24 to 32 mm Hg). His cup/disc ratio is 0.7 with a notch inferotemporally in both optic nerves. Despite extensive patient education, fields are totally unreliable. A goal of 30% lowering gives a target pressure of 20 mm Hg. β-Blocker use is contraindicated because of severe asthma. Treatment of one eye with pilocarpine 1% results in pressures of 22 mm Hg in the treated eye and 31 mm Hg in the untreated eye. A trial of 2% pilocarpine produces intolerable symptoms. Treatment with pilocarpine 1% is begun in both eyes and dipivefrin is added in one eye; resulting pressures are 18 mm Hg in the eye with both drugs and 22 mm

TABLE 4-7 *Follow-up of Mild Glaucoma in a Person Who Cannot Perform Reliable Fields*

Baseline

- At least three IOP measurements at different times of day
- At least two threshold visual field examinations to determine that patient cannot do reliably
- Gonioscopy
- Disc photographs

Obtain within 2 months

Initial treatment

- Pressure checks and medication adjustments at 1-4-week intervals until treatment regimen is established

Complete within 2 months if possible

Follow-up

	Months									Years 4 through 6		Years 6 and after	
	1	3	6	9	12	18	24	30	36	Every 9 months	About year 6	Every year	Every 2 or 3 years
IOP	X	X	X	X	X	X	X	X	X	X	X	X	X
Visual field	Unable to perform reliably												
Gonioscopy*					X		X		X	X	X	X	X
Undilated disc examination	X	X		X									
Dilated disc and fundus examination			X		X	X	X	X	X	X†	X	X†	X†
Disc photos									X		X		X

*If the patient is treated with miotic drops, repeat gonioscopy promptly.
†If the patient is using miotic drops and is seen less than twice a year, he or she may use dilating drops at home to avoid posterior synechiae formation.

Hg in the eye with only pilocarpine. Treatment with both medications is started for both eyes.

- When should this patient be reexamined?
- What should be tested on follow-up?

This patient has a distinctly abnormal optic nerve that makes the diagnosis of glaucoma highly likely, but he is very unlikely to show measurable optic nerve changes within only a few months. At the initial follow-up examination, check that the pressure remains low and that the angle remains open. Schedule a pressure check and gonioscopy a month or so after beginning bilateral treatment with the two drugs. This time course should allow for stabilization of the effect of the dipivefrin. Arrange a follow-up pressure check in another 2 months. If the pressure is stable, recheck the pressure and dilate the patient's pupils to examine the nerve in 3 more months (6 months into follow-up). Test the pressure in 3 more months, and repeat tonometry, gonioscopy, and dilated fundoscopy in 3 more months (now 12 months into follow-up). If stable, lengthen the follow-up intervals to every 6 months and perform a disc examination through a dilated pupil at every visit henceforth. On every other visit, perform gonioscopy. Repeat the nerve photographs and compare them to initial photographs every 2 years (Table 4-8). If the pressure rises above the goal, treat as described above.

- What should be done if this patient's condition worsens?

If the patient's nerves show progressive damage, reset the pressure level 25% below the level at which the progression occurred and treat on the frequency schedule for severe glaucoma. Proceed through laser and filtration surgery if needed to achieve the goal.

CASE EF—MARGINALLY CONTROLLED SEVERE GLAUCOMA

A 64-year-old man has pressures averaging 26 mm Hg (range, 23 to 29 mm Hg), with a cup/disc ratio of 0.8 and loss of the inferotemporal rim in both eyes. The patient cannot perform reliable fields. Baseline photographs are of good quality. The target pressure, if the patient had been able to do good fields, would have been 16 mm Hg. However, following the guide in Chapter 3 for a person who cannot perform reliable fields and has severe disease, the goal is either a pressure of 15 mm Hg or a 50% lowering, whichever is lower. Thus the goal is 13 mm Hg. With use of a nonselective β-blocker in one eye, the pressure falls to 19 mm Hg in the treated eye and is 27 mm Hg in the untreated eye. Treatment is begun in both eyes, and 2 weeks later the pressure is 19 mm Hg in each eye. With the addition of pilocarpine 1% to one eye, the pressure falls to 16 mm Hg in the eye treated with both drops and is 20 mm Hg in the eye with only β-blocker treatment. Use of pilocarpine 4% in one eye and β-blocker in both eyes gives pressures of 14 mm Hg and 20 mm Hg. Both eyes are treated with pilocarpine 4% and β-blocker, and the pressure 1 month later is 14 mm Hg in both eyes. Gonioscopy shows that the angle is still open.

A laser trabeculoplasty in one eye in conjunction with medication achieves a pressure of 12 mm Hg a month after completion of the treatment; laser surgery is performed in both eyes. Initial treatment involves about 5 months, after which the nerve appears stable on dilated examination.

- When should this patient be reexamined?
- What should be tested on follow-up?

This patient has severe disease and a low pressure goal, which has been achieved. Examine the patient in about a month to determine whether the pressure remains low. If the pressure is still controlled, recheck the pressure in another 2 months. If the patient's condition seems stable, check the pressure

TABLE 4-8 *Follow-ɴp of Moderate Glaucoma in a Person Who Cannot Perform Reliable Fields*

Baseline	• At least three IOP measurements at different times of day • At least two threshold visual field examinations to determine that patient cananot do reliably • Gonioscopy • Disc photographs	Obtain within 2 months
Initial treatment	• Pressure checks and medication adjustments at 1- to 4-week intervals until treatment regimen is established	Complete within 2 months if possible
Follow-up		

	Months					Years 2 and after		
	1	**3**	**6**	**9**	**12**	**Every 6 months**	**Every year**	**Every 2 years**
IOP	X	X	X	X	X	X	X	X
Visual field	Unable to perform reliably							
Gonioscopy*					X		X	X
Undilated disc examination	X	X		X				
Dilated disc and fundus examination			X		X	X	X	X
Disc photos								X

*If the patient is treated with miotics drops, repeat gonioscopy promptly.

TABLE 4-9 *Follow-up of Severe Glaucoma in a Person Who Cannot Perform Reliable Fields*

Baseline	• At least three IOP measurements at different times of day • At least two threshold visual field examinations to determine that patient cannot do reliably • Gonioscopy • Disc photographs	Obtain within 2 months
Initial treatment	• Pressure checks and medication adjustments at 1- to 4-week intervals until treatment regimen is established	Complete within 2 months if possible

Follow-up

	Months									Years 2 and after	
	1	3	6	9	12	15	18	21	24	Every 6 months	Every year
IOP	X	X	X	X	X	X	X	X	X	X	X
Visual field					Unable to perform reliably						
Gonioscopy*					X				X		X
Undilated disc examination	X	X		X		X		X			
Dilated disc and fundus examination			X		X		X		X	X	X
Disc photos†					X				X		X

*If the patient is treated with miotic drops, repeat gonioscopy promptly.
†If the discs are too cupped to notice a change, do not repeat photos.

every 3 months for 24 months. Examine the nerve after the patient's pupils are dilated every 6 months, and obtain nerve photographs every year and compare them to the initial photographs. Perform gonioscopy yearly. If the patient's condition is stable for 2 years, check the pressures and examine the patient after the pupils are dilated every 6 months thereafter. Obtain photographs every year (Table 4-9). If the pressure rises above the target pressure, add carbonic anhydrase inhibitors. If they are either not tolerated or not effective, we recommend filtration surgery in one eye, even if progression has not been documented.

• What should be done if this patient's condition worsens?

If a patient demonstrates progressive nerve damage or has convincing subjective worsening despite a pressure in the low teens, check carefully for the possibility of another process as outlined in Chapter 6. Assuming that none is found, the only treatment is to lower the pressure if at all possible. If the patient has not had filtration surgery, perform filtration surgery, with a pressure goal of less than 10 mm Hg. We prefer to pursue this course in one eye at a time because the side effects of surgery to maximally lower pressure can be significant. If the goal is achieved in one eye without significant side effects, we perform surgery in the other eye.

The Patient Whose Fundus Cannot Be Seen Well Because of Miosis, Cataract, or Other Media Opacity

Provided the visual field on such patients remains stable, management follows the routine guidelines. However, if the field worsens, it is necessary to decide whether the worsening is related to media opacity or to glaucomatous damage. A generalized depression of the field is more likely to be media related than glaucoma related. Deepening of a preexisting scotoma can result from either. If a new scotoma appears in the absence of deepening of preexisting scotomas, the change is probably related to glaucoma in a patient with glaucoma, but it can obviously be caused by any other ocular or nonocular cause of visual field defect. Cataract management is described on p. 120.

Regular dilation of patients on chronic miotic therapy will diminish the incidence of glaucoma patients whose fundi cannot be visualized.

The Patient Who Has Advanced Cupping and Visual Field Loss on Initial Examination

Use the schedule in Tables 4-5 and 4-6 for follow-up of patients with severe glaucoma.

5

Glaucoma Suspects I: Elevated IOP

A glaucoma suspect is someone who, for one or more reasons, is at higher than usual risk of developing glaucomatous optic nerve damage and visual deficiency and therefore warrants careful follow-up. The most common conditions that place a person at risk are the following:

- Elevated IOP
- Large or asymmetric optic cups
- Presence of a disc margin splinter hemorrhage
- Unexplained visual field defect consistent with glaucoma
- Strong family history of glaucomatous field loss

Chapter 6 discusses the management of patients with nerve or field changes suggestive of glaucoma who also have normal eye pressure. Those with a strong family history of glaucoma are discussed in Chapter 11.

Individuals with elevated pressure form the largest group of glaucoma suspects. If the evaluation described in Chapter 2 does not reveal fully manifest glaucomatous damage, then the patient is a glaucoma suspect. The term *ocular hypertensive* is best avoided for these patients because it implies that they have a specific condition that is not glaucoma.

Our recommended regimen for the care of glaucoma suspects with elevated IOP differs little from that for individuals with manifest mild glaucoma. After establishing a baseline, decide whether to treat to lower the IOP by comparing the risk of future glaucoma damage if the pressure is not lowered to the risk, bother, expense, etc. of treatment to lower the pressure. If treatment is chosen, set a pressure goal and attempt to achieve it. Finally, regardless of whether the pressure is lowered, follow up on the patient's course to determine if it is worsening (see box below).

Management Steps for Glaucoma Suspects

1. Establish a baseline.
2. Determine the risk of glaucomatous damage.
3. Decide whether to treat the IOP. If treatment is chosen, set a pressure goal and attempt to achieve it.
4. Continue to observe all patients for evidence of worsening.

ESTABLISHING A BASELINE

The initial evaluation for patients with elevated eye pressure is described in Chapter 2. Obtain at least three IOP measurements, preferably at different times and on different days.

DETERMINING THE RISK OF GLAUCOMATOUS DAMAGE

Categories of Suspects

The decision to treat or not to treat a patient with elevated pressure depends on the relative risk of damage from pressure and the risks, costs and difficulty of treatment. Some glaucoma suspects have mild glaucoma — an optic nerve or visual field may have subtle damage and still be within normal limits — but it is not possible at the outset to distinguish them from other suspects whose condition will not progress. The major question to ask about any glaucoma suspect is, "How likely am I to recognize a small enough amount of glaucomatous damage that I can start treatment without hurting the patient's function?" Thus a questionable central visual field defect and a 0.7 cup, even if associated with a pressure of 22 mm Hg, is more worrisome than a pressure of 35 mm Hg with a healthy looking, minimally cupped optic nerve and a full visual field.

To simplify our recommendations for managing glaucoma suspects who have high pressure but no definite field loss, we have constructed an arbitrary and admittedly imperfect risk table (Fig. 5-1). The following assumptions were considered in constructing the risk table:

- The pressure at the time a person becomes a glaucoma suspect has probably been present for some years.
- The greater the pressure for any given degree of damage, the higher the threshold for damage in that patient.
- The higher the pressure, the greater the risk of glaucomatous damage.
- The larger the cup, the more likely it is that the cupping is not entirely physiologic.

Factors Affecting Risk Categories

FAMILY HISTORY OF GLAUCOMA

A first-degree relative with glaucoma increases the risk by one category.

VASCULAR OCCLUSION

Treat a person who has elevated pressure and has had a retinal vein occlusion as a high-risk suspect.

DISC HEMORRHAGE

The presence of a disc hemorrhage increases risk by one category.

HIGH MYOPIA

High myopia (<6 D) increases risk by one category.

AGE

Age greater than 70 years increases risk by one category.

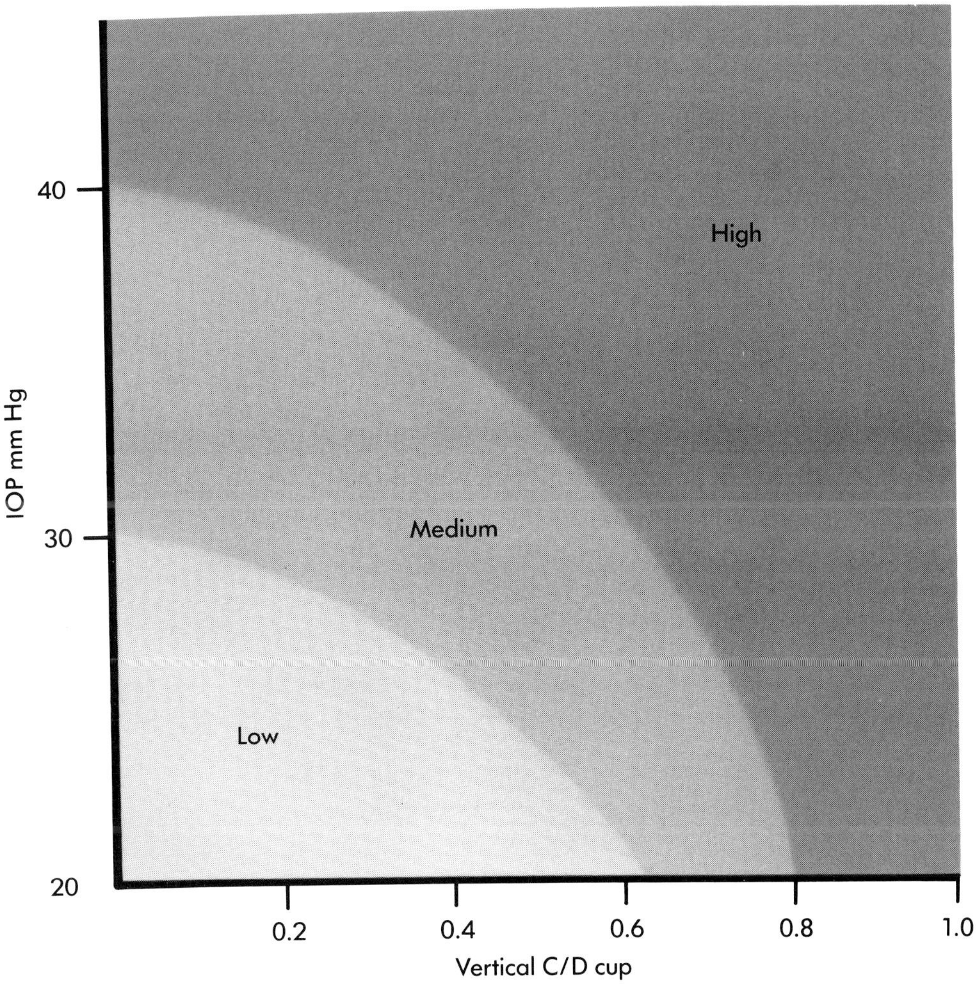

FIG. 5-1 Risk categories in patients with elevated pressure without fully developed glaucoma.

DECIDING WHETHER TO TREAT, DETERMINING GOALS, AND PLANNING FOLLOW-UP

Low-Risk Suspects

Low-risk patients may experience worsening of their conditions over time, but such changes are unlikely to happen quickly. We recommend follow-up without treatment. Any progression is likely to appear very slowly, with adequate time to undertake therapy before the damage is severe enough to be symptomatic. We do not believe that allowing early damage to occur before starting therapy weakens the nerve and makes it more susceptible to further harm from pressure. We think that the benefit of "preventive" treatment in this group is outweighed by the expense, inconvenience, and medical side effects of therapy. We discuss this philosophy with the patient and do rarely treat low-risk patients who request such therapy. Regular observation should not be considered nontherapy, but rather therapy that is delayed until it is needed. A reasonable schedule for follow-up is outlined in Table 5-1.

TABLE 5-1 ***Follow-up of a Low-risk Glaucoma Suspect***

Baseline	• At least three IOP measurements at different times of day • At least two threshold visual field examinations • Gonioscopy • Disc photographs	Obtain within 2 months
Initial treatment	• Treat only if the patient strongly prefers treatment	

Follow-up

	Months		Yearly thereafter
	6	**12**	
IOP	X	X	X
Visual field	X	X	X
Gonioscopy		X	X
Undilated disc examination	X		
Dilated disc and fundus examination		X	X
Disc photos	Repeat only if the patient's condition is suspected of worsening.		

Medium-Risk Suspects

These individuals challenge the doctor to balance the risks and benefits of ocular hypotensive treatment. If a patient's pressures can be lowered, his or her chance of developing glaucomatous damage will decrease. However, not all medium-risk patients need treatment; and, once begun, treatment usually continues for life.

Although we recommend discussing the advantages and disadvantages of treatment with the patient, few patients in our practice have strong opinions and most want a recommendation. If the fields are reliable and consistent and if the nerve is easily examined, we usually follow up without treatment. If the patient prefers treatment, we recommend a therapeutic trial of topical medicine. If the fields are only fair or if it is difficult to examine the nerve, we generally recommend a trial of pressure lowering.

If the patient tolerates a therapeutic trial of simple medication, which is generally a β-blocker once or twice a day, and if the pressure decreases at least 20%, we continue treatment. If the pressure does not decrease at least 20%, we usually discontinue treatment and follow up on the patient's course without treatment.

A sample follow-up schedule for a medium-risk patient is presented in Table 5-2.

TABLE 5-2 *Follow-up of a Moderate-risk Glaucoma Suspect*

Baseline	• At least three IOP measurements at different times of day • At least two threshold visual field examinations • Gonioscopy • Disc photographs	Obtain within 2 months
Initial treatment	• Most people do not need treatment if they can be followed up • Consider a therapeutic trial based on the findings and the patient's desires. If medication is chosen, it should be easily tolerated.	

Follow-up

	Months							Years 3 and after
	4	8	12	18	24	30	36	Yearly
IOP	X	X	X	X	X	X	X	X
Visual field	X	X	X	X	X	X	X	X
Gonioscopy*			X		X		X	X
Undilated disc examination	X	X		X		X		
Dilated disc and fundus examination†			X		X		X	X
Disc photos	Repeat only if the patient is suspected of worsening							

*If the patient begins to use miotic drops, perform gonioscopy promptly to assess for increased pupillary block.

†If the patient uses miotic drops, dilate the pupil at least every 6 months. The patient may use dilating drops at home if he or she would not otherwise need examination.

High-Risk Suspects

High-risk suspect patients have large cups, pressures substantially above normal, or both. Although not everyone with very high pressure has glaucoma, the greater the IOP, for any given degree of nerve cupping, the greater the chance a person will demonstrate progressive disease. The assumption that the pressure at the time of diagnosis has been present for some time applies to high pressures as well; patients with highly elevated pressure without definite damage usually have high thresholds for damage. However, the potential damage, if the assumption proves false, increases with increasing pressure. Initially we consider everyone with a pressure above 40 mm Hg to be at high risk for damage.

Try to lower the pressure in these high-risk individuals unless, after a discussion of their condition, they specifically oppose it. The goal of treatment is to decrease the risk of rapid damage, not to achieve some normal pressure reading. Be careful not to pursue a course of expensive, annoying, or risky therapy for a clinical condition that is less threatening than mild, but full manifest, glaucoma. As when treating other glaucoma suspects, we use medication only if it is well tolerated. Our first choice is β-blocker treatment. In a person at high risk who cannot tolerate a β-blocking agent, try either dipivefrin or weak pilocarpine. A sample follow-up plan for a high-risk patient is shown in Table 5-3.

TABLE 5-3 *Follow-up of a High-risk Glaucoma Suspect*

Baseline	• At least three IOP measurements at different times of day • At least two threshold visual field examinations • Gonioscopy • Disc photographs	Obtain within 2 months
Initial treatment	• Therapeutic trial to lower pressure unless the patient prefers not to use medication • Treatment should be well tolerated	

Follow-up

	Months						Years 2 through 4		Years 5 and after	
	2	4	6	8	10	12	Every 6 months	Every year	Every 6 months	Every year
IOP	X	X		X		X	X	X	X	X
Visual field	X	X		X		X	X	X	*	X
Gonioscopy†						X		X		X
Undilated disc examination	X	X		X			X		X	
Dilated disc and fundus examination‡						X		X		X
Disc photos	Repeat only if the patient's condition is suspected of worsening.									

*If the IOP rises above the level maintained over the first 4 years, repeat the visual fields every 6 months for several years.

†If the patient begins to use miotic drops, perform gonioscopy promptly to assess for increased pupillary block.

‡If the patient uses miotics drops, dilate the pupil at least every 6 months.

MODIFYING TREATMENT

The three major findings on follow-up that prompt modification of treatment are the finding of a disc hemorrhage, a change in the visual field, and a change in the disc.

- If a disc hemorrhage occurs without a disc or field change, consider the patient to be a high-risk suspect at the beginning of the follow-up phase.
- If a glaucomatous visual defect develops on follow-up, repeat the field examination; if the defect is confirmed, treat the patient for glaucoma.
- If the nerve appears to have developed increased cupping, repeat the photographs and compare the two sets. If the progression is confirmed, treat the patient for glaucoma.

6

Glaucoma Suspects II: Cupping or Field Loss without Elevated Pressure (Normal Tension Glaucoma)

All patients with glaucoma have optic nerve damage, but not all optic nerve damage is glaucomatous. The nerve fiber bundle defect is the hallmark of glaucoma, but not every nerve fiber bundle defect is caused by glaucoma. In the absence of elevated pressure, the presence of optic nerve cupping or an unexplained visual field defect warrants a careful evaluation. The diagnostic possibilities of greatest immediate concern when a patient is first seen with an abnormal field or disc are treatable neurologic conditions, particularly tumors, and treatable vascular conditions such as cranial arteritis. Other fairly common conditions include nonarteritic vascular conditions, glaucoma with labile pressures, and past elevated pressure and resultant damage. These conditions must be recognized because their management differs from that of normal tension glaucoma (NTG).

Normal tension glaucoma, also called low tension glaucoma, is defined in various ways. We use the term *suspected NTG* (or *NTG suspect* to refer to a person with the condition) to denote the presence of glaucomalike cupping, field loss, or both, in a person whose pressures always measure less than 22 mm Hg. We use the term *progressive NTG,* or simply *NTG,* to describe suspected NTG that is actually observed to be progressive while the pressure remains normal. Thus on initial presentation a patient can, at most, be called a NTG suspect.

In general, patients suspected of having normal tension glaucoma are identified in one of two ways. The clinician may note abnormal cupping during a routine examination of a person with normal IOP and then obtain a visual field examination that does not clearly point to another explanation. Or the patient may note a visual symptom and come to the doctor, who performs a field examination that shows a field defect. Occasionally an asymptomatic person has a routine screening visual field test that shows a defect.

The following discussion concerns those patients in whom another diagnosis is not immediately obvious and in whom NTG is a possibility. We do not discuss patients in whom a routine evaluation leads to a clear diagnosis, for example those with bitemporal hemianopsia or acute and obvious retinal vascular occlusions. The evaluation of a NTG suspect proceeds as does the evaluation of a person with elevated pressure. The goal is to identify those individuals who have some recognizable condition and particularly to recognize those individuals who have treatable conditions.

EVALUATING THE PATIENT

History: Asymptomatic Patient

The history in an asymptomatic patient may suggest one or more diagnoses, but history will not provide a diagnosis. There are several lines of questioning that relate to various diagnostic possibilities.

HYPOTENSION

Shock or marked hypotension sometimes causes optic nerve damage and field loss that mimic glaucoma. Ask about injuries, previous blood transfusions, hypotensive episodes during surgery, hospitalization with intensive care, etc. Damage caused by hypotension rarely progresses. Because it is usually impossible to be certain, even in a person with a history of shock, that the ocular findings and medical history are related, these patients remain NTG suspects and require follow-up.

POSSIBLE PREVIOUS PRESSURE ELEVATIONS

Prior use of topical or systemic corticosteroids or past injury may have temporarily caused elevated pressure. A patient who is using systemic β-blockers may have had elevated IOP before using the medication. Pigmentary dispersion may have caused a pressure elevation in earlier years.

VASOSPASM

Migraine is associated with NTG. Other vasospastic conditions such as Raynaud's phenomenon also appear to be associated with NTG. Paradoxically, many individuals with vasospastic disorders have relatively low blood pressure.

FAMILY HISTORY

Primary open-angle glaucoma and NTG may mingle within the same family. Ask not only whether relatives have glaucoma, but also try to determine the severity of any disease uncovered.

History: Symptomatic Patient

In addition to checking the history-related points mentioned, question a patient with a symptomatic visual field defect about the onset (date, circumstances, associated symptoms) of the defect and about its subsequent course. A significant visual field defect that had a sudden onset is unlikely to be related to glaucoma, and the major immediate diagnostic concern in this setting is cranial arteritis for which the patient should be evaluated. A visual annoyance noted some time ago that has worsed may be NTG, but compressive lesions also progress.

Examination

VISUAL ACUITY

The best corrected visual acuity guides the evaluation of cupping and field loss. Until late in the disease, glaucoma rarely decreases the Snellen acuity significantly, whereas mass lesions involving the optic nerve often affect the acuity.

VISUAL FIELDS

Perform a central 30° static threshold field examination. If the acuity is unexpectedly reduced or if the patient complains of central visual symptoms, perform an Amsler grid examination before ocular manipulation. Examine the field carefully for atypical features, especially for central scotomas (look at the foveal threshold value) and for asymmetry across the vertical midline.

Typical nerve fiber bundle defects that cross the vertical midline occur in patients with glaucoma, disc drusen, and anterior ischemic optic neuropathy. Central scotomas do not generally occur in glaucoma and suggest optic nerve compression; vertical hemianopic defects cannot be attributed to glaucoma.

SLIT-LAMP EXAMINATION

Look for evidence of conditions that may have elevated the pressure in the past, such as trauma or previous inflammation. Also check for conditions that may be associated with intermittent pressure elevations, such as pigment dispersion or narrow angles.

TONOMETRY

If some method other than applanation was used to check the pressure, repeat the measurement with an applanation tonometer. A number of pressure measurements on different days and different times of day may detect a variable, sometimes elevated pressure. Both for diagnosis and as part of a baseline examination, we suggest that measurements be done on at least 3 different days and that over those 3 days the measurements cover the hours of 8 A.M. to 6 P.M. at 2-hour intervals.

GONIOSCOPY

Examine the angle for evidence of previous events, such as trauma and inflammation, and for evidence of possible intermittent angle closure. If the angle is very narrow or is closed in places and if it appears to be on a pupillary block mechanism, perform laser iridectomy and proceed with the evaluation. A narrow angle can exist coincidentally with any other ocular or systemic abnormality, but significant pupillary block in this setting should be treated.

OPHTHALMOSCOPY

Disc examination. Examine the disc using a magnified binocular system and a slit beam. The disc configuration in NTG is the same as that in primary open-angle glaucoma. Vertical elongation of the cup, focal notching of the neuroretinal rim, hemorrhage along the disc margin, peripapillary halo or crescent, and disc

Disc Findings and NTG

- Disc findings that support a diagnosis of glaucoma
  - Vertical elongation of the cup
  - Focal discrete notching of the neuroretinal rim
  - Splinter hemorrhage on the disc margin
  - Asymmetry of cupping
  - Peripapillary crescent or halo
- Disc findings that support another diagnosis
  - Segmental pallor of the neuroretinal rim
  - Significant pallor without corresponding tissue loss
  - Shunt vessels on the disc
  - Disc drusen
  - Rotation or truncation of the disc

asymmetry not associated with anisometropia are all characteristic of glaucoma. Pallor disproportionate to cupping, especially an area of focal pallor corresponding to a field defect, suggests a nonglaucomatous cause (Plate 9). Drusen of the nerve head may cause field defects, and if suspected but not seen may be confirmed with echography (Plate 10). Shunt vessels on the disc suggest a previous retinal vein obstruction (Plate 11). Anomalous or hypoplastic discs may be associated with visual field defects (Plate 12). The box on p. 136 summarizes the major disc findings and their relationship to likely diagnoses.

Retinal findings. Examine the retina carefully for retinal scars that could produce field defects, for subtle staphylomas, and for signs of previous vascular occlusion, such as vascular attenuation, shunt vessels, and peripheral hemorrhages.

DIAGNOSING NORMAL TENSION GLAUCOMA

Differential Diagnosis

Chart 6-1 summarizes the diagnostic steps in patients suspected of having NTG.

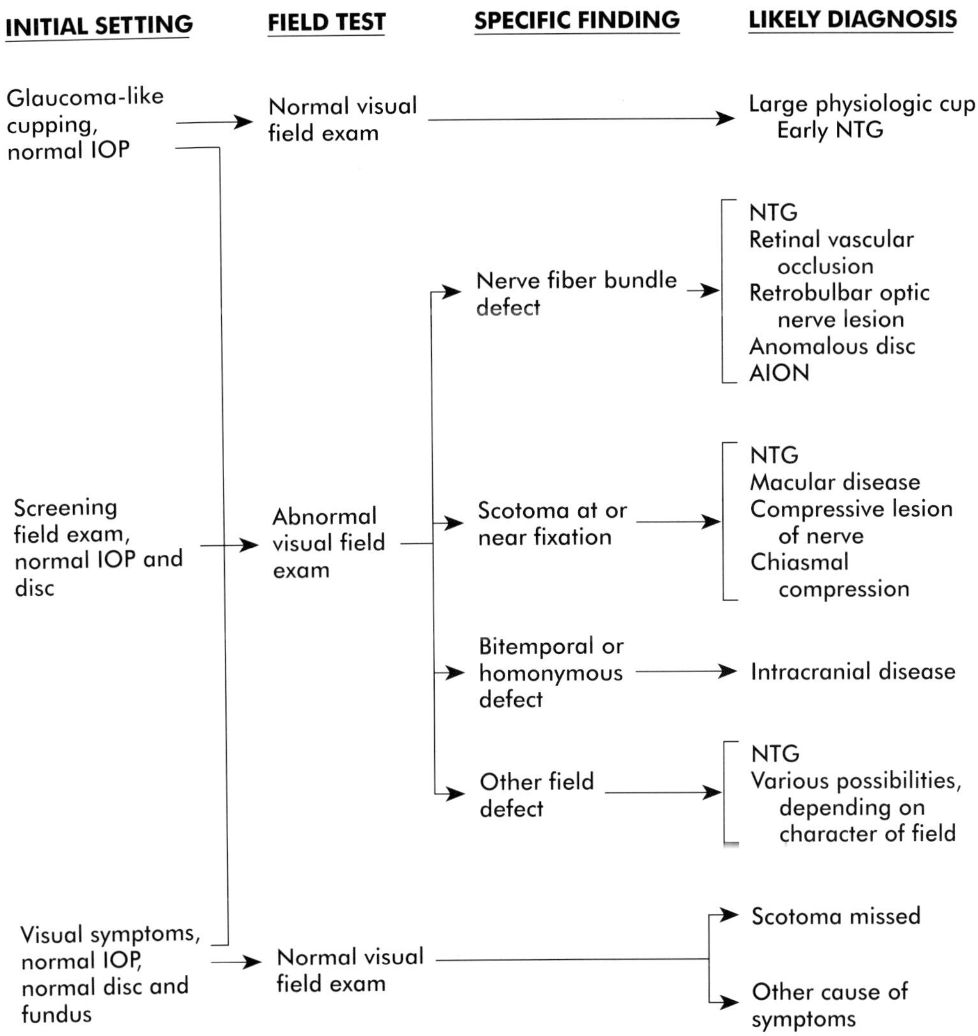

CHART 6-1 Differential diagnosis of NTG suspects.

◆ *Cupping—no field loss*

If there are no other disc findings, such as hemorrhages, and if the neuroretinal rim is intact and of good color, the most likely diagnosis is large physiologic cupping. NTG without detected field loss is more likely if the disc has any of the other findings supporting glaucoma.

Glaucoma-like cupping, normal IOP → Normal visual field exam → Large physiologic cup / Early NTG

◆ *Cupping—field loss—nerve fiber bundle defect*

Nerve fiber bundle defects crossing the vertical midline are always prechiasmal and usually indicate a lesion at the nerve head or in the retina. Retinal vascular causes, such as branch arterial occlusions and anterior ischemic optic neuropathy (AION), are visible on fundus examination when acute, but after the early signs resolve they may be difficult to recognize. These conditions mimic NTG when they occur in patients with large physiologic cupping. Examine the vessels for thinning and the retinal pigment epithelium for local derangement. Segmental pallor of the nerve in the area corresponding to the field defect suggests a vascular accident, as does a history of acute field loss. Bilateral cupping and nerve fiber bundle defects are more likely to be related to glaucoma than to any other cause, whereas strikingly unilateral cases with symmetric IOP are more likely not glaucoma.

Glaucoma-like cupping, normal IOP → Abnormal visual field exam → Nerve fiber bundle defect →
- NTG
- Retinal vascular occlusion
- Retrobulbar optic nerve lesion
- Anomalous disc
- AION

◆ *Cupping—field loss—scotoma at or near fixation*

Although paracentral scotomas occur frequently in individuals who have NTG, central scotomas are not common. Central scotomas associated with cupping may be caused by compression of the optic nerve. Pallor of the nerve disproportionate to the cupping also suggests nerve compression in the presence of generous physiologic cupping. If neither the Amsler grid examination nor a careful macular examination reveals maculopathy to explain central field loss, it is appropriate to investigate the optic nerve with echography, neuroradiologic imaging, or both, particularly in unilateral cases. Myopic eyes (perhaps with a temporal crescent) may have scotomas affecting fixation early in the course of NTG.

Glaucoma-like cupping → Abnormal visual field exam → Scotoma at or near fixation →
- NTG
- Macular disease
- Compressive lesion of nerve
- Chiasmal compression

◆ *Cupping—field loss—bitemporal or homonymous hemianopia*

These defects indicate disease at or behind the chiasm. Although pallor alone generally accompanies descending optic atrophy, cupping may also develop, or generous physiologic cupping may have been present beforehand.

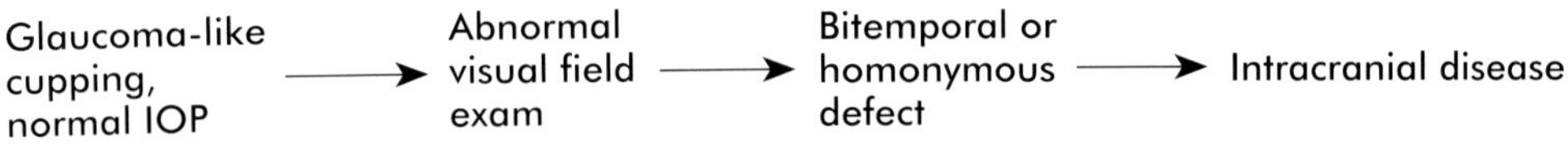

◆ *Cupping—other field loss*

The character of the field loss determines the diagnostic possibilities. Atypical field loss *may* develop in NTG, but individuals with such field loss should be thoroughly evaluated.

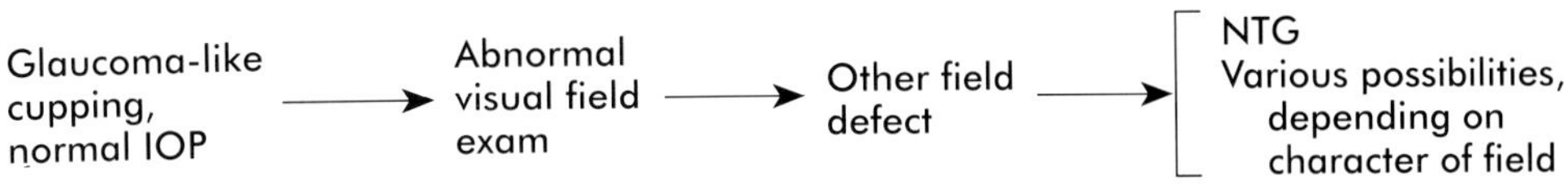

◆ *Field loss—with or without symptoms—no obvious cupping*

The possible causes of field loss without abnormal cupping are the same as those with cupping, but NTG is much less likely than other conditions. Buried disc drusen may present in this fashion. Echography confirms or rules out the presence of drusen. In other cases, the nature of the field loss guides the diagnostic considerations.

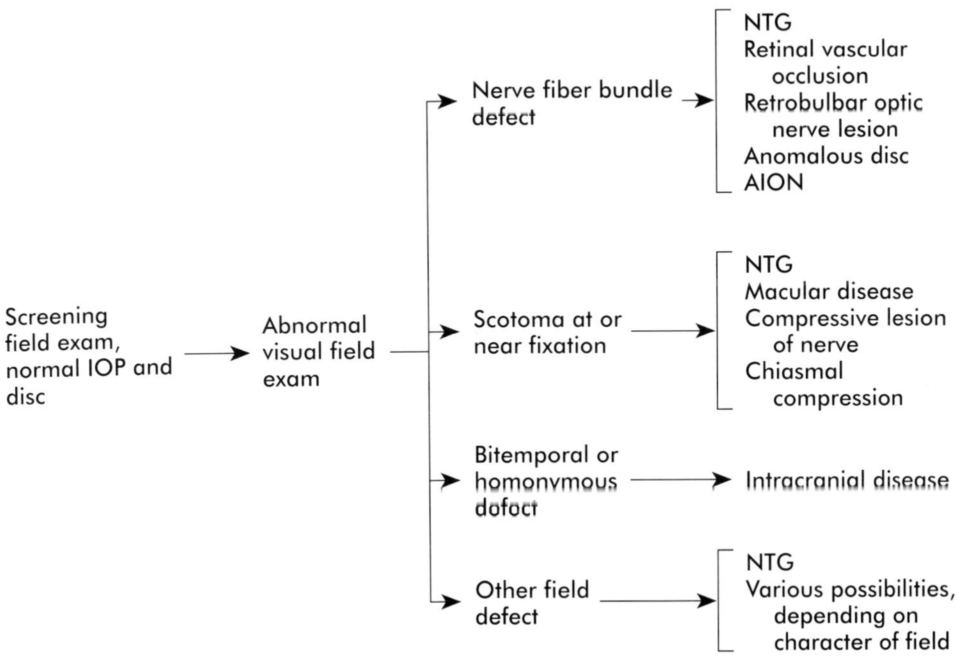

◆ *Symptoms suggesting scotoma—no field loss*

Routine perimetry may miss small scotomas that fall between test points. Symptomatic scotomas are generally central, and sometimes a patient can draw his or her scotoma on an Amsler grid chart. Depending on the character of the scotoma drawn, consider the above possibilities. If the patient has NTG, it will become apparent over time.

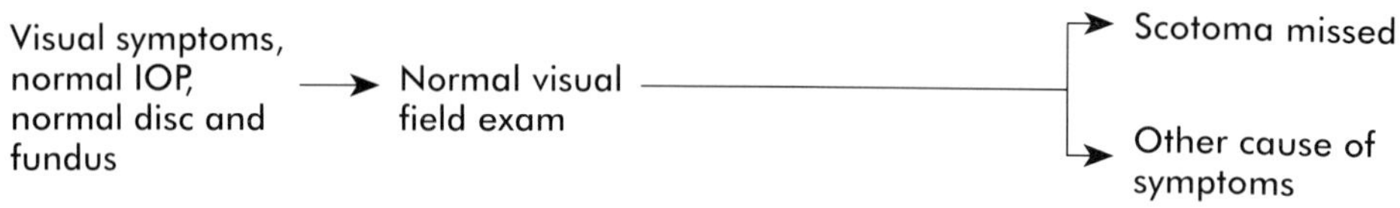
Visual symptoms, normal IOP, normal disc and fundus
Normal visual field exam
Scotoma missed
Other cause of symptoms

Positive Signs of NTG

The previous paragraphs emphasize the importance of ruling out conditions that mimic NTG, but the diagnosis of NTG is not solely a process of exclusion. The following findings support NTG as the explanation of disc and field findings for which another explanation is not apparent:

- A high normal pressure, perhaps 18 to 20 mm Hg (rather than 12 to 15 mm Hg) on the average
- Typical glaucomatous configuration to the excavation of the nerve
- Bilaterality of nerve fiber bundle defects in the visual field that do not respect the vertical meridian
- A peripapillary crescent or halo on the disc margin
- Splinter hemorrhages across the disc margin
- Migraine, other forms of vasospasm, or low blood pressure
- Family history of glaucoma
- Significant myopia

A past history of a major hemodynamic crisis favors the diagnosis of nonprogressive damage but does not rule out NTG.

Neuroradiologic Investigation

In the setting of an NTG evaluation, we recommend CT or MRI scanning for the following indications:

- Unexplained decrease in visual acuity (central scotoma)
- Unusual visual field loss — field loss other than nerve fiber bundle defects or paracentral scotomas
- Possibly bitemporal or homonymous hemianopic defects (clear defects also need evaluation, but they are not NTG diagnostic dilemmas)
- Pallor disproportionate to cupping, unless the pallor is clearly confined to either the upper or lower half of the nerve (and thus likely related to a vascular event)
- Uniocular field loss not explained by obvious ocular asymmetry or concurrent unilateral disease

In the more common typical presentation of a patient with normal Snellen acuity, glaucomatously cupped nerves, and bilateral nerve fiber bundle defects, we do not obtain imaging studies (Fig. 6-8).

Medical Evaluation

General medical evaluation is usually unrewarding. It may reveal some treatable medical condition such as hypertension, and perhaps patients are well served by finding a condition that deserves treatment in its own right. Only rarely is there a finding (such as a carotid occlusion of the side with worse visual loss) that seems related to the suspected NTG.

MANAGING SUSPECTED NORMAL TENSION GLAUCOMA

Opinions differ regarding the appropriate management of suspected and progressive NTG because theories about the cause of the condition also differ. The two poles of opinion are, on the one side, that NTG is a primary nerve degeneration without significant relation to intraocular pressure, or conversely, that NTG is the same condition as ordinary open-angle glaucoma but that the nonpressure risk factors are so pronounced that the nerve is damaged at pressure in the normal range. If pressure is not involved, then lowering the IOP will not help the patient's condition. If pressure is involved, then lowering the IOP should halt or slow the glaucomatous damage.

Both types of NTG may exist. We believe that many, or even most, cases of progressive NTG are pressure related and result from the same pathophysiologic process as POAG — they are part of the same spectrum of disease. However, we do not know whether the benefits of lowering pressure substantially enough to halt glaucomatous damage outweigh the risks. The lower the pressure is at baseline, the more difficult it is to achieve a substantial pressure decrease; thus aggressive surgical measures may be needed. Some NTG suspects on follow-up have nonprogressive conditions, and these patients are certainly not helped by ocular hypotensive therapy.

There has been interest over the years in attempting to improve the health of the optic nerve in individuals with suspected NTG by increasing blood flow to the optic nerve. Drugs such as calcium channel blockers are sometimes used in desperate individuals who are losing vision at an alarming rate despite the best pressure lowering that can be achieved. There is no documentation of ultimate benefit (better retention of vision) or documentation that any drug achieves an improved blood flow in the optic nerve head.

Normal tension glaucoma suspects are currently managed much the same as glaucoma suspects with elevated pressures. The clinician should establish a baseline and then determine the risk of progressive symptomatic glaucomatous damage. Decide whether to treat the patient, and if treating, set a pressure goal and attempt to achieve it. Continue to observe all patients for evidence of worsening, and modify the goals and treatment depending on the patient's course (see box below).

Baseline Examination

The baseline examination for NTG suspects is the same as for POAG suspects and includes disc photographs and a baseline set of threshold field examinations (Chapter 3). Obtain numerous pressure readings at different times in the day as mentioned on page 136.

Normal Tension Glaucoma Suspects—Management Steps

1. Establish a baseline.
2. Determine the risk of progressive symptomatic glaucomatous damage.
3. Decide whether to treat the patient; if treating, set a pressure goal and attempt to achieve it.
4. Continue to observe all patients for evidence of worsening.
5. Modify the goals and treatment depending on the patient's course.

Determination of Risk

For purposes of determining risk and deciding whether to treat, there are two categories of individuals suspected of having normal tension glaucoma: those who have no field loss and those with abnormal fields. Risk in this context refers to the risk of having symptomatically significant damage develop without first having an asymptomatic defect develop that both alerts the clinician to the progressive nature of the condition and indicates the pace of damage. Risk does not mean something that can necessarily be changed by changing the pressure; the relative risks of untreated NTG versus the treatment necessary to lower pressure in indivduals with the condition are not known. Table 6-1 summarizes the risk categories in individuals with suspected NTG.

SUSPECTS WITHOUT FIELD LOSS

All patients without field loss are low-risk suspects. Even if field loss develops, symptomatic field loss is unlikely to develop. Any change in such patients' conditions is likely to be slow.

SUSPECTS WITH FIELD LOSS

Even if there are findings suggestive of progressive disease, such as a splinter hemorrhage, the risk to the patient relates to the pace of disease, which is not apparent at onset. When an NTG suspect has field loss, the location of the field loss guides assessment of risk. The more severe the field loss, and particularly the closer a scotoma is to fixation, the greater the risk that detectable worsening from baseline will be visually critical; thus we are more aggressive in such cases.

It is occasionally possible to be fairly confident that a condition is not progressive. For example, if a patient gives a history of a symptomatic scotoma that has been stable for some time, we would categorize the patient to be at low risk for progression. Convincing historical information is generally absent, and we usually rely on field criteria.

TABLE 6-1 *Risk of Symptomatic Progression Related to Position of Scotoma and Size of Cup in NTG*

		Cupping			
		C/D* < 0.4	C/D $\geq 0.4 < 0.6$	C/D $\geq 0.6 < 0.8$	C/D ≥ 0.8
Field loss	None	Low risk	Low risk	Low risk	Low risk
	Mild	Low risk	Low risk	Moderate risk	Moderate risk
	Moderate	Moderate risk	Moderate risk	Moderate risk	High risk
	Severe	High risk (Look for another explanation)	High risk	High risk	High risk

*C/D, cup:disc ratio.

Establishment of a Plan: Goals and Treatment

LOW-RISK NTG SUSPECTS

If low-risk NTG suspects in time have progressive NTG, symptomatic damage is unlikely to develop rapidly. Follow up with these patients without therapy using the schedule for low-risk glaucoma suspects in Chapter 5.

MEDIUM-RISK NTG SUSPECTS

Medium-risk glaucoma suspects have either mild field loss and significant cupping or significant visual field loss, although the relationship of their findings to the IOP remains uncertain. In the absence of other explanations for field loss, we recommend treating one eye to lower the IOP at least 30% and observing the other eye. In this manner, whichever course has the better risk/benefit ratio in a given person, the patient will have it in one eye. Treat these patients by the guidelines for moderate glaucoma in Chapter 4. This includes attempting to lower the pressure using well-tolerated topical and laser therapy but does not include oral or surgical treatment unless the pressure is lowered less than 20%. If the IOP does not decrease at least 20% with topical and laser treatment, proceed with additional medical and surgical treatment in the chosen eye with a goal of 30% IOP lowering. The second eye may ultimately be treated if it progresses, while the treated eye does not.

HIGH-RISK NTG SUSPECTS

Regardless of whether high-risk NTG suspects have pressure-related damage, they certainly have vision-threatening disease. After ruling out other treatable conditions as best as possible, treat both eyes with topical, laser, and oral therapy as needed to lower the IOP by at least 30%. If the pressure does not decrease at least 30%, perform filtering surgery in one eye in pursuit of the pressure goal. We do not do filtration surgery in the other eye until it is apparent that the eye with surgery has fared better.

These guides usually result in low-risk suspects being followed up without medication. Moderate-risk suspects usually achieve at least a 20% pressure lowering with drops and laser. High-risk suspects require filtration surgery about half the time, and it usually achieves the pressure goal.

Follow-Up Schedule

LOW-RISK SUSPECTS

Use the follow-up schedule described in Chapter 5 for the follow-up of low-risk open-angle glaucoma suspects (Table 5-1).

MEDIUM-RISK SUSPECTS

Follow up with medium-risk suspects according to the schedule for moderate glaucoma in Tables 4-3 and 4-4.

HIGH-RISK SUSPECTS

Follow up with high-risk suspects according to the schedule for severe glaucoma in Tables 4-5 and 4-6.

Modification of Treatment

If a patient, either treated or untreated, demonstrates progressive damage, evaluate the patient to ensure that the progression does not suggest some nonglaucomatous process. If no other explanation is found and the findings are consis-

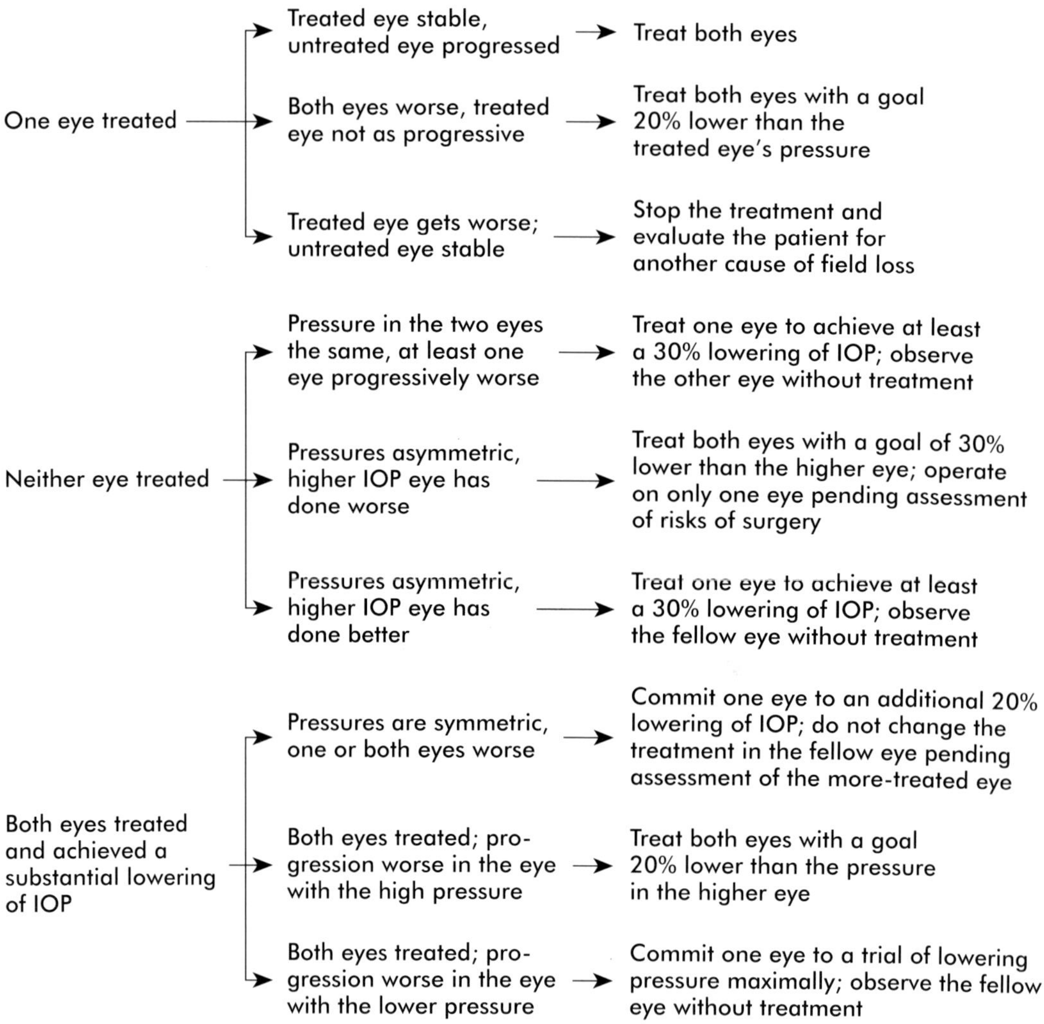

CHART 6-2 Management of progressive NTG.

tent with glaucoma, then the patient has progressive NTG. Progressive NTG does not mean that pressure is a causative factor. As discussed previously, the relationship between IOP and damage in this condition is uncertain.

However, progression of disease under observation does mean that a person's condition is at very high risk to continue to worsen. If the patient has had unilateral treatment or has consistently asymmetric pressures, then the comparative courses in the two eyes help to guide therapy. Unless it is evident that *not* treating the IOP in a given person is better than treating it, we continue to treat at least one eye to lower the pressure. Chart 6-2 outlines a management plan to follow if progression occurs.

◆ *One eye was treated and achieved a substantially lower pressure*

The purpose of unilateral therapy is to give one eye the better treatment, if indeed one is better. If a patient's condition shows convincing progression, confirmed on repeat examination, then the treatment should be adjusted accordingly.

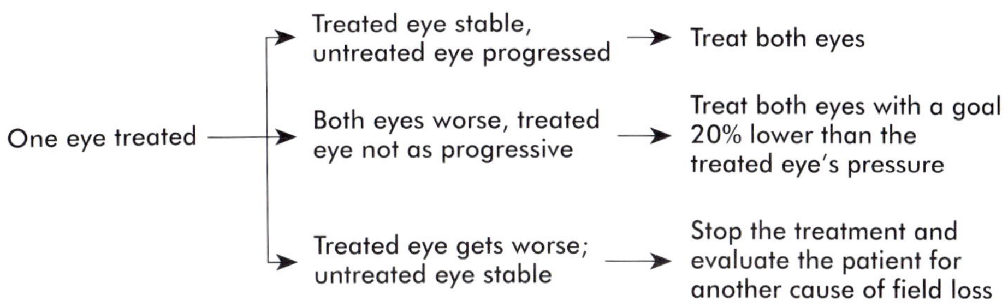

- If the treated eye is stable, while the untreated eye is worse, then treat both eyes to achieve at least the pressure of the treated eye. Continue to follow up with the patient.
- If both eyes are worse, but the treated eye is not as much worse as the untreated eye, then treat both eyes with a goal 20% lower than the pressure already achieved by treatment in the treated eye.
- If the untreated eye has fared *better* than the treated eye, stop the treatment and reevaluate the patient for some other cause for visual loss.
- If a treated eye has no glaucomatous progression but loses vision related to treatment, for example, from complications following surgery for a cataract that developed after filtration surgery or from hypotony maculopathy, while the untreated eye develops progressive glaucomatous damage, treat the previously untreated eye up to the point at which the complications occurred, in the hope that with submaximal treatment the initially untreated eye fares better overall than the eye treated first. This can be a difficult decision at times.

◆ *Neither eye was treated*

- If the pressures in the two eyes are symmetric, commit one eye to achieving a 30% lowering of IOP by whatever means are necessary. Continue to observe the patient's other eye without treatment and decide whether to treat it depending on the course in the treated eye.
- If the pressures are consistently asymmetric, and if the eye with the higher pressure has fared *worse* than the other eye, this supports a pressure-

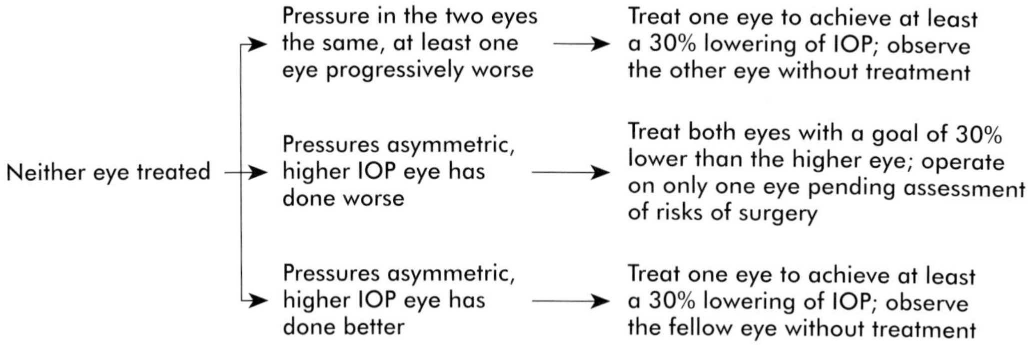

related element to the damage. Treat both eyes with a goal of 30% lowering of pressure. If surgery is required, do it in only one eye initially and continue to observe the condition of both eyes. Proceed with surgery in the opposite eye after sufficient time has elapsed that the clinician can be confident of a favorable course in the first eye.

- If the pressures are consistently asymmetric, and if the eye with the higher pressure has fared *better* than the other eye, commit one eye to achieving a 30% lowering of IOP using whatever means are necessary. Continue to observe the other eye without treatment. Pressure may be a factor in this situation, but the evidence is less compelling than if the eye with the higher pressure worsened.

◆ ***Both eyes were treated and achieved substantially lower pressures***

- If the pressures in the two eyes are symmetric and one or both are worse, commit to achieving an additional 20% lowering of IOP in one eye using whatever means necessary. Continue to observe the other eye and decide whether to treat it depending on the course in the more aggressively treated eye.

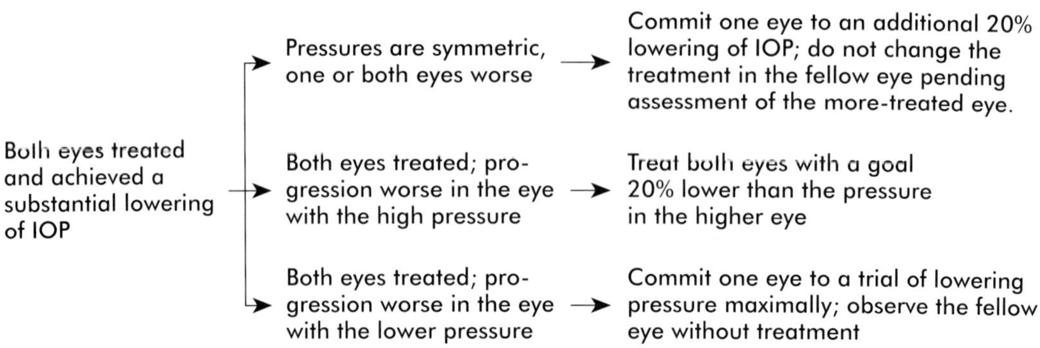

- If the pressures are consistently asymmetric, and if the eye with the higher pressure is *worse* than the other eye, treat both eyes with a goal of 20% additional lowering of pressure. If (additional) surgery is required, do it in only one eye initially. Proceed with the other eye depending on the course in the first eye.
- If the pressures are consistently asymmetric, and if the eye with the higher pressure has fared *better* than the fellow eye, commit to achieving a 20% additional lowering of IOP in one eye using whatever means necessary. Continue to observe the other eye without treatment. This course commits one eye to each course of treatment, although the initial response does not support pressure-related damage.

The management of NTG is frustrating for the patient and for the doctor. We recommend explaining to the patient — early, emphatically, and repeatedly — that the best course is not known and that the purpose of treatment is to provide the best chance possible of having appropriate treatment in at least one eye.

7

Glaucoma Suspects III: The Abnormal Angle

This chapter discusses patients who have not had surgery in whom the gonioscopic findings alone suggest that glaucoma may develop. We discuss gonioscopic findings in individuals with pressure, disc, or field abnormalities elsewhere. Although there are many possible abnormal gonioscopic findings, the common conditions that fit this category are as follows:

- Narrow angle
- Dense pigmentation of the trabecular meshwork
- Congenital anomalies such as the Axenfeld-Rieger syndrome
- Angle recession

NARROW ANGLE

Most patients with narrow angles do not develop primary acute angle closure glaucoma. However, such glaucoma almost always occurs in eyes with narrow angles. None of the various provocative tests introduced over the years accurately predicts who will have spontaneous closure. We perform iridectomy on asymptomatic individuals with narrow angles and no other suggestion of glaucoma who fit any of the following categories:

- Angle closure glaucoma in the other eye
- Peripheral anterior synechia
- History of transient episodes of visual blur, halos, or pain that are typical for self-limited attacks of angle closure
- Elevated IOP and angle closure that develops when the pupils are dilated (The purpose of the iridectomy is to allow for prompt and safe dilation if the patient develops an ocular complaint, not because closure after pharmacologic dilation predicts spontaneous angle closure.)
- Inability to be evaluated promptly if symptoms develop
- Significant patient anxiety about the risk of spontaneous angle closure glaucoma

Chart 7-1 summarizes the evaluation and decision process for treating a patient with a narrow angle.

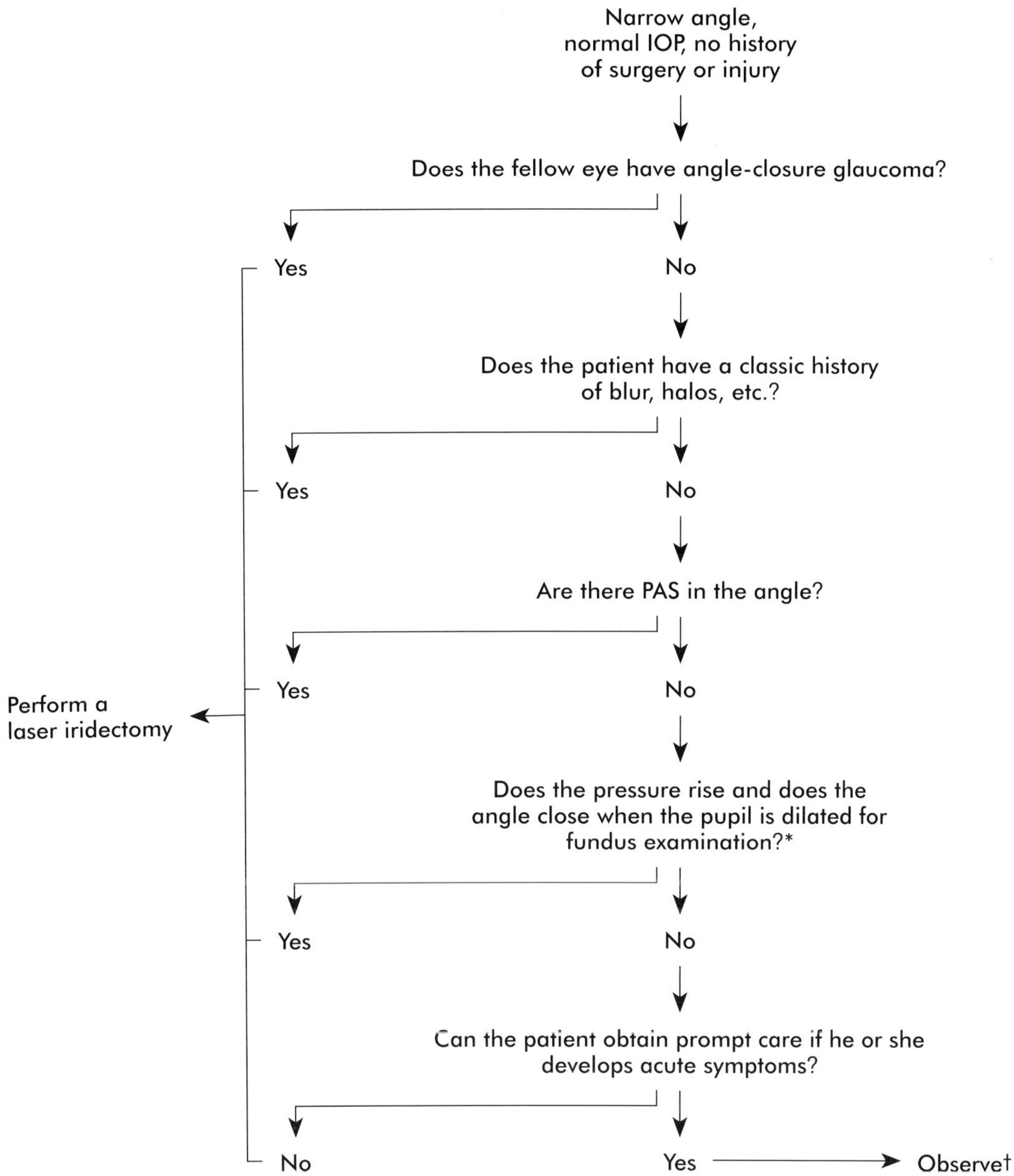

CHART 7-1 Management of an asymptomatic person with a narrow angle.
*Angle closure after dilation does not accurately predict spontaneous angle closure. However, dilation-induced angle closure may impede evaluation of subsequent ocular problems. If the patient does not want to have an iridectomy, it is acceptable, although less desirable, to avoid dilation.
†If the patient suffers from anxiety about his or her risk of angle closure, perform an iridectomy.

DENSE PIGMENTATION OF THE TRABECULAR MESHWORK

Pigmentary dispersion and pseudoexfoliation are the most common causes of increased pigmentation. As noted in Chapter 2, unilateral pigmentation is sometimes caused by a lens implant that chafes against the iris and is very rarely caused by a tumor that sheds cells into the eye. In the absence of other indication of glaucoma, neither pigmentary dispersion nor the pseudoexfoliation syndrome without elevated pressure demands special treatment.

CONGENITAL ANOMALIES SUCH AS AXENFELD/RIEGER SYNDROME

Individuals with congenital anomalies of the anterior segment who do not have glaucoma or elevated pressure should have an ophthalmic examination at least yearly.

ANGLE RECESSION

A patient who is noted to have an angle recession on routine examination has a higher chance of developing glaucoma than a similar person without a recession. The likelihood depends on the degree of the initial trauma to the anterior segment as well as on the patient's underlying outflow dynamics. There is no precise amount of angle recession that decrees glaucoma in the future, nor is there a degree of recession below which the practitioner need not worry.

Always examine the rest of the eye for other evidence of trauma. We recommend a diagnostic visual field examination to identify possible visual field effects related to the injury. Reexamine the patient yearly.

8

Acute Symptomatic Elevated Intraocular Pressure

The patient who is initially seen with a sudden onset of symptoms (other than field loss) caused by high IOP may have any type of glaucoma that produces markedly elevated pressure. Corneal edema, which causes blurring and halos, and ciliary spasm, which causes deep, aching pain, may result from either an acute process that produces a sudden, severe pressure increase or from a chronic pressure elevation that eventually becomes high enough to produce anterior segment ischemia.

Although the *possible* diagnoses include almost all types of glaucoma, there are only a few *likely* diagnostic possibilities. The most common are:

- Primary acute angle closure glaucoma
- Primary chronic angle closure glaucoma with acute anterior segment decompensation
- Neovascular glaucoma
- Pseudoexfoliation with glaucoma
- Pigmentary dispersion with glaucoma
- Glaucoma resulting from old trauma
- Glaucomatocyclitic crisis

The use of the term *glaucoma* is conventional for these conditions even if glaucomatous nerve or field damage is absent. Patients with these conditions usually have acute symptoms in only one eye, and the history and physical examination usually allow accurate diagnosis and identification of those patients who do not "fit" one of the usual categories.

MAKING A DIAGNOSIS

History

Although the diagnosis depends on the physical examination in this group of patients, the history and circumstances of presentation provide clues that may suggest a specific cause of high pressure. None of these clues is absolute, but they are helpful. The typical presentation for each of the likely conditions follows.

PRIMARY ANGLE CLOSURE GLAUCOMA (ACUTE AND CHRONIC)

This condition is more common in women than men. Most patients are older than 60 years of age. Almost all patients with acute angle closure glaucoma are hyperopic. Some have histories of transient episodes of pain or blurred vision in one or both eyes. If these symptoms occurred in relation to pupillary dilation, such as while sitting in a darkened theater, and resolved with pupillary constriction, such as entering the lobby, the diagnosis is very likely. Patients with chronic angle closure glaucoma do not have histories of such episodes.

NEOVASCULAR GLAUCOMA

Most previously undiagnosed people who have neovascular glaucoma have either diabetic retinopathy or have had a central retinal vein occlusion. Those with diabetic retinopathy usually know that they have diabetes, but may be unaware of any eye disease. Individuals with juvenile onset diabetes usually have had their disease more than 10 years. Those with central retinal vein occlusions usually have noticed a decrease in their vision within the previous 2 to 4 months. Many of these patients have hypertension.

PSEUDOEXFOLIATION WITH GLAUCOMA

These patients are rarely younger than 65 years of age. They may have any refractive error and any other medical problems.

PIGMENTARY GLAUCOMA

This condition generally occurs in young (<50 years old), moderately myopic men. They often describe transient episodes of blurred vision or of seeing halos around lights, particularly after exercise. (These episodes are probably caused by elevated pressure related to a shower of pigment in the anterior chamber.)

OLD TRAUMA

Trauma is more common in men than in women. The injury may have occurred decades before presentation and may be forgotten.

GLAUCOMATOCYCLITIC CRISIS

Patients with this condition may be of any age, but most patients are seen before the age of 60. There is no refractive or gender predilection. Patients may have a history of previous episodes of blurring, but neither pain nor redness, sometimes in the eye not involved in the episode that prompts medical attention.

Examination

The physical examination allows accurate diagnosis of most cases of acute pressure elevation. The salient points of the various aspects of the examination are as follows:

VISION

Corneal edema may decrease the acuity markedly. If the acuity is good, central retinal vein occlusion with neovascular glaucoma is highly unlikely.

PUPILS

When the pressure is high, the pupil often is somewhat dilated and nonreactive or sluggish because of iris ischemia. The presence or absence of an afferent defect does not provide useful differential diagnostic information.

SLIT-LAMP EXAMINATION

If corneal edema obscures the view, topical glycerine may allow adequate biomicroscopy and gonioscopy.

Cornea. The presence of a Krukenberg spindle suggests pigmentary glaucoma or pseudoexfoliation.

Anterior chamber. Note the depth of the central anterior chamber and compare it with the opposite eye. If the lens has moved forward and caused angle closure while the opposite eye has a deeper chamber and seemingly nonoccludable angle, consider pseudoexfoliation, traumatic subluxation of the lens, or ciliary block glaucoma. To supplement gonioscopy, it is often helpful to examine the peripheral anterior chamber with a narrow, well-focused slit beam. Even when the cornea is edematous, it may be possible to detect that the peripheral iris is in tight contact with the peripheral corneal endothelium, confirming angle closure. If the peripheral iris is distant from the cornea, this finding suggests secondary open-angle glaucoma.

If there is mild inflammation in conjunction with a normal iris and an open angle in this setting, the most likely diagnosis is glaucomatocyclitic crisis. The evidence of inflammation in glaucomatocyclitic crisis may be minimal initially, with only a mild flare and a few cells on presentation. The typical keratic precipitates may not appear until several days into the course. If there is substantial anterior segment inflammation, refer to Chapter 9.

Iris. Neovascularization is usually visible around the pupillary border if anterior segment neovascularization is the cause of acutely elevated pressure.

If there is evidence of trauma (sphincter rupture is probably the most common finding) associated with an open angle, then glaucoma related to angle contusion is the likely diagnosis.

Lens. Phacodonesis suggests either old trauma or, occasionally, pseudoexfoliation. Pseudoexfoliative material may be visible on the lens surface.

Gonioscopy. Many patients have corneal edema, which renders gonioscopy difficult. If application of topical glycerine does not clear the view, it is often useful to perform gonioscopy on the uninvolved eye. If the angle is closed, perform indentation gonioscopy, which not only helps confirm that the angle is closed by revealing the structures in the artificially opened angle, but may reveal peripheral anterior synechiae, which indicate a chronic process causing the acute symptoms.

FUNDOSCOPY

Fundus evaluation, particularly if it precedes dilation, is often difficult in a photophobic patient who has corneal edema. If it is possible to see the fundus, note if the disc is swollen from an acute pressure rise or is cupped from a chronic pressure elevation with acute symtoms related to anterior segment decompensation. Try to determine the retinal causes of rubeosis iridis in cases of neovascular glaucoma.

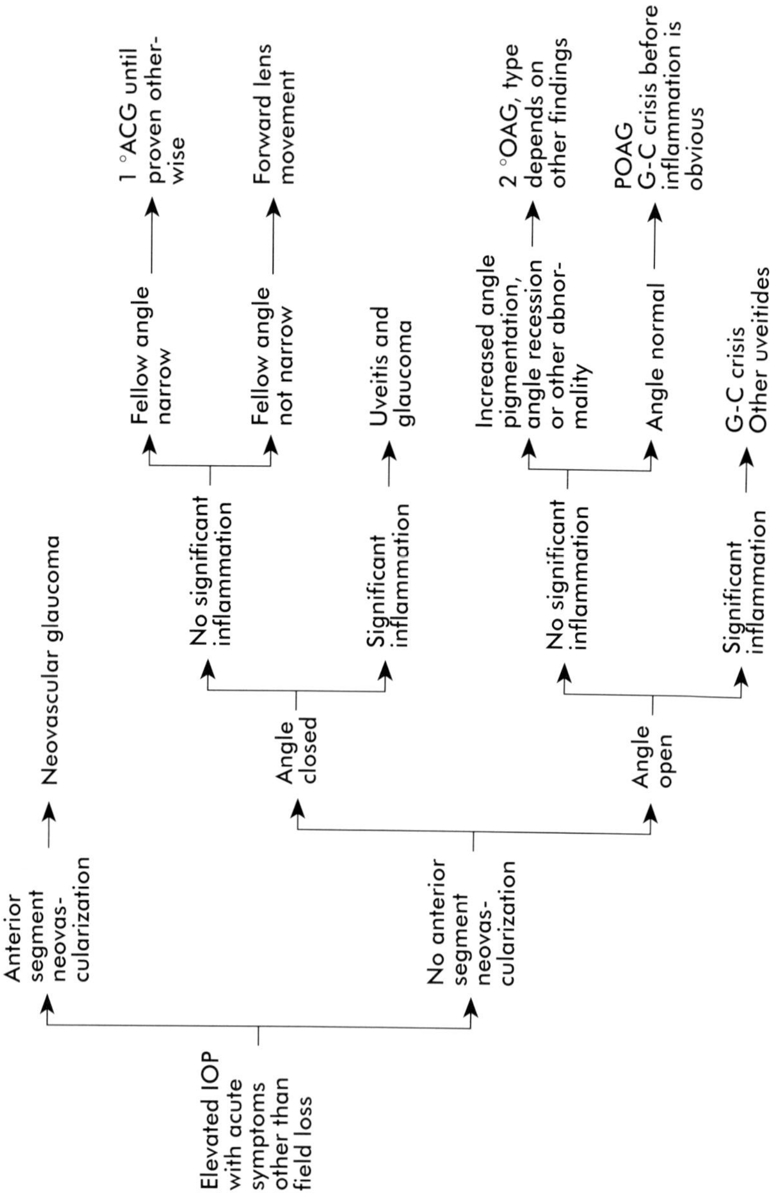

CHART 8-1 Differential diagnosis of the common causes of acute symptomatic elevated IOP.

Differential Diagnosis

Chart 8-1 outlines the differential steps in gonioscopic diagnosis with the conditions that commonly present with symptomatic pressure elevation.

◆ *Angle neovascularization*

If the angle is either closed with neovascularization or is open but contains a neovascular network over the trabecular meshwork, evaluate the posterior segment (fundoscopy, echography) to clarify the cause of the neovascular glaucoma.

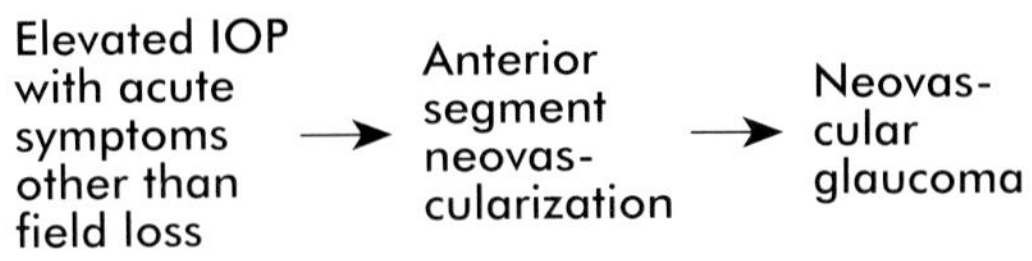

◆ *No neovascularization, angle closed*

Angle closure in an eye without significant anterior chamber reaction usually indicates primary acute angle closure glaucoma. Unless the patient has, for example, anisometropia, the other eye usually has a very narrow angle. If the opposite eye has a narrow angle and peripheral anterior synechiae, then chronic angle closure with acute decompensation is likely. If the opposite angle is not narrow, then seek another explanation since other types of angle closure *may* present in this setting. If the central anterior chamber depth in the involved eye is distinctly more shallow than in the other eye, the patient probably has a component of forward lens movement. This occurs in pseudoexfoliation, following trauma with lens subluxation, and occasionally as an isolated finding. In practice, forward lens movement, even if suspected, is usually confirmed after peripheral iridectomy.

Angle closure in an eye with significant anterior segment inflammation is discussed in Chapter 9.

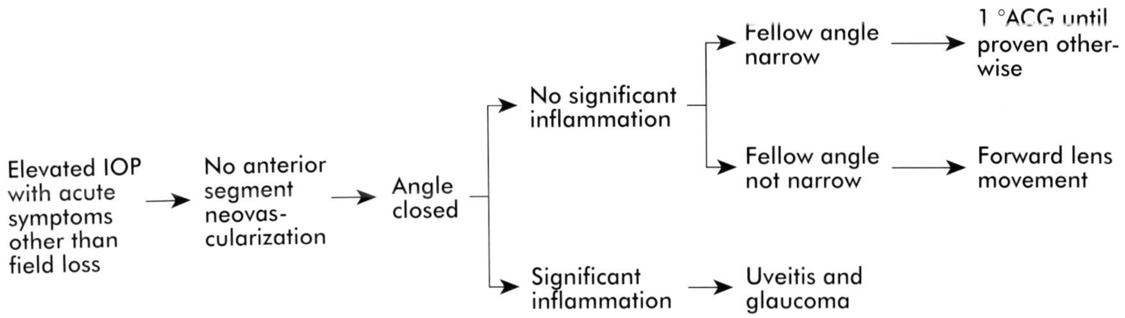

◆ *No neovascularization, angle open*

If the angle is open without neovascularization and the anterior chamber is quiet, look carefully for pigmentation and for evidence of trauma. A densely pigmented trabecular meshwork is always found in pigmentary glaucoma and is often seen to a slightly less striking degree in pseudoexfoliation. Examine the eye carefully for evidence of trauma; compare the two eyes for help in distinguishing asymmetry in angle depth and pigmentation.

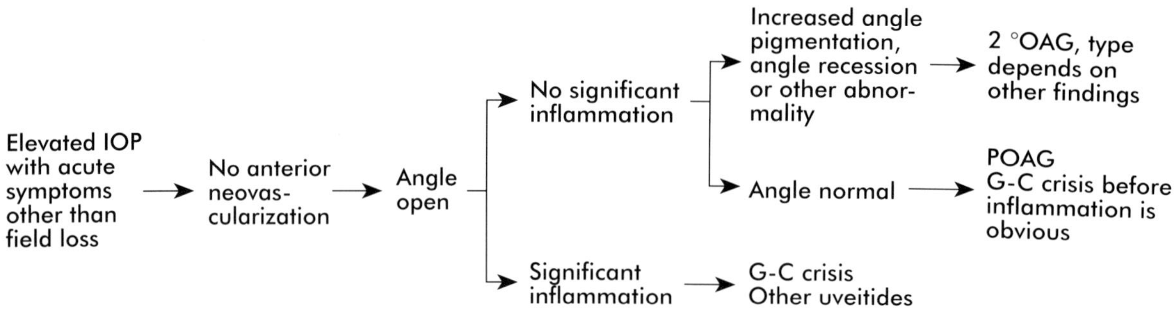

Mild anterior segment inflammation suggests glaucomatocyclitic crisis and at times the inflammation is not apparent initially. Other uveitides may present acutely and are discussed in Chapter 9.

PATIENT TREATMENT

Neovascular Glaucoma

DETERMINATION OF MECHANISM

Proliferative diabetic retinopathy and recent central retinal vein occlusion are straightforward diagnoses in most cases. If neither of these possibilities seems reasonable, and if the physical examination reveals no cause, such as a choroidal tumor, it is likely that there is no clear explanation. Neovascularization occurs secondarily to chronic marked pressure elevation, as with untreated angle closure; it is important to examine the opposite eye for diagnostic clues. If none of the likely explanations appears to be accurate, the ocular ischemia syndrome is a default diagnosis in people with vascular disease. We avoid neuroradiologic diagnostic maneuvers to search for surgically treatable vascular conditions until after consulting with the patient's internist to determine whether corrective action could be taken if such a lesion is found.

TREATMENT OF UNDERLYING CAUSES

Retinal ablation by either photocoagulation or cryoablation is the treatment of choice for both proliferative diabetic retinopathy and neovascularization related to central vein occlusions. Medical therapy before ablation and while awaiting regression of the neovascularization includes antiinflammatory agents and suppressants of aqueous humor formation. The following is a typical regimen:

- Atropine 1% bid
- Prednisolone acetate 1% qid
- β-blocker bid
- Methazolamide 50 mg bid

After ablation, the degree of inflammation determines the duration of treatment with cycloplegic and corticosteroid drops. Management of the IOP is discussed in the next section.

If the neovascularization does not have an apparent explanation, we usually treat the patient medically for a few days to attempt to lower the pressure slightly and quiet the eye. If the neovascularization remains unexplained, we obtain a fluorescein angiogram. If there is substantial retinal nonperfusion, we recommend retinal ablation. If the cause of neovascularization is ocular ischemia related to vascular disease, then there is no well-established means to promote regression of the neovascularization, although such individuals often do have retinal ablation.

TREATMENT OF THE IOP

Once the treatable causes of neovascularization have been managed, the residual eye pressure must be treated. The management depends on the response of the eye to ablation (if done) as well as to the pressure.

Regressed neovascularization. If the neovascularization regresses and the pressure falls to below 40 mm Hg, treat the patient as a glaucoma suspect as outlined in Chapter 5, but avoid using miotics. If the pressure remains above 40 mm Hg or if the optic nerve appears to be glaucomatously cupped, treat the patient as if he or she has manifest glaucoma; however, avoid miotics and do not perform laser trabeculoplasty. If surgery is indicated, perform either a filtration procedure with antimetabolities or use a seton drainage procedure.

Persistent neovascularization. Active neovascularization bodes ill for an eye. Manage such patients according to the guidelines for the chronic care of uveitis with elevated pressure described in Chapter 9.

Primary Angle Closure Glaucoma

The management of primary angle closure glaucoma involves immediate, early, and chronic steps.

IMMEDIATE TREATMENT

The first treatment step is to lower the severely elevated IOP and open the angle. The most common course is to lower the pressure to allow perfusion of the iris sphincter so it can respond to miotic drops. Two ways to lower the IOP are the administration of hyperosmotic agents and corneal indentation to force the angle open for several minutes. Three or four instillations of pilocarpine over 30 minutes will constrict the pupil if the pressure has been lowered. We treat patients with corticosteroid drops to quiet the eye, relieve symptoms, reduce synechiae formation, and prepare the eye for iridectomy.

During an acute episode of angle closure glaucoma, the aqueous inflow almost ceases and suppressants of aqueous humor formation alone do not stop the attack. After the pressure decreases and aqueous humor production resumes, such agents may be unnecessary if the angle is open. However, it is reasonable to treat patients with β-blockers, carbonic anhydrase inhibitors, or both until the functional status of the outflow system is known.

If a patient has acute angle closure glaucoma and forward lens movement is suspected, treat the patient to lower the IOP but do not give miotic drops. Cycloplegic agents are appropriate treatment for forward lens movement, but it is reasonable to perform an iridectomy to remove any possible pupillary block contribution before such drugs are used.

EARLY TREATMENT

Relieve pupillary block. Perform a peripheral iridectomy in both the involved eye and, if it has a narrow angle, in the opposite eye. Even if this cannot be done in the involved eye immediately because of corneal edema, it can usually be done immediately in the other eye. Examine the patient frequently while waiting for the cornea in the involved eye to clear sufficiently to allow laser treatment.

Gonioscopy. After performing the iridectomy, study the angle for clues to the patient's future course. Peripheral anterior synechiae may have formed over an extended period of chronic angle closure or may have formed during a prolonged acute congestive attack. Synechiae directly block the egress of aqueous humor and raise the outflow pressure by about the same percentage as the angle is closed (see Chapter 3 for a discussion of outflow pressure). Thus if the ordinary outflow pressure is 5 mm Hg (IOP of 15 mm Hg), then a closure of 50% of the angle would be expected to double the outflow pressure and raise it to about 10 mm Hg, or an IOP of about 20 mm Hg.

If forward lens movement caused the angle closure, the gonioscopic appearance after iridectomy remains unchanged.

Dilate the pupil and examine the angle. If peripheral iridectomy does not relieve the angle closure and if forward lens movement is suspected, administer a cycloplegic agent, such as Cyclogyl 1%, and reexamine the eye. If the angle opens, the diagnosis is confirmed. If iridectomy relieves angle closure, plateau iris syndrome must still be ruled out. This is an uncommon condition in which the angle remains closed or closes with dilation, despite the presence of a patent iridectomy (Fig. 8-1). It is often difficult to diagnose this condition without checking the angle before and after dilation. Treatment of a patient with plateau iris syndrome includes long-term miotic therapy and peripheral iris retraction (laser iridoplasty), which is described in standard surgical texts.

Examine the fundus. After angle closure has been treated, all patients should have a complete fundus examination if one has not already been performed.

CHRONIC TREATMENT

After an attack of acute angle closure glaucoma, the production of aqueous humor may be unusually low. This may be related to inflammation, but it resolves. Particularly if there are extensive peripheral anterior synechiae, it is important to carefully continue to observe the patient's condition to determine whether the IOP rises as the formation of aqueous humor resumes. Appropriate follow-up depends on the intraocular pressure and the extent of peripheral anterior synechiae formation.

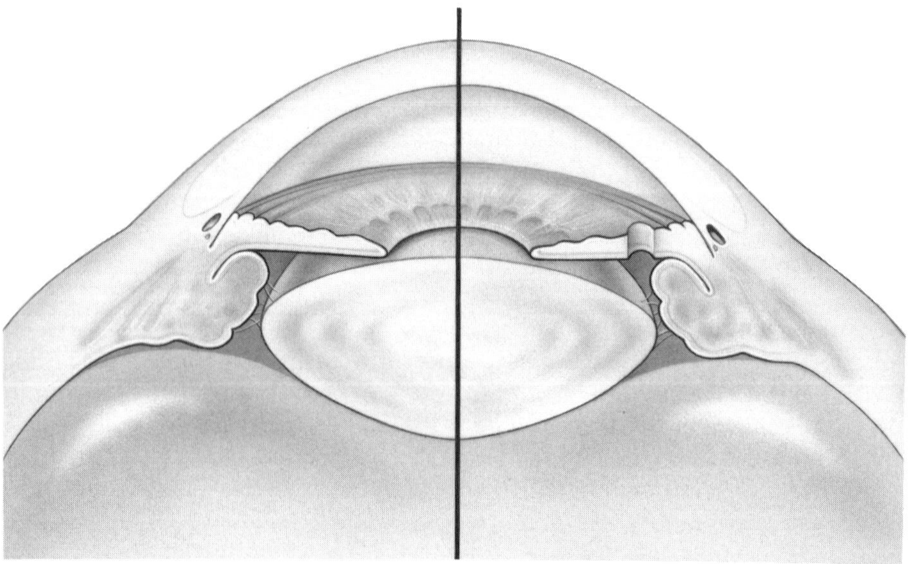

FIG. 8-1 Plateau iris and angle closure, proposed anatomic basis. The ciliary processes are more anterior than usual, and the peripheral iris drapes over them, *left*. Iridectomy does not alter the configuration because ciliary processes continue to support the iris, *right*.

Normal pressure after early treatment. Peripheral anterior synechiae increase resistance to aqueous humor outflow and probably increase a patient's chance of developing elevated pressure with time. Even eyes with no synechiae may have damaged outflow systems. Thus we consider such patients as suspects for developing high pressure (or glaucoma suspect-suspects) and examine them frequently early after the attack of angle closure. Disc photographs and visual fields should be obtained for all patients to document the effects of the acute episode. We suggest the following graded management based on the extent of peripheral anterior synechiae:

- Low risk: Less than 25% peripheral anterior synechiae

Examine the patient 6 and 18 months after the acute attack. If the pressure remains low and the eye appears stable, examine the patient every 1 to 2 years thereafter; further visual field examinations are not necessary.

- Medium risk: Between 25 and 75% peripheral anterior synechiae

Examine the patient 4, 8, 12, and 24 months after the attack. If the pressure remains low and the eye appears stable, examine the patient every 1 to 2 years thereafter. The patient does not need to repeat the visual field examination.

- High risk: Greater than 75% peripheral anterior synechiae

Examine the patient 3, 6, 9, 12, and 24 months after the attack. If the pressure remains low and the eye appears stable, examine the patient every 1 to 2 years thereafter. Visual fields need not be repeated.

Elevated pressure after early treatment. If the pressure is elevated after iridectomy, determine the extent of peripheral anterior synechiae. Extensive synechiae may be treated with incisional or laser synechialysis, and such maneuvers are appropriate if the pressure is elevated because of synechial closure. Establish a baseline and begin chronic follow-up after such treatment.

One of the assumptions involved in managing individuals with asymptomatic elevated IOP — that they have had the same pressure as they have at diagnosis for some time — is clearly false in individuals after acute angle closure glaucoma. The pressure has *not* been elevated for an extended time. Most have had very high pressure for a short period and now have a lower but still elevated pressure. They may have fully manifest glaucoma, but their IOP without treatment, although still elevated, may now be safe for them. The follow-up phase is thus similar to follow-up of glaucoma suspects as described in Chapter 5.

However, uncertainty regarding a patient's sensitivity to pressure dictates that the patient should have frequent examinations in the early years of follow-up. We suggest that the follow-up guides in Chapter 5 be used with the adaptation that *everyone* be considered to be at high risk for the first year. If the patient's condition remains stable, observe those patients who are at low or moderate risk by the recommended schedules.

Pseudoexfoliation or Pigmentary Dispersion with Acute Open-Angle Glaucoma

Both pseudoexfoliation and pigmentary dispersion are generally treated the same as primary open-angle glaucoma. However, when the presentation is that of an acute symptomatic pressure elevation, there are a few differences in the evaluation and management.

- It is not necessary to obtain several different pressure readings before starting treatment, because the IOP may be highly labile and the symptoms demand attention.
- It is reasonable to postpone obtaining a full threshold visual field until the acute episode is resolved. Then begin to establish a baseline.

- If both eyes have symptomatically elevated pressures, it is acceptable to begin treatment at the same time without a unilateral trial.

Even if the pressure is very high, avoid beginning more than one medication at a time. A person with corneal edema and pressures of 50 mm Hg and 55 mm Hg may need to have a lower pressure in each eye, but the patient does not need to achieve a pressure of 15 mm Hg immediately. The higher the initial pressure, the greater will be the expected drop in pressure from the first medication. We usually administer a β-blocker and have the patient stay in the office until the pressure starts to decrease. Within a day or so we reexamine the patient and consider whether to add more treatment. We obtain baseline fields and photographs after the acute episode is resolved.

Many patients with pseudoexfoliation or pigmentary glaucoma who are seen initially with acute symptomatic glaucoma require laser or filtration surgery in the reasonably short term. However, we generally use the medication steps because some patients respond quite well. The chronic care of individuals with these conditions follows closely the guides for patients with primary open-angle glaucoma (POAG) with a few modifications discussed in Chapter 11.

Old Trauma

The medical management of acute open-angle glaucoma associated with old trauma is almost the same as that of POAG. Patients with a sufficiently elevated pressure to have acute symptoms often require surgery, but we treat them medically initially. Such patients do not need multiple IOP readings and visual fields before treatment. The clinician should treat to lower the pressure, usually with a β-blocker (miotics may work poorly) and then establish a baseline, etc. Treatment is much like that of patients with POAG with differences discussed in Chapter 11. If the IOP does not respond to initial topical medical treatments, we proceed with carbonic anhydrase inhibitors and filtration surgery since laser treatment is rarely beneficial.

Glaucomatocyclitic Crisis

Treatment for glaucomatocyclitic crisis is discussed in Chapter 9.

9

Uveitis and Elevated Pressure

Uveitis encompasses a large, diverse group of conditions, many of which are accompanied by elevated IOP at some point in their clinical course. In a particular patient with uveitis, the IOP may range from quite low to very high, because inflammation decreases both the rate of aqueous humor formation and the ease of aqueous humor exit from the eye. The balance between these two effects determines the pressure at any given time. The major causes of impaired outflow and thus elevated pressure are as follows:

- Temporary blockage of trabecular meshwork by inflammatory debris
- Peripheral anterior synechiae formation related to organization of debris in the angle and gradual incorporation of the iris
- Appositional and then synechial angle closure caused by pupillary block from posterior synechiae formation
- Steroid-induced pressure elevation related to the treatment of ocular inflammation

The differential diagnosis, particular clinical features, and specific management of the various uveitides are beyond the scope of this book. Most patients with nontraumatic uveitis and elevated pressure have either idiopathic inflammation or a recognized syndrome that is managed in the same manner as idiopathic uveitis. Those with traumatic uveitis, following either surgical or nonsurgical trauma, are discussed in Chapter 10 and are managed similarly. However, management of the following syndromes is distinct from that of idiopathic uveitis:

- Glaucomatocyclitic crisis
- Fuchs' heterochromic iridocyclitis
- Herpes zoster or simplex associated uveitis
- Phacolytic glaucoma
- Ciliary body inflammation and rotation with angle closure glaucoma

One of the goals of the evaluation of patients with uveitis and elevated pressure is to recognize these conditions. A second goal is to recognize those patients who have one of the chronic uveitis syndromes, most commonly sarcoidosis and juvenile rheumatoid arthritis, so that their care can be planned for the long term from the outset.

RECOGNIZING PARTICULAR UVEITIS/GLAUCOMA SYNDROMES

Glaucomatocyclitic Crisis

Glaucomatocyclitic crisis (Posner-Schlossman syndrome) typically presents as an acute unilateral pressure elevation associated with mild inflammation. The patient's complaints relate to corneal edema—either blurring or halo vision.

Pressures often reach the range of 40 to 55 mm Hg, and the anterior chamber has a modest cellular response with little or no flare. The eye is not red. The usual error in diagnosis is to attribute the signs and symptoms to acute glaucoma caused by angle closure. Gonioscopy of both the involved eye and the opposite eye differentiates the two. Keratic precipitates may be absent initially but usually develop within a few days, when the anterior segment appearance resembles idiopathic iridocyclitis. A distinguishing feature is the lack of posterior synechiae in glaucomatocyclitic crisis.

Glaucomatocyclitic crises resolve spontaneously within a few weeks, with or without treatment. The crises often recur, and, although generally unilateral at any one episode, they may develop in both eyes. Both cupping and field loss may develop with recurrent or prolonged episodes.

Patients with a typical history and typical physical findings do not need uveitis work-ups. Treat each episode with suppressants of aqueous humor formation. Corticosteroids are generally not necessary. Follow the guidelines on page 166 for the management of recurrent episodes of inflammation. Some individuals have elevated, albeit less elevated, pressure between episodes, which is managed by the routine guidelines for elevated IOP.

Fuchs' Heterochromic Iridocyclitis

This syndrome classically involves unilateral heterochromia (lighter on the involved side), inflammation, and cataract formation. Approximately 10% of cases are bilateral and may be difficult to diagnose. The cornea has characteristic small keratic precipitates that may be connected by fine filaments. The inflammation does not cause anterior or posterior synechiae (except at a rare Koeppe nodule), although it may be associated with mild anterior segment neovascularization. Pressure elevation develops in about 15% to 20% of patients. Because heterochromia, inflammation, and unilateral cataract formation usually precede pressure elevation, the condition often presents as elevated IOP in a unilaterally pseudophakic patient with mild inflammation.

The inflammation associated with Fuchs' heterochromic iridocyclitis is generally mild and does not improve with antiinflammatory medication. Treatment with corticosteroids does not decrease the eye pressure. Medical treatment of the high pressure proceeds as described in the section for chronic uveitis and glaucoma, but treatment often fails to control the pressure. If patients with this condition require surgery, we perform filtration surgery and use supplemental 5-fluorouracil injections.

Herpes Zoster or Simplex Uveitis with Elevated Pressure

Both herpes zoster ophthalmicus and herpes simplex keratouveitis are treated with antiviral agents. The routine guidelines for treating elevated IOP apply to both conditions.

Phacolytic Glaucoma

Lens protein leaks through the capsule of some mature and hypermature lenses. Macrophages ingest the protein and clog the trabecular meshwork, causing acute pressure elevations that may reach the range of 60 to 80 mm Hg. The protein-laden macrophages are visible as large cells in the anterior chamber where they have been reported to glisten on slit-lamp examination. (We have not found the glistening to be obvious). The patient's vision is poor.

After obtaining an echographic screen of the fundus, we treat a patient with no history of uveitis who has high pressure, large cells in the anterior chamber, and a mature or hypermature cataract as if he or she has phacolytic glaucoma. We perform prompt extracapsular extractions and have implanted posterior chamber lenses with good results.

Ciliary Body Rotation and Angle Closure Glaucoma

Inflammation of the ciliary body may cause the lens to move forward and close the angle by a posterior pushing mechanism (Fig. 9-1). Symptoms include blurred vision (from increased myopia, corneal edema, or both) and photophobia. The central chamber has cells and flare. It is shallow and quite asymmetric to the opposite eye. Peripheral iridectomy does not resolve the angle closure, and the condition is treated with cycloplegics and corticosteroids. It is unusual among the uveitis/elevated pressure conditions in that angle closure is present at the onset and in that it is usually successfully treated.

GENERAL MANAGEMENT OF PATIENTS WITH ELEVATED PRESSURE AND UVEITIS

The management of patients with elevated pressure associated with uveitis will be discussed as if patients could be divided according to three general categories:

- Patients with a single, short (<6 months) period of inflammation and high pressure; for example, idiopathic anterior uveitis, inflammation following surgery, or associated with blunt trauma
- Patients with recurrent episodes of inflammation and elevated pressure separated by intervals without inflammation, such as recurrent anterior uveitis and glaucomatocyclitic crisis
- Patients with chronic uveitis associated with elevated pressure

In practice, even if a patient does fit neatly into one of these groups, it may not be apparent at presentation. We recommend treating new patients according to the guidelines for a single episode unless they clearly belong in one of the other groups.

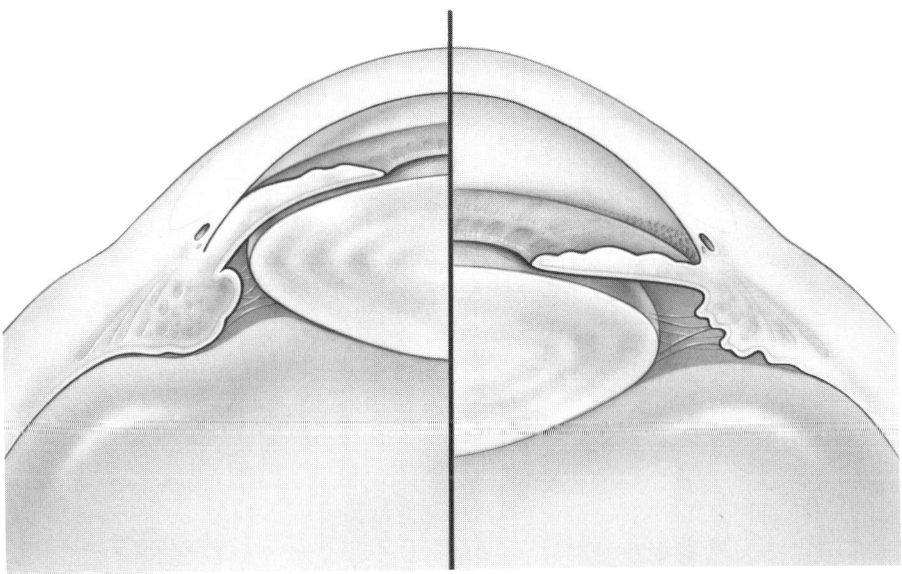

FIG. 9-1 Ciliary body rotation and inflammation with angle closure, left; normal for comparison, right.

For all three groups, there are two major constant recommendations that also apply to patients with uveitis who do not have elevated pressure: prevent or relieve pupillary block, and treat with as small a dose of corticosteroid as possible to control the inflammation.

Prevention or Relief of Pupillary Block

Posterior synechiae develop in inflamed eyes. If they entirely close the pupil, pupillary block ensues. Synechia formation is related to the degree of inflammation and to the size and mobility of the pupil. Except for cases of glaucomatocyclitic crisis and Fuchs' heterochromic iridocyclitis (which do not tend to develop posterior synechiae), cycloplegic drops are used in patients with iridocyclitis to prevent synechiae formation. If an eye is treated with chronic long-acting cycloplegics such as atropine, homatropine, or hyoscine, intermittent use of a mydriatic agent to move the pupil further decreases synechia formation. Depending on the degree of inflammation, we suggest use of phenylephrine 10% once a day to once a week. To increase intraocular penetration and decrease systemic absorption, advise the patient either to close his or her lids or to use nasolacrimal obstruction for 5 minutes after the drops are instilled. Miotic drops exacerbate posterior synechia formation and should be avoided.

If posterior synechiae are already present but there is no pupillary block, attempt to break as many as possible. Daily use of phenylephrine for 1 or 2 weeks in conjunction with either a short- or long-acting cycloplegic breaks many early adhesions.

When pupillary block and elevated pressure related to 360° posterior synechiae develop in a patient with uveitis, it is reasonable to perform a laser iridectomy to decompress the eye temporarily. However, laser procedures may exacerbate inflammation, and the small holes achieved with laser treatment often close within a short time. We therefore generally recommend prompt surgical sector iridectomy in such patients with active inflammation.

Use of Minimum Corticosteroids

Standard uveitis treatment involves use of sufficient corticosteroids and cycloplegics to control the inflammation, with medications then tapered to as low a dosage as maintains control of inflammation. Inflamed eyes often have low pressures that rise as the inflammation is treated and the aqueous humor production rises. In addition to this indirect effect on pressure, corticosteroid use can also cause a direct pressure elevation in some individuals. It may be impossible to determine whether patient's pressure rises because of increased aqueous humor production or because of decreased outflow from corticosteroid use, but provided the patient is being treated with as small a dose of steroid as possible (but enough to control the inflammation), the distinction is not clinically relevant.

MANAGEMENT OF A SINGLE EPISODE OF INFLAMMATION AND HIGH PRESSURE

A patient who is expected to have a single episode of elevated pressure does not generally need a formal disc and field baseline. We do examine the disc to determine whether the patient has evidence of cupping to suggest a chronic but unrecognized problem. We also examine the retinal periphery carefully because of the occasional association between peripheral retinal detachment, mild inflammation, and elevated pressure (Schwartz's syndrome). At every follow-up visit we check the disc for hemorrhages or obviously increased cupping, but neither the inconvenience nor the expense of multiple visual fields and disc photographs seems warranted for most people. Not every patient has a brief and limited inflammation, and if the inflammation and elevated IOP persist for 6 months, then we proceed to the guidelines for chronic care.

We suggest arbitrary and unproved management guidelines in patients with an initial episode of inflammation and high pressure. We prefer to treat with topical medication only; since miotics are relatively contraindicated, we use β-blockers if possible. Carbonic anhydrase inhibitors are a second choice. Most patients tolerate short-term modest elevations of pressure. (Most people also tolerate short-term marked elevations of pressure, but we do not assume that a patient's nerve can tolerate elevated pressure until the passage of time provides some information.) We are reluctant to consider surgical intervention for what will probably be a temporary condition.

If the patient's history or physical examination suggests preexisting glaucoma, then we modify the following guidelines for pressure goals as indicated by the state of the disc and field.

IOP >21 mm Hg ≤ 30 mm Hg

- Treat the inflammation.
- Taper corticosteroids as soon as reasonable.
- If pressure remains elevated after inflammation resolves and steroids are withdrawn, manage the patient as a glaucoma suspect.
- If inflammation and elevated pressure remain at 6 months, follow the guidelines for the management of chronic uveitis and glaucoma.

IOP >30 mm Hg ≤ 40 mm Hg

- Treat the inflammation.
- Taper corticosteroids as soon as possible.
- Treat with β-blocker if tolerated.
- Obtain disc photographs and field examination if the IOP does not decrease to <30 mm Hg after the β-blocker is begun.
- Follow at weekly intervals for 2 weeks and then at monthly intervals if the IOP does not fall below 30 mm Hg. If the disc on any examination appears different from the photographs, use the management guidelines for patients with chronic uveitis and glaucoma.
- If pressure remains elevated after inflammation resolves and steroids are withdrawn, manage the patient as a glaucoma suspect.
- If inflammation and elevated pressure remain at 6 months, follow the guidelines for the management of chronic uveitis and glaucoma.

IOP >40 mm Hg

- Treat the inflammation.
- Taper steroids as soon as possible.
- Treat with β-blocker, if tolerated, and, if needed and tolerated, with carbonic anhydrase inhibitor to lower the IOP below 40 mm Hg.
- Obtain disc photographs and field examination if the IOP does not fall to <30 mm Hg.
- Follow at weekly intervals for 2 weeks and then at monthly intervals if the IOP does not fall below 30 mm Hg. If the disc on any examination appears different from the photographs, use the guidelines for management of chronic uveitis and glaucoma.
- If the IOP cannot be lowered below 40 mm Hg, consider surgery. We

avoid laser trabeculoplasty because it is ineffective and aggravates the inflammation. Filtration surgery on an inflamed eye has a lower chance of success, and unsuccessful surgery does not help the patient's condition. If the disc and field can be followed serially, we sometimes observe patients who have pressures in the 40 mm Hg range until there is evidence of progression. We generally operate on patients with pressures above 50 mm Hg; we almost always recommend prompt surgery in individuals who have pulsatile central retinal arteries.

MANAGEMENT OF RECURRENT EPISODES OF INFLAMMATION AND ELEVATED PRESSURE SEPARATED BY INTERVALS WITHOUT INFLAMMATION

When it is expected that the patient will have multiple episodes of inflammation and elevated pressure, establish a full baseline as described in Chapter 2 as soon as the first episode has quieted. Treat each episode's pressure as described for the initial single episode. After each bout of inflammation, repeat the visual field and disc examination and compare the findings to the baseline. If the patient develops progressive disc or field damage, then set a lower pressure goal for treatment during subsequent episodes.

Some individuals who have recurrent inflammation with elevated IOP develop higher-than-normal pressures between episodes. Between episodes use the follow-up schedule for glaucoma suspects for such patients (see Chapter 4). They may require treatment only during the episodes of inflammation and higher pressure if progressive damage only occurs at these times; however, if the pressure between episodes also produces harm, chronic treatment for glaucoma is required.

MANAGEMENT OF CHRONIC UVEITIS ASSOCIATED WITH ELEVATED PRESSURE

Some types of uveitis, for example those associated with sarcoidosis and juvenile rheumatoid arthritis, are chronic. In addition, apparently acute conditions may fail to resolve. After an arbitrary limit of 6 months, we assume that the uveitis will be chronic. When a person has elevated pressure and chronic uveitis, we attempt to lower the pressure even if there is no damage. In our experience, the risk of damage is sufficient to justify treatment in such cases. The principles of glaucoma care in patients with chronic uveitis are much the same as those for primary open-angle glaucoma:

- Correct the correctable.
- Establish a baseline.
- Set a pressure goal and treat to achieve the goal.
- Continue to observe the patient to assess the stability of his or her condition.
- Modify goals and treatment as indicated.

Correction of the Correctable

Rule out or treat pupillary block. Control the inflammation, usually with corticosteroids and cycloplegics. Treat the pressure initially according to the guidelines listed under the single episode management section while the inflammation is controlled.

Establishment of a Baseline

As soon as the inflammation is reasonably controlled, establish a baseline. Waiting until the inflammation is controlled usually increases the quality of the baseline studies. In a significantly inflamed eye, the nerve may be swollen and the cup falsely small. Photophobia, corneal edema, and inflammatory debris impede fundoscopy and interfere with examination of the visual field. If the inflammation at the time of presentation is very mild, the vision is good, and the patient is comfortable, then start immediately to obtain baseline studies (see Chapter 2).

Determination of a Pressure Goal

When the patient has uveitis and elevated pressure on presentation, it is not possible to assume (as when dealing with asymptomatic pressure elevation) that the pressure has probably been at its level for a reasonably long period. Determine the pressure goal as described in Chapter 4, but recognize that it is only an estimate.

Treatment to Achieve the Pressure Goal

Treatment involves control of inflammation and suppression of aqueous formation with β-blockers and carbonic anhydrase inhibitors. Avoid use of miotics because of their tendency to exacerbate inflammation and promote posterior synechiae formation. Laser trabeculoplasty is not generally successful in inflammatory glaucoma, and surgery is both more difficult and less successful than in primary glaucoma.

We usually begin with a β-blocker once a day with the appropriate antiinflammatory treatment. If the pressure does not decrease to the target level, we increase β-blocker usage to twice a day. If the IOP remains higher than the goal, we decide whether to prescribe a trial of carbonic anhydrase inhibitors, depending on the height of the pressure and the degree of cupping or field loss. If cupping is mild and there is either no field loss or mild loss, we usually add oral medication if the pressure is 40 mm Hg or higher. If the cupping is moderate, and field loss, if present, is mild or moderate, we add oral medication at a pressure of about 32 mm Hg or if the pressure has fallen less than 20%. If the cupping or field loss is severe, we prescribe carbonic anhydrase inhibitors when the pressure is greater than about 26 mm Hg or has decreased less than 30%. We begin treatment with methazolamide 25 mg bid, and, if needed, increase to methazolamide 50 mg bid. If the pressure is still above the carbonic anhydrase inhibitor threshold, and the patient tolerates methazolamide well, we change the regimen to acetazolamide 250 mg qid or to Diamox Sequels bid. In any case, if the patient does not tolerate the medication, we discontinue it. Chart 9-1 summarizes these recommendations.

Follow-Up

Because of the potential complications of uveitic glaucoma, we recommend using the follow-up schedule for severe primary open-angle glaucoma described in Chapter 4. *On each examination* examine for and, if found, treat posterior synechiae and pupillary block. Perform gonioscopy frequently. Progressive peripheral arterior synechiae formation related to inflammatory debris generally dictates increased antiinflammatory treatment and increases the probability that the pressure may rise.

Modification of Goals and Treatment

The principles of goal modification are described in Chapter 4. The usual practical question that arises in the chronic care of uveitic patients is if and when to move from medical to surgical management. In our experience, laser surgery has failed, and we no longer perform trabeculoplasty in individuals with uveitis.

Unless there is advanced damage to the nerve, we generally accept whatever

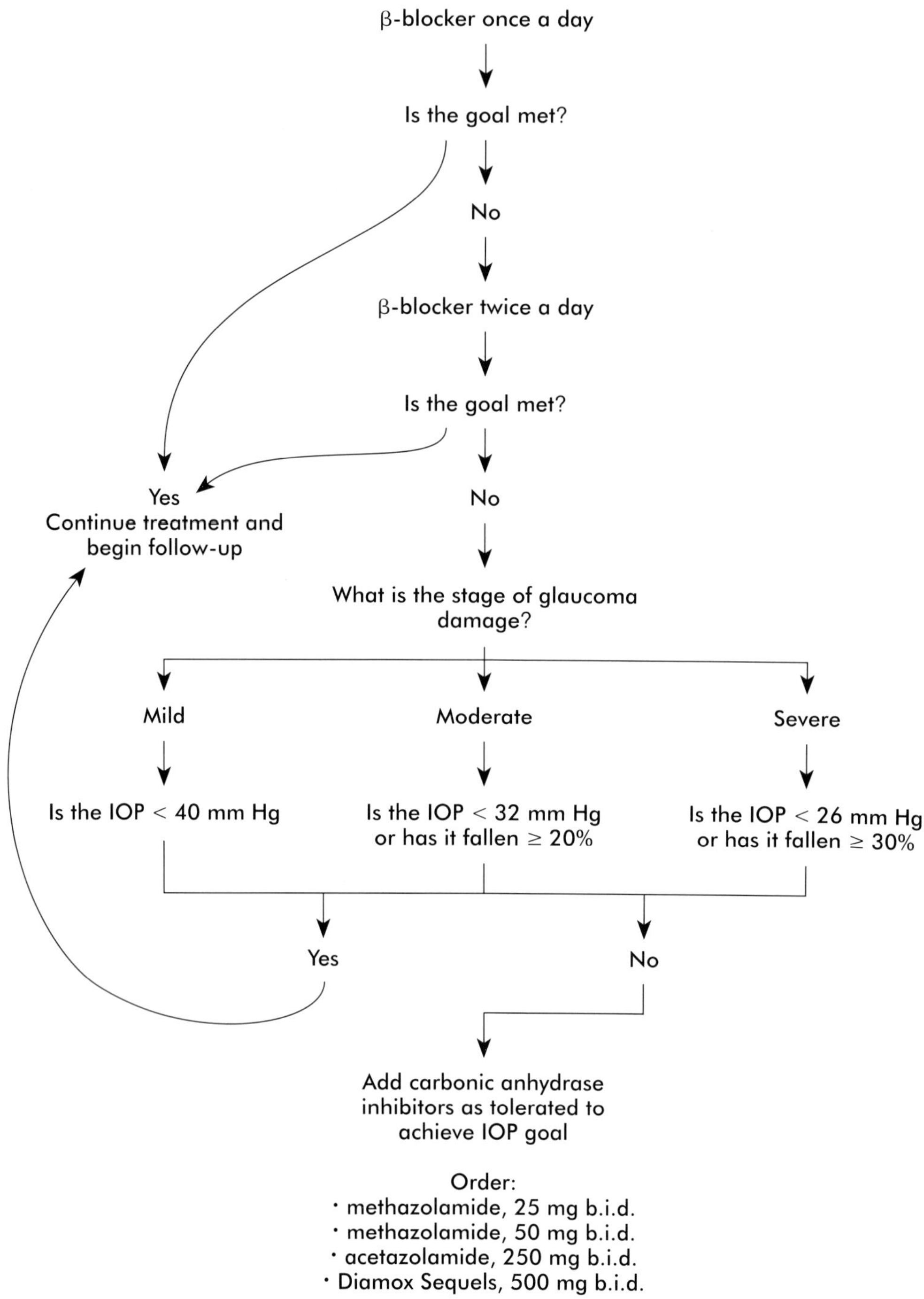

CHART 9-1 Medications to lower the IOP in patients with uveitis.

pressure is achievable with aqueous suppressants and antiinflammatory medication. If the nerve is severely cupped and the pressure has decreased less than 30% and is above 26 mm Hg, or if progressive damage develops at a rate likely to affect the patient's function, we generally operate on one eye and compare the course of the two eyes. Before surgery, we consult with a uveitis specialist to help manage the ocular inflammation.

The details of performing surgery on individuals with uveitis are discussed in standard surgery texts. In our experience, filtration surgery supplemented with 5-fluorouracil treatment is only briefly successful when performed on people with chronic uveitis. (Most filters fail within 2 years.) We have limited experience with mitomycin-C. Seton drainage procedures, such as Molteno or other implants, have sometimes provided good results and are currently the most common procedure in our patients with chronic uveitis and glaucoma.

COMMON PROBLEMS IN THE CARE OF GLAUCOMA AND UVEITIS

Although it is easy to offer guidelines for the care of patients with glaucoma and uveitis, in practice it can be difficult to decide the best course for an individual patient. Two common problems that arise in the management of these patients are the following:

- Steroid-related pressure elevation
- Cataract interference with visual fields and fundus visualization

Steroid-Related Pressure Elevation

As noted, treating with as small a dose of steroid as possible to control the inflammation is one of the general guides in managing glaucoma and uveitis. If a patient appears to have a significant pressure elevation that might be steroid related, the question sometimes arises of whether to change to a different drug, for example an antimetabolite, for control of the uveitis. Usually a patient in whom this course is considered has bilateral uveitis that corticosteroids can control, but also has glaucoma related to the steroid treatment. We refer these patients to a uveitis specialist for consultation.

Cataract Interference

When cataract precludes adequate fundus evaluation and field examination in a patient with chronic uveitis and glaucoma, our treatment recommendation depends on the type of uveitis and the degree of pressure elevation. We use a routine surgical approach in patients with glaucomatocyclitic crisis and with Fuchs' heterochromic iridocyclitis when the patient considers his or her disability sufficient to warrant the risk of surgery. When cataract surgery is elected in individuals with idiopathic chronic uveitis or in chronic uveitis associated with sarcoidosis or juvenile rheumatoid arthritis, we recommend pars plana lens extraction and vitrectomy without intraocular lens implantation. In individuals with herpetic disease associated with glaucoma and chronic uveitis (either idiopathic or part of a recognized syndrome), we encourage the patient to wait for surgery until he or she is no longer able to function well. Then we usually perform routine extracapsular cataract surgery.

10

Elevated Pressure and Surgical and Nonsurgical Trauma

The mechanisms of elevated pressure after surgery, accidental penetrating trauma, and blunt trauma are, with a few exceptions, the same. Evaluation and management of high pressure after trauma follow four straightforward steps:

- Determine the probable mechanism(s) of the pressure elevation.
- Manage the emergent and treatable causes of elevated IOP—infection and angle closure.
- Manage residual pressure elevation as the eye recovers.
- Proceed to chronic care of elevated IOP if the pressure elevation does not resolve.

After describing the mechanisms of elevated pressure after trauma, we present algorithms for the evaluation of patients with high pressure in two prototype situations: high pressure following cataract extraction and high pressure following blunt trauma. We briefly discuss elevated pressure after other anterior segment and posterior segment surgery. For simplicity, we refer to nonsurgical injury as *accidental,* regardless of whether the injury was purposeful, and assume that blunt trauma has not caused scleral rupture. Ruptured globes and eyes that have sustained penetrating accidental trauma generally have low pressure initially. If the pressure becomes elevated after surgical repair, they are included in the category of postoperative pressure elevation.

Most high pressures resolve within a few weeks after surgery or other trauma. If the pressure remains elevated after the first month, reevaluate the patient for one of the causes of late pressure elevation. If no reversible cause is found and the pressure is still high after 3 months, follow the guides for routine treatment of chronic high pressure: establish a baseline, decide if treatment is indicated and, if it is, set a pressure goal, treat to achieve the goal, continue to observe the patient, and modify the goal and treatment if indicated.

IDENTIFYING THE MECHANISMS OF ELEVATED PRESSURE IN PENETRATING AND NONPENETRATING TRAUMA

Table 10-1 summarizes the major causes of IOP elevation after surgical trauma and accidental nonpenetrating trauma. Several conditions may occur concurrently.

TABLE 10-1 ***Major Causes of Elevated Pressure after Trauma***

	Surgical trauma	Blunt trauma
Acute causes of elevated IOP		
Infection	X	—
Inflammation	X	X
Pupillary block	X	X
Other types of angle closure	X	X
Hyphema	X	X
Residual viscoelastic material	X	—
Direct damage to the outflow system	X	X
Late causes of elevated IOP		
Chronic infection	X	—
Corticosteroid-induced elevated IOP	X	X
Peripheral anterior synechiae	X	X
Ghost cell and hemolytic glaucoma	X	X
Outflow system scarring	X	X
Epithelial ingrowth	X	—

Early Mechanisms of Pressure Elevation

ACUTE INFECTION

Endophthalmitis may cause pressure elevation, perhaps because inflammatory debris blocks aqueous outflow. Once appropriate antimicrobial treatment is begun, examine the eye regularly to identify other mechanisms of pressure elevation.

INFLAMMATION

Inflammation raises eye pressure by the mechanisms discussed in Chapter 9. In addition to nonspecific inflammation related to trauma, retained lens material incites inflammation that generally persists until the lens material is resorbed, removed, or encapsulated. Inflammation related to lens material may explode, as does phacoanaphylactic endophthalmitis, or it may smolder, as does most inflammation from retained lens cortex after cataract surgery. An intact but subluxed or dislocated lens does not generally cause inflammation.

PUPILLARY BLOCK

Pupillary block may be seen early or it may develop, with or without symptoms, some time after surgery or injury. Pupillary block rarely develops in eyes that have undergone peripheral iridectomy. It is particularly common in eyes with anterior chamber lenses and no iridectomy.

Adhesions of the iris to the vitreous face, lens, or lens implant may block passage of aqueous humor toward or through the pupil. Figure 10-1 illustrates some variants on pupillary block that may develop after surgical or accidental trauma. If only the pupil margin is adherent to underlying structures, the iris leaf bows forward, giving a typical iris bombé appearance as posterior chamber pressure increases. If much of the posterior iris surface is adherent, only the mobile peripheral iris may protrude forward, and iris bombé may be apparent only in the peripheral anterior chamber. (Before complete blockage develops,

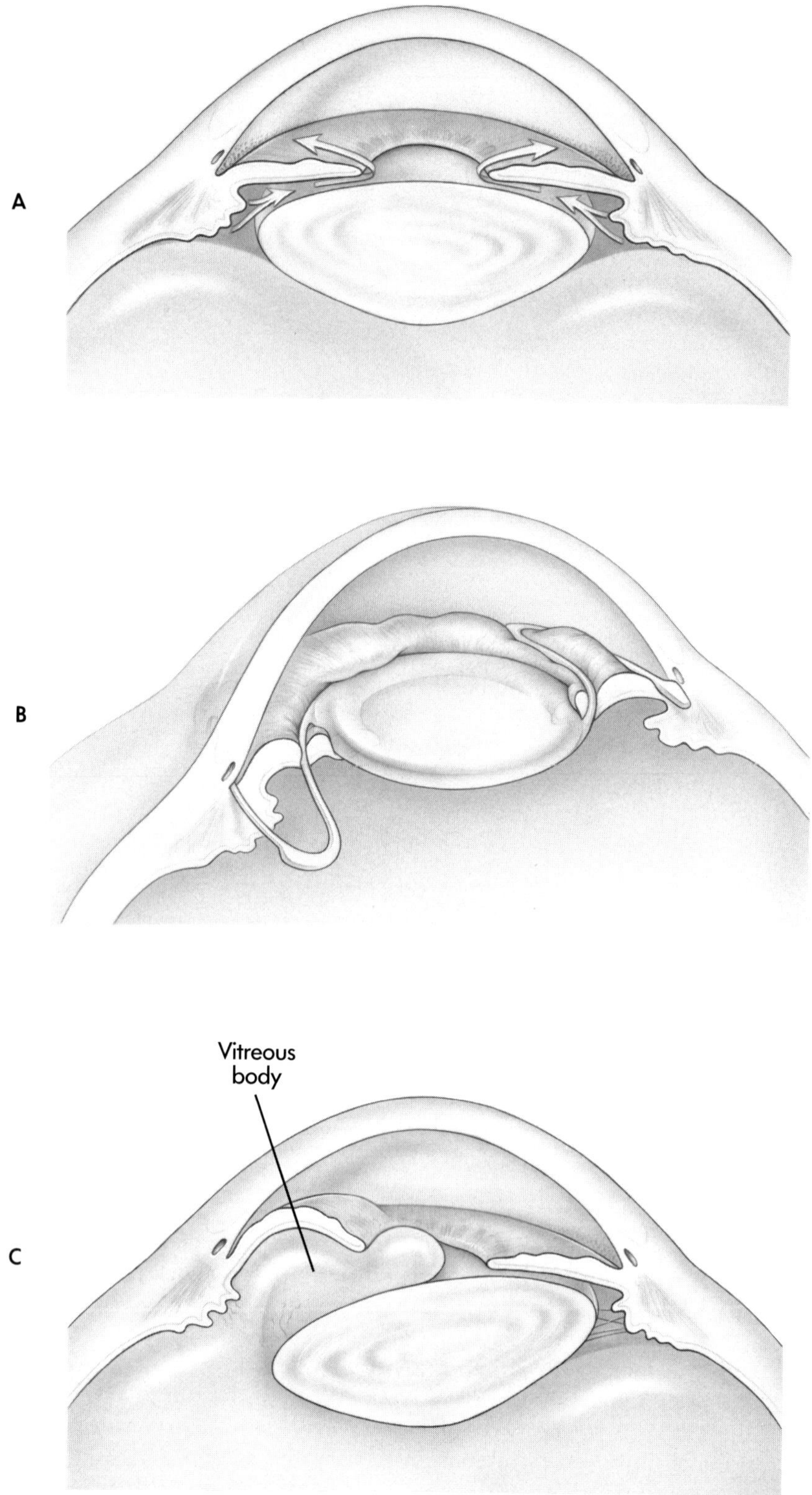

FIG. 10-1 Variations on pupillary block after trauma. **A,** Normal aqueous humor flow. **B,** Anterior chamber intraocular lens causing pupillary block. **C,** Herniated vitreous humor causing pupillary block.

Continued.

D

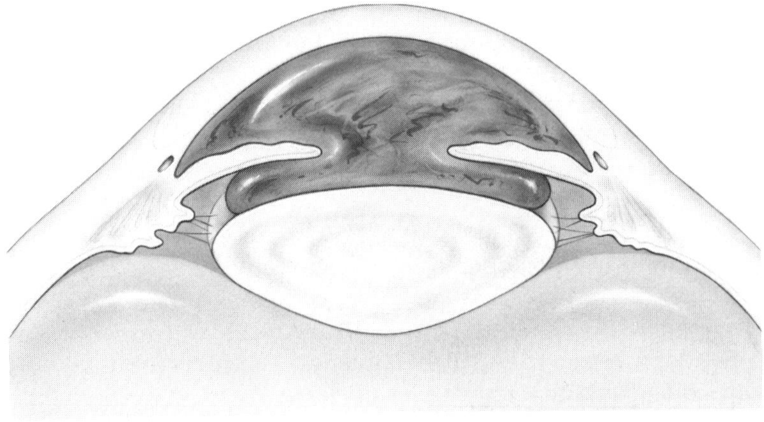

E

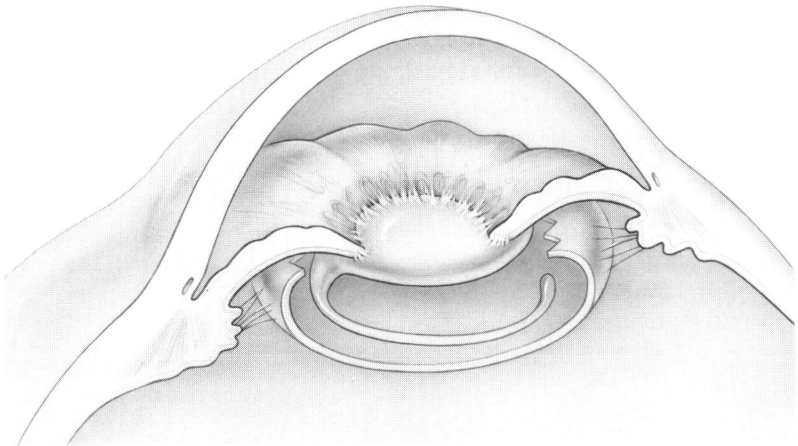

F

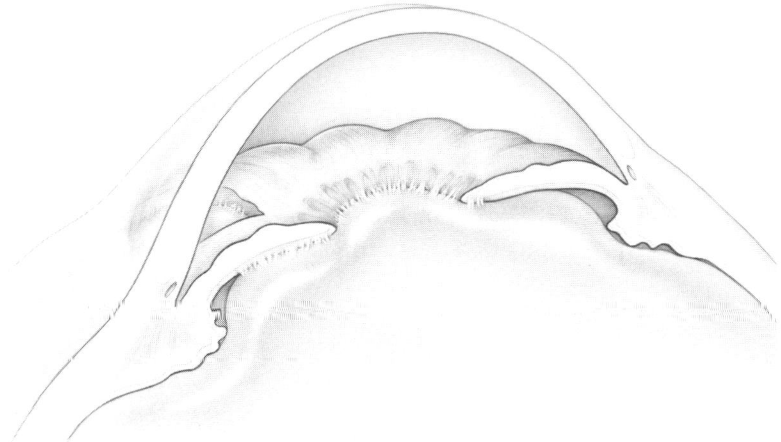

FIG. 10-1, cont'd. **D,** Collar button clot causing pupillary block. **E,** Synechiae to lens causing pupillary block. **F,** Synechiae to vitreous face causing pupillary block.

the bulging peripheral iris may crowd the angle without closing it and producing an elevated pressure; peripheral iris bulge without high IOP should be treated if noted.)

Lens subluxation, which may occur from blunt trauma, causes relative pupillary block related to forward movement of the lens and may, in combination with vitreous gel, cause pupillary block.

POSTERIOR PUSHING ANGLE CLOSURE

In the early postoperative or posttraumatic period, angle closure with elevated pressure may develop in several ways other than pupillary block. For discussion, we divide these into ciliary block and forward rotation of the iris-lens diaphragm. These distinctions are arbitrary and the underlying pathophysiologic mechanism is often unclear.

Ciliary block. Ciliary block, also known as malignant glaucoma and aqueous humor misdirection, is a condition in which aqueous humor does not freely enter the posterior chamber because of resistance somewhere in the zonular/capsular/hyaloid face junction. The central anterior chamber is shallow because the lens or vitreous face is pushed forward, and peripheral iridectomy neither prevents nor resolves the angle closure. Ciliary block most typically occurs in an eye with a small anterior segment and anatomically narrow angle. The precise mechanism of ciliary block is not understood, but a model that explains the central chamber shallowing and its resolution with cycloplegia is illustrated in Figure 10-2. As ciliary block begins to develop, the lens moves forward, and relative pupillary block may cause the iris to bulge forward and close the angle. At this stage, we believe that iridectomy may sometimes reverse the process. With fully developed ciliary block the lens or vitreous body itself (not the posterior chamber aqueous humor) pushes the iris onto the trabecular meshwork surface; at this stage iridectomy is of no benefit.

Forward rotation of the iris-lens diaphragm. Ciliary body inflammation, ciliary body or suprachoroidal hemorrhage, and scleral buckling may each cause the ciliary body to rotate inward around its attachment to the scleral spur. This moves the iris-lens diaphragm forward (Figs. 9-1, 10-6, and 10-8). The angle closure that results does not generally resolve after iridectomy, although the angle may widen with cycloplegia. Suprachoroidal hemorrhage also acutely raises the IOP by a mass effect, but after compensatory exit of aqueous humor the eye returns to equilibrium; a nonexpanding mass does not cause persistent elevated pressure in the absence of angle closure.

HYPHEMA

Blood in the anterior chamber may raise the pressure in at least two ways. A clot that spans the pupil will cause pupillary block (Figs. 10-1, *D,* and 10-3). As serum and aqueous humor exit through the meshwork, the posterior chamber expands because the aqueous humor cannot pass the pupil. The iris thus moves forward to close the angle while the red cells become compacted.

Even in the absence of pupillary block, red blood cells may block the trabecular meshwork. The red cells of patients with sickle cell trait or sickle cell disease may sickle in the anterior chamber and, being inflexible, block outflow for longer than nonsickled cells. Vitreous hemorrhage without hyphema does not cause elevated IOP acutely, although blood in the vitreous cavity may later cause both ghost cell and hemolytic glaucoma (discussed in a later section).

A

B

C

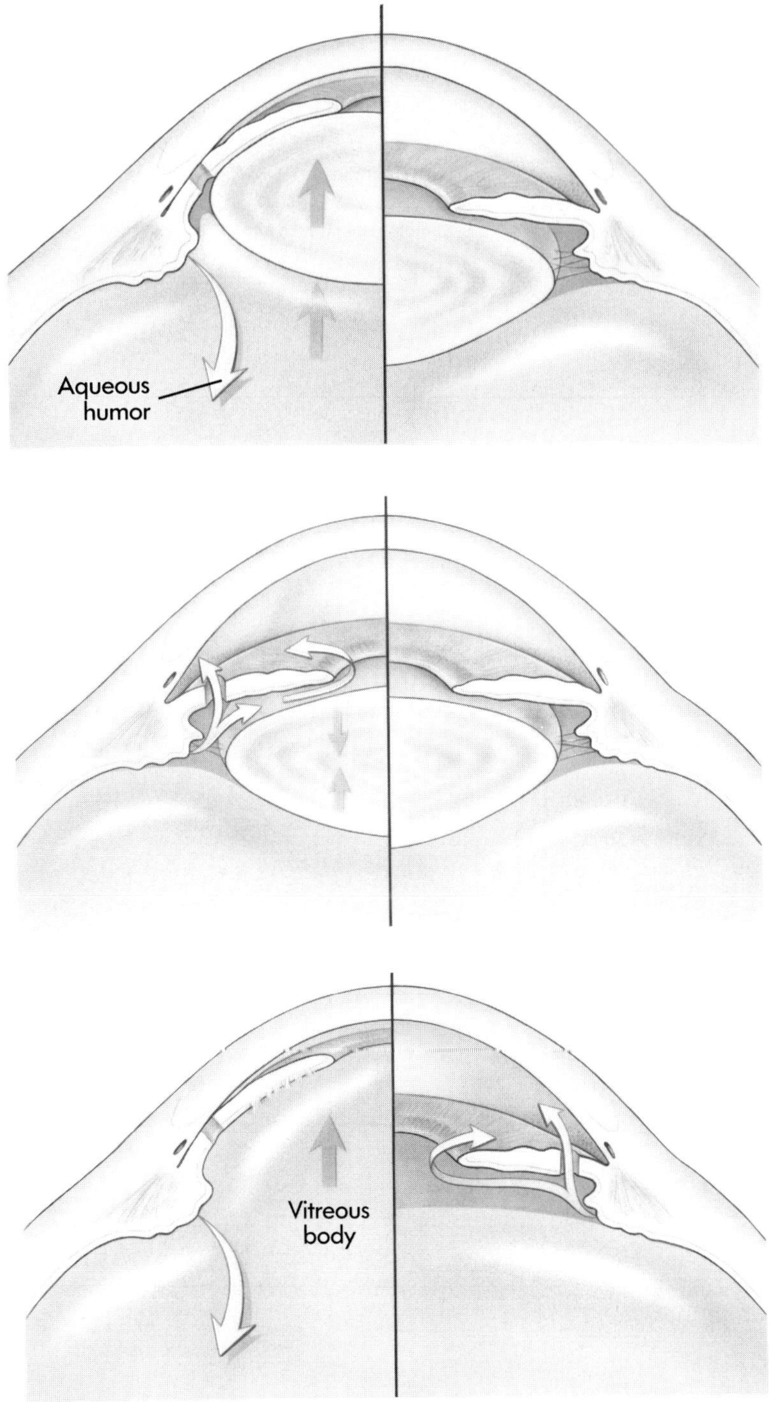

FIG. 10-2 **A,** Ciliary block, left; normal for comparison, right. The lens moves forward, pressing the iris against the cornea, and aqueous humor flows backward into the vitreous body, thus pushing the vitreous face forward. **B,** Resolution of ciliary block after atropine administration, left; normal for comparison, right. Atropine pulls the lens back and decreases the lens thickness. The iris falls back, and aqueous humor flows into the anterior chamber. **C,** Aphakic ciliary block, left; normal for comparison, right. For an unknown reason, despite the presence of an iridectomy aqueous humor flows backward into the vitreous body, thus pushing the vitreous face forward.

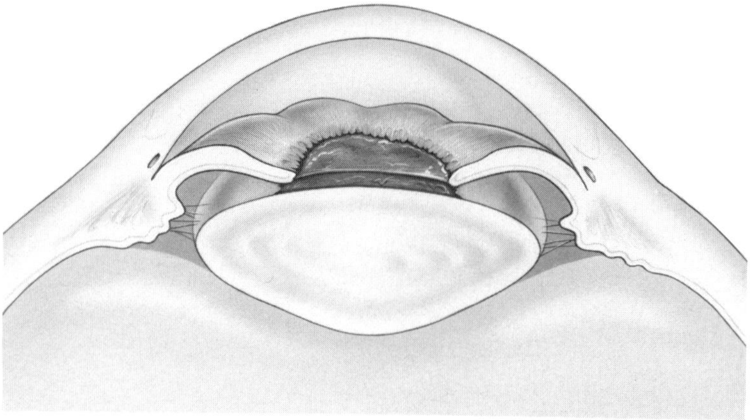

FIG. 10-3 Small clot causing pupillary block. See also Fig. 10-1, *D*.

VISCOELASTIC MATERIAL IN THE EYE

Mechanical blockage of the trabecular meshwork by viscoelastic material can raise the pressure until the substance dissolves. Dissolution generally occurs within 48 hours.

DIRECT TRAUMA TO THE OUTFLOW SYSTEM

Blunt ocular trauma indents the eye at the point of impact, transiently raising the IOP to very high levels and stretching the intraocular structures and the ocular coat (Fig. 10-4). Ciliary muscle rupture results in "angle recession" and bleeding, which present as hyphema. Stretching of the ocular coat causes microshredding of the trabecular meshwork and flap tears in the meshwork. Ciliary muscle and trabecular meshwork damage lead to swelling (early) and scarring (late), which impair aqueous humor outflow and result in high pressure. The incision in cataract surgery may likewise damage the trabecular meshwork and the posttrabecular collector channels.

Later Causes of Elevated Pressure

CHRONIC INFECTION

Subacute and chronic infection may elude diagnosis for months. The most common organism to cause low-grade infection is *Propionibacterium acnes* infection, which sometimes causes pressure elevations associated with smoldering inflammation.

CORTICOSTEROID-INDUCED PRESSURE ELEVATION

Corticosteroids directly affect IOP by decreasing the ease of aqueous humor outflow. They may indirectly raise pressure in inflamed eyes by decreasing inflammation, thereby increasing aqueous humor production. After uncomplicated surgery or mild trauma, corticosteroids can generally be discontinued if they are suspected of elevating the pressure. Following complicated surgery or significant trauma associated both with outflow system damage and lingering inflammation requiring continued corticosteroid use, it may be difficult to determine the precise contribution of corticosteroids to high pressure.

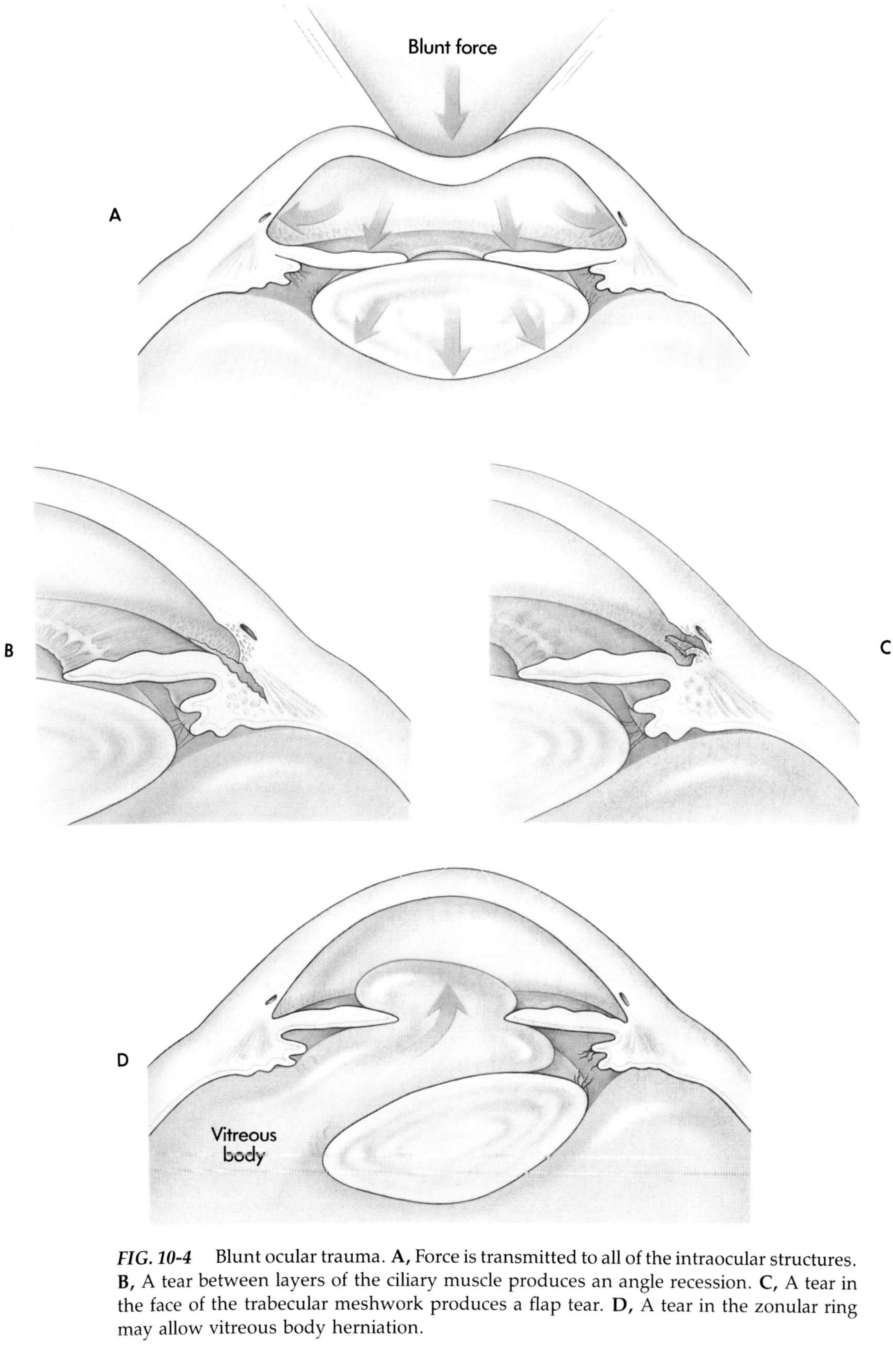

FIG. 10-4 Blunt ocular trauma. **A,** Force is transmitted to all of the intraocular structures. **B,** A tear between layers of the ciliary muscle produces an angle recession. **C,** A tear in the face of the trabecular meshwork produces a flap tear. **D,** A tear in the zonular ring may allow vitreous body herniation.

BLOOD-INDUCED GLAUCOMA

Blood enters the vitreous cavity in two ways: a hyphema may move backward through a rent in the zonule-posterior capsule diaphragm, or the patient may have a hemorrhage from a posterior structure directly into the vitreous cavity. Blood in the vitreous cavity resorbs slowly. Red cells may degenerate, and, if degenerated cells or their breakdown products move into the anterior chamber, may cause either ghost cell glaucoma or hemolytic glaucoma.

Ghost cell glaucoma. Ghost cells are degenerated red blood cells, which have become spherical rather than disc-shaped and appear tan or khaki colored. Like sickled cells, they are inflexible and may block the trabecular meshwork and increase resistance to outflow.

Hemolytic glaucoma. This condition is caused by trabecular meshwork blockage by fragments of hemolyzed red cells and by macrophages laden with these blood breakdown products. The cells in the anterior chamber are red.

ANGLE CLOSURE

Peripheral anterior synechiae. Peripheral anterior synechiae develop from the healing of ruptures in the trabecular meshwork and face of the ciliary body, from healing of an incision, or from prolonged contact between the iris and the trabecular meshwork, especially in an inflamed eye. The peripheral anterior synechiae directly block outflow and raise outflow pressure in proportion to the extent of meshwork covered.

Epithelial ingrowth. In epithelialization of the anterior chamber, the epithelial sheet first covers the trabecular meshwork and then pulls the iris up over the meshwork.

TRABECULAR MESHWORK DAMAGE

Blunt ocular trauma may produce immediate and persistent pressure elevation, or may be followed by normal pressure for many months to decades before the pressure increases. An acute pressure elevation may not occur, even in the presence of substantial outflow system damage, because of other effects of trauma such as decreased aqueous humor production. Thus a history of normal pressure in the early stages after an injury does not rule out subsequent pressure elevation related to trabecular meshwork damage.

EVALUATING THE PATIENT

History

PREEXISTING OCULAR DISEASE

If the condition of the patient's eye before surgery or accidental injury is not known, try to determine by history the preexisting vision and question the patient regarding previous glaucoma. In the absence of better information, the status of the opposite eye indicates the likely previous status of the involved eye.

PAIN

Severe pain generally accompanies acute endophthalmitis and suprachoroidal hemorrhage.

HEMATOLOGIC HISTORY

Determine whether the patient has any known hematologic conditions, particularly a bleeding disorder or sickle hemoglobinopathy.

OPERATIVE HISTORY

If the media are clear, the physical examination—revealing what *is* present rather than what *might be* present—is more useful than the operative history. However, if blood, corneal edema, or inflammatory debris obscure the view, the operative history may suggest diagnostic possibilities. If the capsule ruptured during a phacoemulsification, both nucleus and cortex may be present within the eye. If the nucleus was removed intact in an extracapsular extraction, capsular rupture generally means that cortex remains. Vitreous loss does not itself increase the IOP, but it is usually associated with additional manipulation and inflammation. If no peripheral iridectomy was performed, particularly if an anterior chamber lens was inserted, consider pupillary block.

Examination

VISION

Profoundly decreased vision (less than hand movements) in the absence of hyphema suggests either infection or significant posterior segment injury.

PUPILLARY EXAMINATION

Test for an afferent defect and record the findings. The consensual pupil response (Marcus Gunn sign) is helpful if the response of the pupil in the injured eye is indeterminant.

EXTERNAL EXAMINATION

Periorbital edema and marked conjunctival swelling or injection suggest a possible infection.

SLIT-LAMP EXAMINATION

Hypopyon or marked inflammation, particularly if inflammation involves the vitreous body, strongly suggests infection. Hyphema following blunt trauma is evidence of a tear in the uveal tissue of the angle and indicates likely trabecular meshwork damage. The clinician should examine the eye specifically with a narrow beam to see if the peripheral iris is in contact with the peripheral cornea, in which case the angle is obviously closed, or if a visible space extends as far to the peripheral anterior chamber as can be seen. If the peripheral anterior chamber is shallow or if the angle appears to be closed, determine if the central chamber is shallow. Check for iris bombé (bulging of the iris further anterior than the pupil plane); if it is present, study the pupil to see if blood, vitreous humor, fibrin, or a fibrous adhesion is blocking the passage of aqueous humor. Note if there is a peripheral iridectomy (surgery) or iridodialysis (accident) and, if one is present, whether it appears to be patent or clogged, for example, with vitreous humor.

GONIOSCOPY

Iris bombé indicates pupillary block and may preclude gonioscopy until after relief of the block. If the iris does not show bombé, and if the view is adequate, perform gonioscopy to rule out angle closure glaucoma.

FUNDOSCOPY

Vitreous inflammation suggests infection or lens material in the vitreous. If the eye is inflamed and the capsule was broken, look carefully for retained lens material.

Vitreous blood indicates that either a hyphema moved backward through a rent in the zonule-posterior capsule diaphragm or that the patient had a hemorrhage directly into the vitreous. Unless the cause of vitreous blood is clear, evaluate the patient for evidence of unrecognized penetrating injury (as with a retrobulbar needle) despite the usual association of hypotony with penetration. Look for a choroidal detachment, which in an eye with high pressure, usually indicates suprachoroidal hemorrhage.

LABORATORY EXAMINATION

If possible, echography should be performed in patients who have unexplained angle closure or in patients whose fundus cannot be visualized.

We obtain a sickle preparation for a black patient who has a hyphema and elevated pressure; we also obtain a sickle preparation for any patient who has hyphema without pupillary block and an otherwise unexplained pressure elevation that is disproportionate to the amount of blood. Hemoglobin S is most common among blacks, but it occurs in all races.

DIAGNOSIS AND MANAGEMENT OF HIGH PRESSURE AFTER SURGICAL AND ACCIDENTAL TRAUMA

We describe our diagnostic approach to elevated pressure in these prototypical situations: immediately after cataract extraction, weeks to a few months following cataract extraction, and promptly following blunt trauma. The common causes for elevated pressure after other surgical procedures are discussed in later sections.

Elevated IOP Early After Cataract Surgery

Chart 10-1 summarizes the diagnosis of high pressure in the early postoperative period after cataract surgery.

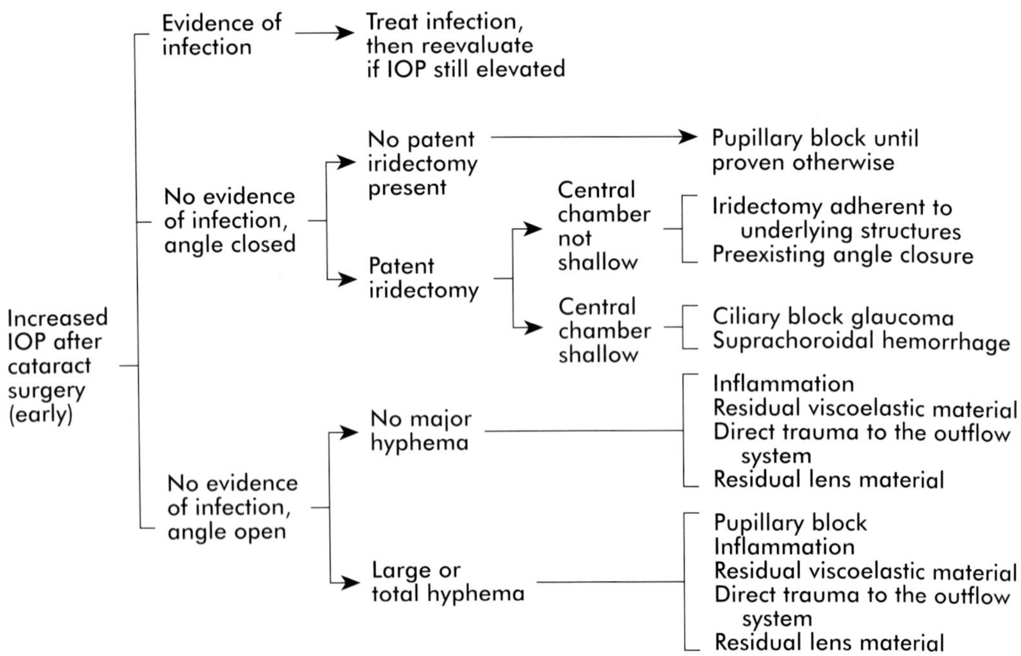

CHART 10-1 Differential diagnosis of elevated IOP after cataract surgery.

◆ ***Early elevated IOP—significant inflammation, other evidence of possible infection***

Acute postoperative intraocular infection causes impressive pain, decreased vision, and both intraocular and extraocular inflammation. The infection, not the pressure, requires emergent care. Treat the pressure elevation according to the guidelines in Chapter 9 for a single episode of inflammation. If the pressure remains elevated after the infection has been treated appropriately, manage it like any other postoperative pressure elevation.

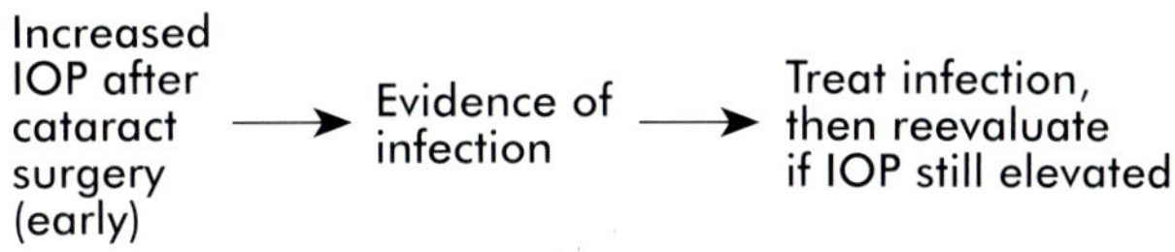

◆ ***Early elevated IOP—closed angle***

Angle closure that develops in the immediate postoperative period is usually obvious on slit-lamp examination. Pupillary block caused by adhesions of the pupil margin to the underlying intraocular lens, vitreous, or capsule, or by apposition of the pupil to an overlying anterior chamber lens is the most common cause of early angle closure. Ciliary block accounts for a smaller number of closure cases. It is usually possible to distinguish between the two conditions at presentation. In an eye with pupillary block, the central chamber is of normal depth and the iris bulges forward from the pupil plane. In cases of ciliary block, the central anterior chamber is shallow or flat (Fig. 10-5).

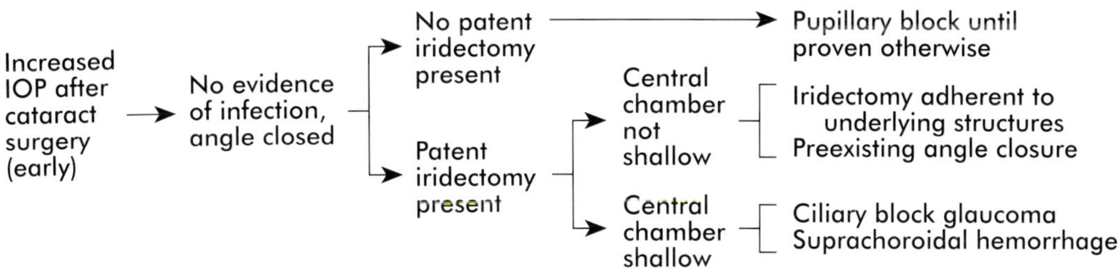

PUPILLARY BLOCK

Perform a laser peripheral iridectomy promptly if the cornea is sufficiently clear. It may be necessary to perform the iridectomy in the midsection or even near the pupil because of iridocorneal touch peripherally. If so, perform a second iridectomy in the periphery after the bombé is relieved if inflammation persists and the more central opening is draped on a posterior structure in such a way that it might become closed by a new adhesion.

If the view is inadequate or if a laser is not immediately available, pupillary dilation will, in many cases, break fresh synechiae and relieve pupillary block. Use of phenylephrine, to pull actively on the pupil, is important, since simple paralysis of the pupil with a cycloplegic agent will not tug on adhesions. Even if the blockage is lysed to produce a clear channel, perform a prompt laser peripheral iridectomy. If there are peripheral anterior synechiae or if elevated pressure persists after relief of the pupillary block, manage the patient's condition according to the guidelines in Chapter 8 for chronic care after angle closure glaucoma.

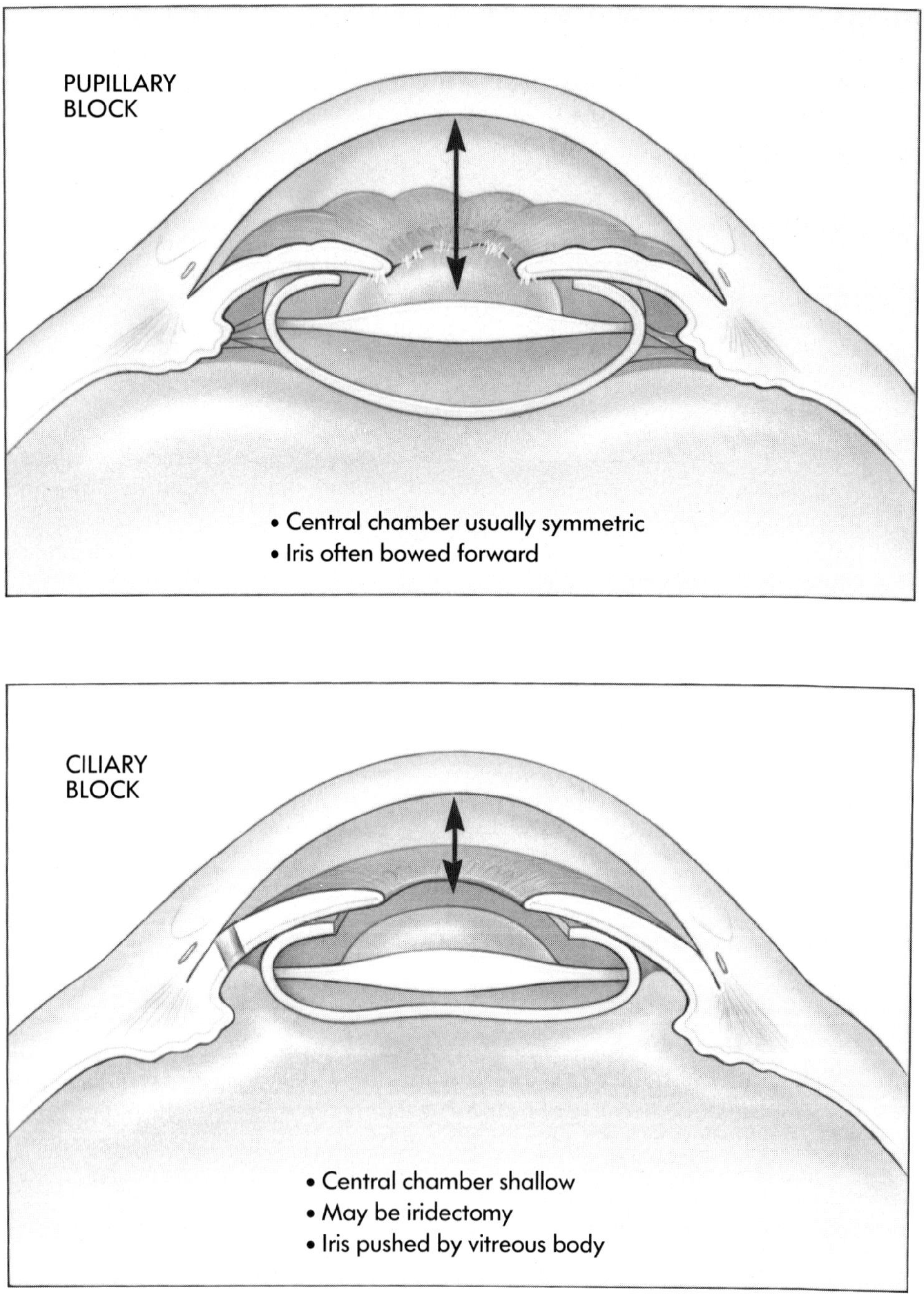

FIG. 10-5 Comparison of usual presentations of pseudophakic pupillary block versus pseudophakic ciliary block.

Timetable for Ciliary Block Management after Cataract Surgery

Immediate (Not all of these can be done at the same time, but they should all proceed as promptly as possible.)	• Laser peripheral iridectomy • Atropine 1%, 1 drop q 5 minutes × 3 • Hyperosmotic agent of choice • β-blocker, 1 drop • Oral acetazolamide, 250 mg • YAG laser disruption of the posterior capsule and anterior hyaloid face
Before surgery (If fundus cannot be seen)	• Echography to rule out posterior lesions
Within several hours (If the block does not resolve)	• Refer to vitreous surgeon for pars plana vitrectomy.

CILIARY BLOCK

When managing presumed ciliary block after cataract surgery, we recommend following several courses simultaneously to lower the pressure and reverse the mechanisms of angle closure. If the patient does not have a patent iridectomy, perform a laser iridectomy as soon as possible to remove the pupillary block element that is always present if the lens or implant is forward. Treat the eye with a strong cycloplegic agent, usually atropine, and give the patient a hyperosmotic agent to lower the pressure acutely. Treat the patient with suppressants of aqueous humor formation to help maintain a low pressure when the underlying process is interrupted, but do *not* use miotics. Disrupt the posterior capsule and the anterior hyaloid face with the yttrium-aluminum-garnet (YAG) laser if possible. If the fundus is not visible, obtain an echographic exam to rule out a posterior lesion, such as suprachoroidal hemorrhage. If these measures do not resolve the ciliary block within a few hours, we refer the patient to a vitreous surgeon for pars plana vitrectomy (see box above).

OTHER CAUSES

Suprachoroidal hemorrhage sometimes causes angle closure, probably by rotating the ciliary body forward, as illustrated in Figure 10-6. Perform a laser iridectomy if no iridectomy is present to remove any component of pupillary block. Treat the patient with cycloplegics, β-blockers, and carbonic anhydrase inhibitors. The pressure usually decreases, and the posterior segment findings rather than the IOP usually guide decisions about drainage of hemorrhage. If the angle does not open and the pressure does not fall, the blood may be surgically drained.

◆ *Early elevated IOP—open angle*

Causes of elevated pressure with an open angle include sterile inflammation, retained lens material, residual viscoelastic material, hyphema, and direct trauma to the outflow mechanism from the surgical incision. Retained nuclear material should generally be removed surgically, but the other possibilities are treated by the guidelines for treatment of inflammation and elevated pressure described in Chapter 9. If there is a total hyphema, refer to page 190.

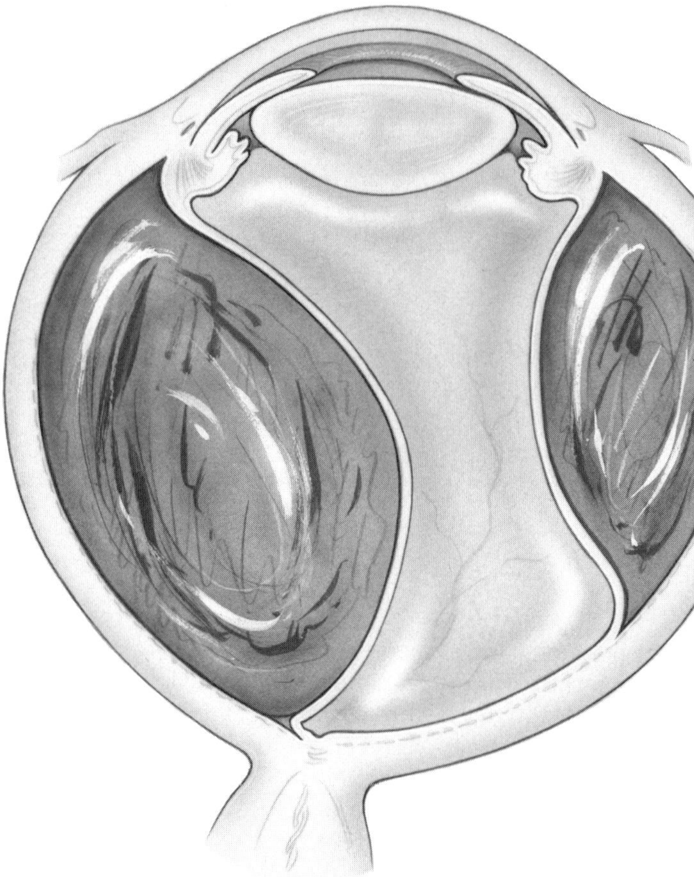

FIG. 10-6 Suprachoroidal hemorrhage causing forward rotation of the iris and ciliary body with angle closure.

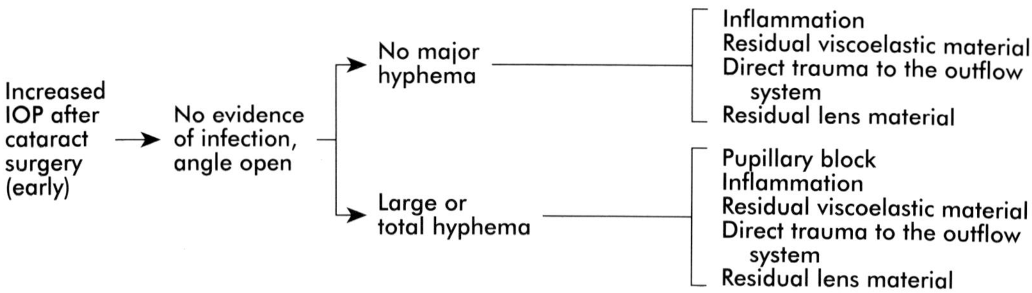

Elevated IOP Later After Cataract Surgery

Chart 10-2 summarizes the diagnostic steps for a patient who has either persistent or newly noted elevated pressure several weeks or months after cataract surgery. The primary division, into eyes with cells in the anterior chamber and eyes without cells, serves to divide eyes that have not stabilized postoperatively from eyes that have stabilized. When the eye is free of inflammation (without use of corticosteroids) and any active pupillary block is relieved by iridectomy, the guidelines for treating any chronic elevated IOP also apply to the postoperative eye.

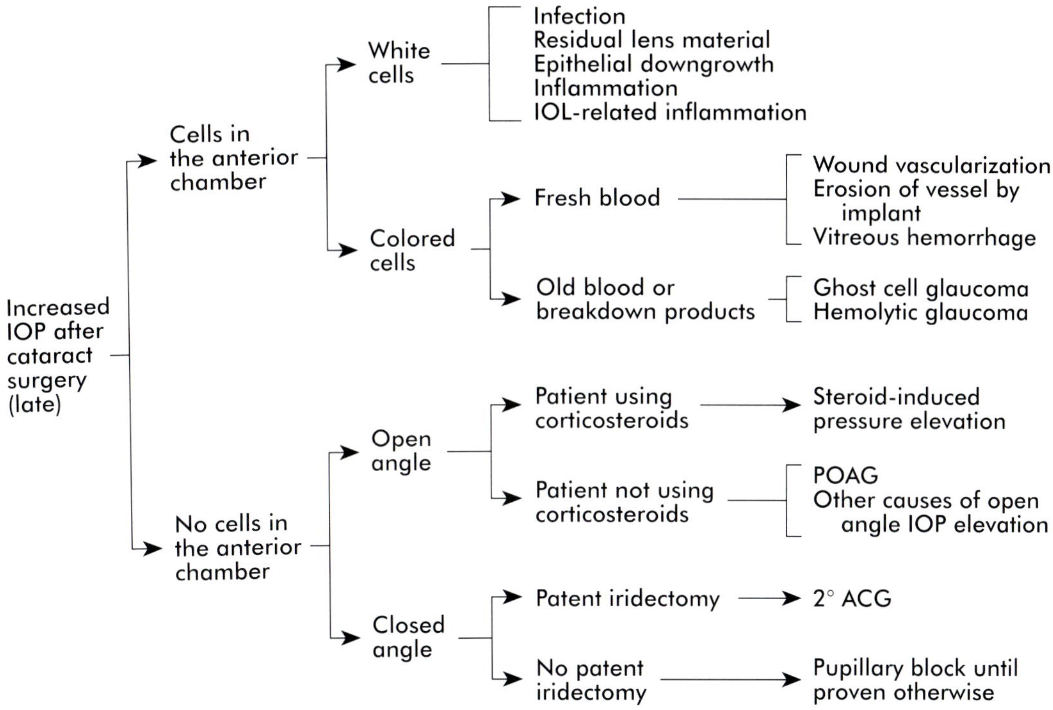

CHART 10-2 Differential diagnosis of elevated pressure in the later postoperative period after cataract retraction.

◆ *Later elevated IOP—cells in the anterior chamber*

Inflammatory cells, red cells, denatured red cells, and epithelial cells may be found in the anterior chambers of eyes with postoperative pressure elevation. The cells usually appear either white or colored. (Even if the color is not clear, associated signs allow the clinician to distinguish among the various likely conditions in this setting.) Always perform gonioscopy to rule out concurrent angle closure.

Persistent inflammation develops only rarely after cataract surgery and often indicates a significant problem. The specifically treatable condition—and thus the most important to diagnose—is low-grade infection.

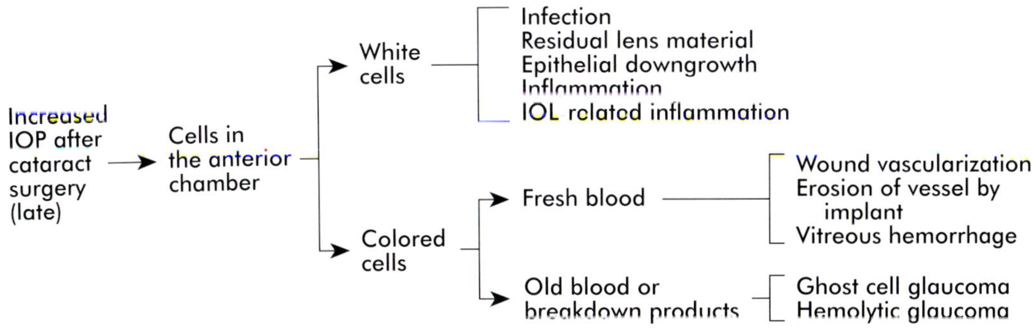

WHITE CELLS

Infection. Low-grade smoldering infection may cause secondary inflammation and high pressure. Anterior chamber tap and culture, if positive, confirm this diagnosis. However, culture results may be negative in the most common recognized situation, that of *Propionibacterium acnes* infection, because the bacterium may be sequestered in residual cortex. Treatment depends on the organism found or suspected and often includes removal of residual lens and capsule. As with acute endophthalmitis after treatment, any of the other postoperative mechanisms of elevated pressure may also develop.

Residual lens material. Persistent high pressure related to residual cortex raises therapeutic, not diagnostic problems in the late period. We suggest using the guides for IOP management discussed in Chapter 9. If surgery is indicated for IOP control, however, the first surgical approach is usually removal of lens material rather than filtration surgery. If the patient has such significant glaucomatous damage that further loss is likely to cause significant visual impairment, we do simultaneous cortex removal and filtration surgery.

Epithelial ingrowth. A cellular membrane with an obvious line on the posterior cornea, large clumps of cells in the anterior segment, and very high IOP characterize epithelial downgrowth. If epithelial ingrowth is suspected, diagnostic argon laser treatment may help to make a diagnosis because epithelial cells turn white when coagulated. This test is not always easy to interpret, particularly in a blue-eyed individual.

The laser technique is as follows. Use large spots (200 μm), long duration (0.5 sec), and low energy (100 to 400 mW). Apply treatment to the iris in the area of presumed ingrowth, which is usually superior. Increase energy from 100 mW gradually until the iris surface contracts. If the iris surface chars, decrease energy since a charred epithelial membrane closely resembles a charred normal iris surface. If the treated area turns white, then use laser burns to determine the extent of involvement.

Details of surgical treatment of epithelial ingrowth are described in surgical texts and are beyond the scope of this book.

IOL-related inflammation. Some styles of lens implants cause inflammation and elevated pressure in significant numbers of patients. Inflammation related to lens implants may also develop if a lens is not ideally positioned or if foreign material is deposited on the lens during manufacture. The following signs and symptoms support this diagnosis:

- Tenderness of the limbus over the haptics of the lens without tenderness of the globe between the haptics (Fig. 10-7)
- Iris tucking or ciliary body indentation visible by gonioscopy
- Presence of an IOL type that is known to be associated with uveitis and elevated pressure

Initial treatment of inflammation related to implants follows the routine uveitis guides (page 164). If the inflammation and elevated pressure do not resolve, the implant should generally be removed.

COLORED CELLS

Most hyphemas clear from the anterior chamber within the early postoperative period. Fresh blood thus indicates recurrent hemorrhage. Colored cells that do not resemble fresh blood indicate either ghost cell or hemolytic glaucoma. Both of these conditions develop when blood in the vitreous cavity denatures and then moves into the anterior chamber through a broken capsular-zonular diaphragm.

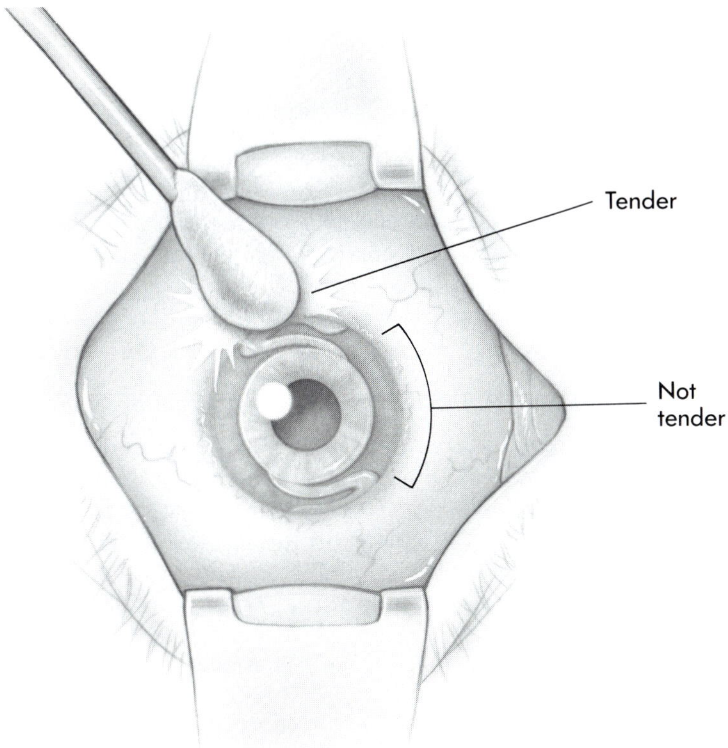

FIG. 10-7 Intraocular lens–related inflammation with limbal tenderness over the haptics.

Fresh hemorrhage. Hyphema without vitreous hemorrhage and without neovascularization of the iris usually indicates either vascularization of the cataract wound or erosion of a uveal vessel by an implant. Diagnosis may be difficult and may be made only after several gonioscopic examinations reveal a very localized clot beneath which a vascular nubbin is seen after the clot resolves. Definitive management of these conditions is discussed in standard surgical texts. The clinician should manage each episode of acute pressure elevation associated with hyphema following the guidelines in Chapter 9 for recurrent episodes of elevated pressure from inflammation. This includes use of corticosteroids to retard synechiae formation while the hemorrhage resorbs.

Ghost cell glaucoma. Tan or khaki colored cells in the anterior chamber of a patient with elevated IOP who has had blood in the vitreous cavity indicate ghost cell glaucoma. The condition is self-limited. Adjust the follow-up frequency and ocular hypotensive therapy using the guides in Chapter 9 for a single episode of inflammation, but do not use corticosteroids. If the pressure does not fall below 40 mm Hg, we generally perform both a vitrectomy and anterior chamber washout.

Hemolytic glaucoma. The cells in the anterior chamber are red. Treatment is the same as that of ghost cell glaucoma.

◆ ***Later elevated IOP, no cells in the anterior chamber, open angle***

If the patient is using corticosteroids, steroid-induced pressure elevation is a possibility. After discontinuing steroid use, the diagnostic possibilities are those

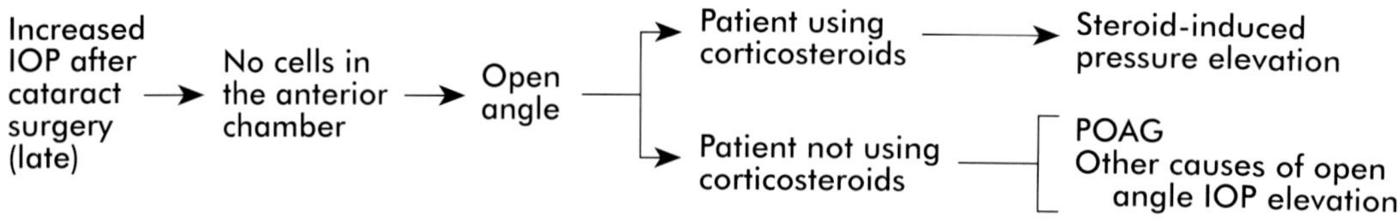

discussed in Chapter 3. Occasionally open-angle glaucoma develops after cataract surgery and persists thereafter. We assume that damage to the outflow channels by the surgical incision in individuals prone to chronic pressure elevation explains some episodes of elevated pressure that do not fall into other categories, although we cannot confirm this assumption.

◆ ***Later elevated IOP, no cells in the anterior chamber, closed angle***

Residual peripheral anterior synechiae may result in chronic pressure elevation despite iridectomy. This must be distinguished from currently active pupillary block, which may have persisted since surgery or may develop in the later postoperative period, particularly in individuals with anterior chamber lenses and in diabetic patients. Iris bombé is usually present. If there is not a patent iridectomy, perform a laser iridectomy. Then evaluate and manage the patient as described in Chapter 8 for the management of patients with primary angle closure glaucoma after relief of pupillary block.

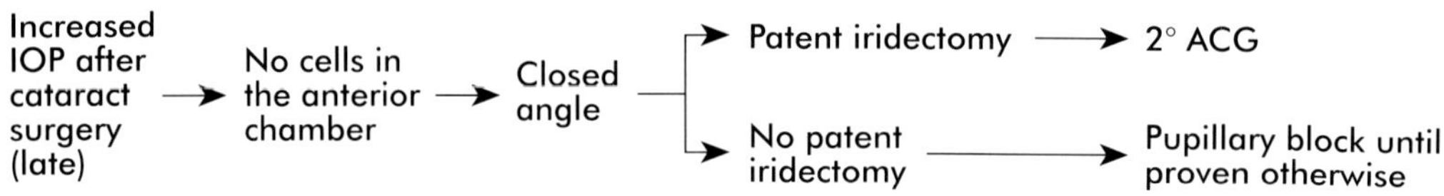

Elevated IOP Early after Blunt Trauma

Chart 10-3 summarizes our recommended approach to patients with high pressure after blunt trauma.

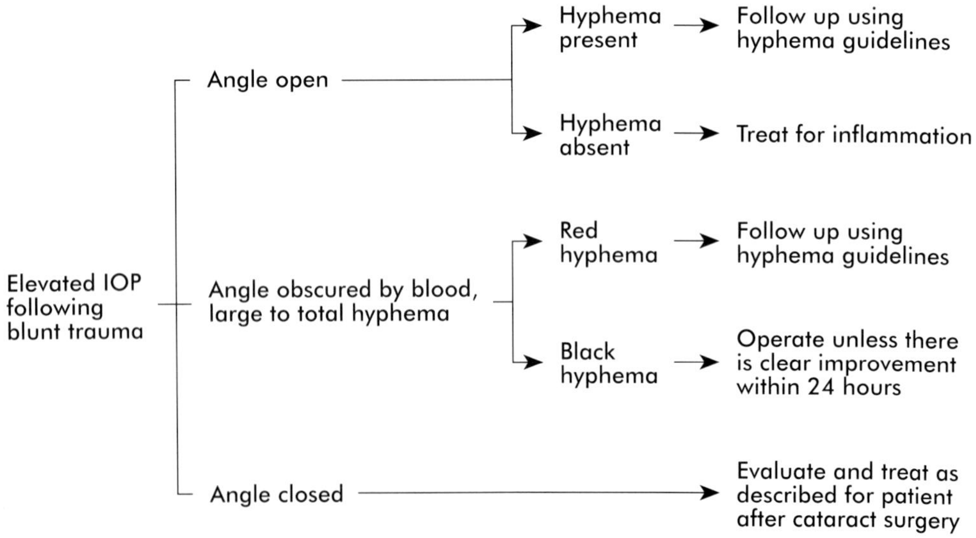

CHART 10-3 Differential diagnosis and management of elevated pressure after blunt trauma.

◆ *Elevated IOP, angle open, partial hyphema*

Direct angle trauma, blockage of the trabecular meshwork by red blood cells, inflammation, and preexisting glaucoma may all contribute to elevated pressure. Because of the risk of recurrent bleeding, various regimens including bed rest, patching, and use of antifibrinolytics are recommended for treatment of hyphema. Our routine treatment is as follows.

Elevated IOP following blunt trauma → Angle open → Hyphema present → Follow up using hyphema guidelines

MEDICAL MANAGEMENT

- Shield the involved eye to prevent additional trauma.
- Treat with long-acting cycloplegic agents (atropine or scopolamine bid) to pull the lens backward, to keep the ciliary muscle immobile, to decrease inflammation, and to relieve discomfort.
- Treat with corticosteroids at least four times a day to increase patient comfort, to decrease inflammation, and to retard synechiae formation.
- Treat with a β-blocker if tolerated and if the pressure is >30 mm Hg.
- Add a carbonic anhydrase inhibitor to the β-blocker if the pressure is greater than 40 mm Hg. We are aware of the concern that the use of carbonic anhydrase inhibitors in individuals with sickle cell trait and disease leads to acidosis and increased sickling. Current data neither confirm nor refute this possibility. We have used carbonic anhydrase inhibitors in individuals with sickle disease but routinely obtain medical consultation.
- Examine the patient daily and assess for afferent defect daily using the consensual pupillary response.

SURGICAL TREATMENT

Occasionally a patient with a partial hyphema and an initially open angle will develop pupillary block (from clot) and iris bombé that is clearly visible above the clot. Laser peripheral iridectomy resolves the bombé.

In a person with a partial hyphema, we do not routinely operate solely for hyphema-associated pressure unless one of the following is present:

- New development of an afferent defect
- Corneal blood staining

When surgery is performed, we perform a trabeculectomy and peripheral iridectomy and do not attempt to remove all the hyphema. The trabeculectomy allows a route for egress of blood, and the iridectomy relieves pupillary block. We expect that a filtering procedure done under these circumstances will fail within a fairly short period. We do not attempt to establish a long-term filtering procedure because of the risks associated with blebs and because of the usually transient nature of the early pressure elevations associated with hyphema.

LATER TREATMENT

Hyphemas generally clear within a few weeks. If the pressure remains elevated after the blood clears and the patient is no longer using corticosteroids, use the management regimen described on p. 191.

◆ *Elevated IOP, angle open, no hyphema*

Inflammation, direct trabecular meshwork damage, and preexisting glaucoma are the most likely possibilities in this situation. Treat the eye presumptively for inflammation and manage the pressure by the guidelines in Chapter 9 for a single episode of inflammation. The detailed regimens for treating persistent high pressure after blunt trauma are discussed in Chapter 11.

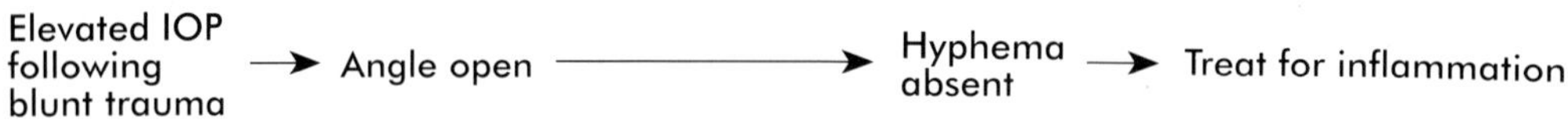

◆ *Elevated IOP, angle obscured by blood, large to total hyphema*

We divide individuals with large to total hyphemas into two groups:

- Those with total or almost total red hyphemas with elevated pressure
- Those with total black hyphemas with elevated pressure

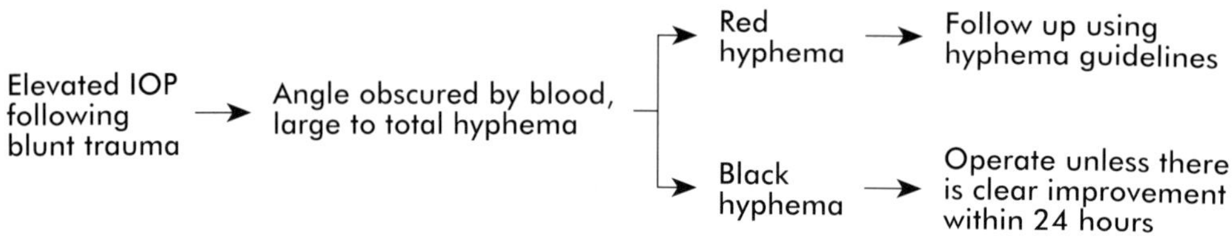

TOTAL RED HYPHEMA AND ELEVATED PRESSURE

Provided a hyphema remains red, it almost always lyses within a fairly short period. We treat the eye as described for partial hyphema with two exceptions. The first is that early peripheral laser iridectomy is impossible, although with a total hyphema the likelihood of pupillary block is high. Until the clot contracts or begins to lyse, it is not possible to visualize the iris. Within a few days, the hyphema contracts and the peripheral iris becomes visible. If it is bowed forward, then perform an iridectomy. The second difference in management is that we recommend surgery if the clot turns from red to black.

TOTAL BLACK HYPHEMA AND ELEVATED PRESSURE

Blood in the eye turns black when the red blood cells are concentrated and compacted by exit of serum. Black clots clear over an extended period, especially when aqueous flow through the anterior chamber is eliminated by pupillary block. When the pressure is elevated in such an eye, it has been our experience that the patient almost always develops either an afferent pupillary defect or corneal blood staining, usually after about a week. Therefore we now operate promptly unless there is a surgical contraindication or the patient's condition clearly improves within 24 hours. We perform a filtering procedure and peripheral iridectomy. We may irrigate the anterior chamber gently, but we do not attempt to remove the clot because of the risks to the corneal endothelium and the chance of lens injury if the anterior segment is instrumented. To date, all the clots that we have treated in this manner have lysed and we have not had to reoperate to clear the hyphema.

◆ *Elevated IOP, angle closed, with or without partial hyphema*

The same general mechanisms of angle closure apply to accidental trauma as to surgical trauma. Once the angle is open, evaluate as previously described.

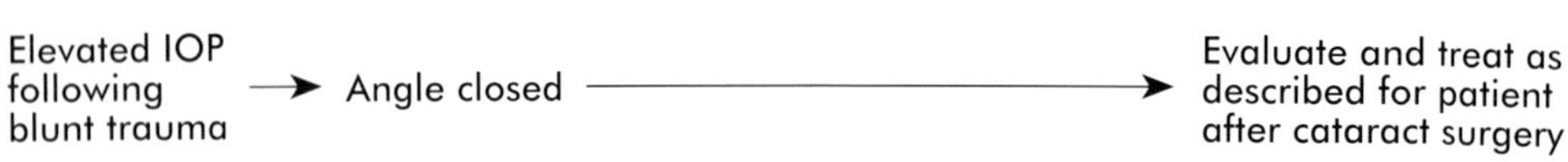
Elevated IOP following blunt trauma
Angle closed
Evaluate and treat as described for patient after cataract surgery

ELEVATED IOP THAT PERSISTS AFTER BLUNT TRAUMA

Blunt trauma that responds to nonsurgical therapy, or at least is not severe enough to require prompt surgery, rarely causes elevated pressure that lasts longer than 1 or 2 months. If the pressure is still elevated 6 months after injury, and if the eye is not inflamed and no corticosteroids have been used for several weeks, we then recommend beginning to establish a baseline for future follow-up of elevated pressure.

The differences in chronic management of elevated IOP related to blunt trauma compared with primary open-angle pressure elevation are discussed in Chapter 11.

High Pressure After Anterior Segment Procedures Other Than Cataract

With minor variations (for example, intraocular lens complications do not occur without an intraocular lens), the discussion of elevated IOP after cataract surgery applies to other anterior segment procedures. The most likely causes vary slightly. The following summarizes our experience in treating high pressure after anterior segment surgery.

PENETRATING KERATOPLASTY

Pupillary block may develop if no peripheral iridectomy is done at the time of the graft. Steroid-related pressure elevation often occurs after the first several weeks, and, if it develops, usually warrants treatment both because of the expected duration of the high pressure and because of the deleterious effect of elevated pressure on the corneal graft. To avoid inflammation that might compromise the corneal graft we avoid use of miotics if possible, but use them in a quiet eye if the alternative is either laser or filtration surgery.

INTRACAPSULAR CATARACT EXTRACTION

When α-chymotrypsin is used, zonular debris may block the angle for several days. The treatment is the same as for a single episode of inflammation.

FILTRATION SURGERY

The following are the most common causes of high pressure immediately after filtering surgery:

- Tight closure of a scleral flap
- Blood under the scleral flap
- Internal blockage of the filtration ostium with blood, lens, or vitreous humor
- Suprachoroidal hemorrhage with rotation of the iris and ciliary body and occlusion of the ostium

Pupillary block is unusual because peripheral iridectomy is usually performed. Ciliary block may develop, usually in eyes with previous angle closure. Hyphema, viscoelastic material, and direct trabecular meshwork damage do not raise the pressure in the presence of a functioning filtration bleb. Treatments are discussed in standard surgical texts. Later, fibrotic closure of the bleb (failure of the procedure) results in pressure elevation.

Elevated Pressure After Posterior Segment Procedures

Most of the major causes of glaucoma after anterior segment surgery may also complicate posterior segment surgery. The major additional conditions related to retina and vitreous surgery are variations on pupillary and ciliary block. We refer to these as buckle-induced ciliary body rotation and bubble-induced pu-

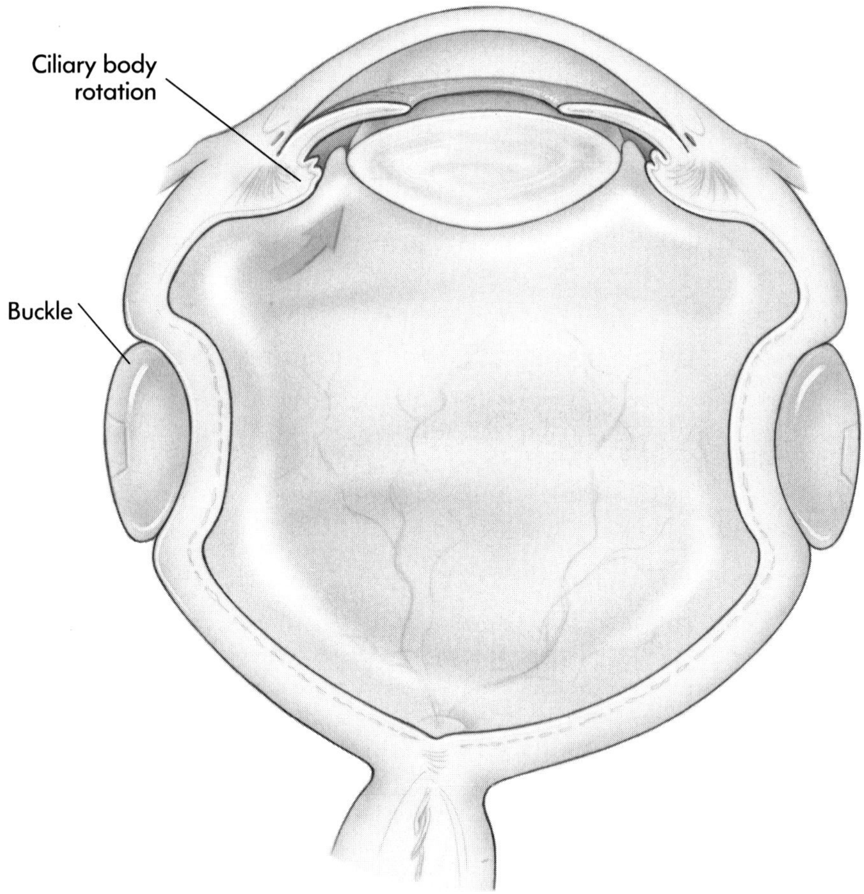

FIG. 10-8 Scleral buckle–induced angle closure.

pillary block. Both conditions can result in elevated pressure in the early postoperative period and in peripheral anterior synechiae formation and persistent glaucoma. In both conditions, the pathophysiology described is presumptive.

BUCKLE-INDUCED CILIARY BODY ROTATION

This condition develops after scleral buckling procedures. The peripheral anterior chamber is usually flat and the central chamber is shallow. Peripheral iridectomy has not been successful in our experience, and we no longer perform it. The presumed pathophysiologic condition is forward rotation of the ciliary body and lens. Figure 10-8 illustrates the presumed mechanism. Our preferred treatment is iridoretraction (laser iridoplasty), accompanied by intense treatment with cycloplegics and corticosteroids.

BUBBLE-INDUCED PUPILLARY BLOCK

A variety of gases remain in eyes after surgery. Some gases expand and some do not; all rise to the anterior part of the eye to block the pupil if the patient lies supine. A gas bubble that occludes the opening(s) between the anterior and posterior chambers causes pupillary block, apposition of the iris to the angle, and high pressure. If the patient is supine, a large bubble lies behind

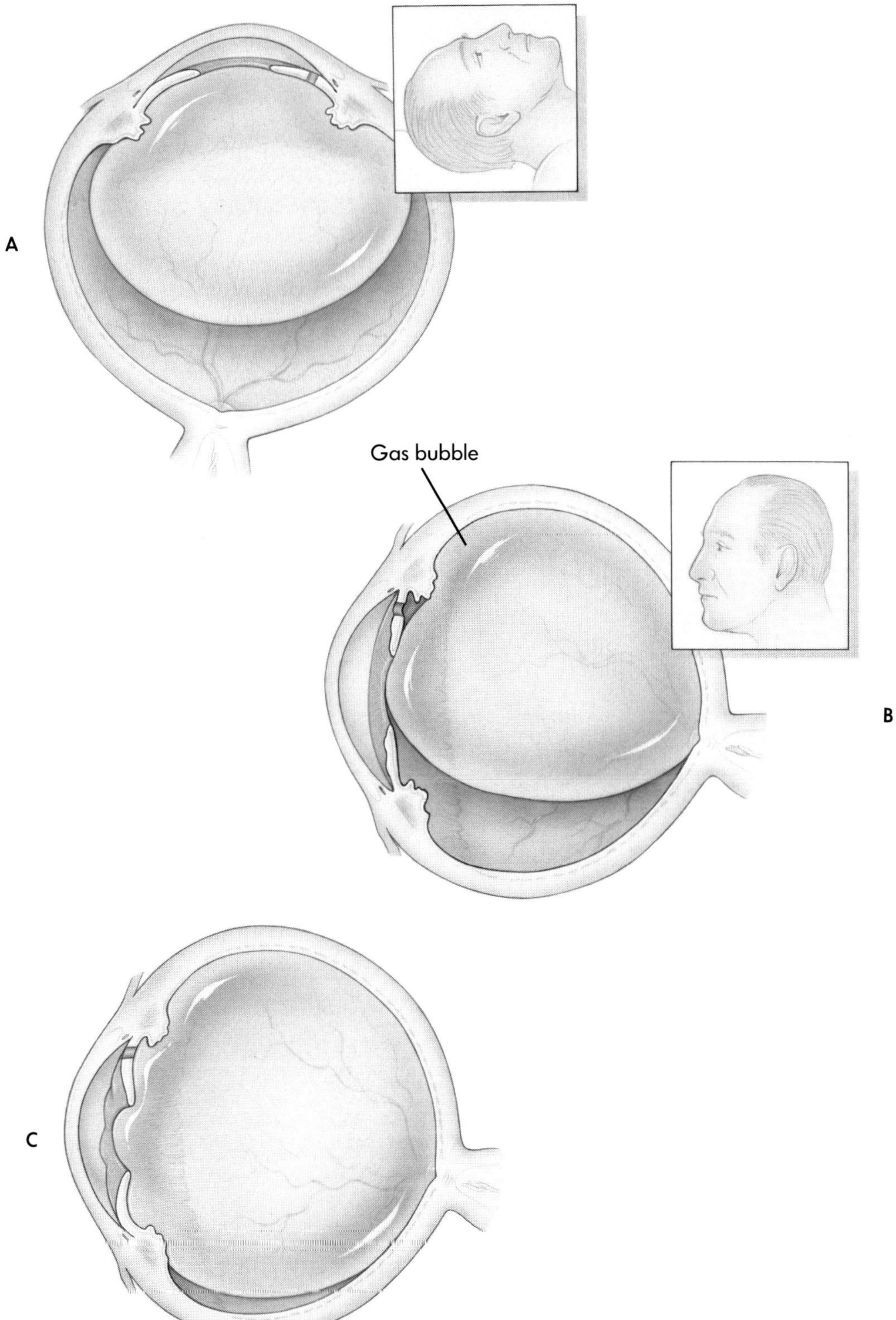

FIG. 10-9 Pupillary block caused by a gas bubble. **A,** With patient supine, the bubble blocks both the pupil and the peripheral iridectomy. **B** and **C,** With the patient upright, the size of the bubble determines whether or not the pupillary block persists.

the angle, and high pressure. If the patient is supine, a large bubble lies behind the pupil, but surface tension prevents it from entering the anterior chamber. As aqueous humor exits through the trabecular meshwork, the iris is lifted forward by the floating bubble until the anterior chamber is flat and the angle is closed. If an iridectomy is present and not covered by the bubble, the anterior chamber can flatten immediately because aqueous humor can pass posteriorly around the bubble and allow it to float anteriorly more freely. If the patient is sitting, the floating bubble can still flatten the anterior chamber if it is large enough (Fig. 10-9). Because eyes are often quite inflamed after procedures associated with gas bubbles, peripheral anterior synechiae may form rapidly; this condition warrants treatment if it is recognized. Face-down positioning of the patient and removal of some of the gas are options. Appropriate treatment should consider both the effects of the pupillary block on the anterior segment and optic nerve and the condition for which the surgery was performed. (A perfect IOP in an eye blinded by a retinal pathologic condition does not benefit the patient.)

11

Miscellaneous Conditions

This chapter discusses some of the particular differences of fairly common glaucomas from primary open-angle glaucoma (POAG) in their care or in their usual course. It also describes an approach to patients who have strong family histories of glaucoma and to patients with large, but apparently normal, cups.

PSEUDOEXFOLIATION WITH GLAUCOMA

Pseudoexfoliation with open-angle glaucoma differs from POAG in a few ways. Probably because the condition is associated with laxity of the zonules, angle closure develops in addition to open-angle glaucoma more commonly than it does in POAG. Perform gonioscopy at least yearly and also promptly after adding use of miotic drops to the patient's treatment regimen.

In our experience, patients with pseudoexfoliation have a tendency to develop rather abrupt increases in pressure even without angle closure. Thus a person whose IOP has been well controlled for years may develop a substantially increased pressure and may have symptoms of acutely elevated IOP. We therefore recommend that individuals with pseudoexfoliation and glaucoma be examined at least every 6 months. Patients with pseudoexfoliation usually respond well to laser trabeculoplasty.

PIGMENTARY GLAUCOMA

This condition is treated in the same manner as POAG. Patients with pigmentary glaucoma are often young and myopic. Ocuserts have proved to be a useful medication for many of our patients. There has been speculation that iridectomy might decrease the friction of the iris on the zonules and improve the condition, but this has not been proved.

ELEVATED EPISCLERAL VENOUS PRESSURE WITH GLAUCOMA

The glaucoma associated with high episcleral venous pressure responds poorly to medical and laser management because the resistance to outflow is beyond Schlemm's canal. Suppressants of aqueous humor formation—β-blockers and carbonic anhydrase inhibitors—are more beneficial than miotics; laser treatment helps little.

We have had good success with filtration surgery in individuals with uncontrolled glaucoma and high episcleral venous pressure. Standard surgical texts describe the use of prophylactic sclerotomies in such cases, and we have followed these recommendations. Because such patients are fairly young, we use postoperative 5-fluorouracil in most cases.

GLAUCOMA ASSOCIATED WITH BLUNT TRAUMA AND ANGLE RECESSION

Acute high pressure after blunt trauma is described in Chapter 10. Glaucoma associated with trauma may also appear as an acute symptomatic elevated IOP as discussed in Chapter 8. The chronic pressure elevation that may follow blunt trauma is managed by the same steps as with primary pressure elevation. Perhaps because the trabecular meshwork is scarred, use of miotic drops often does not lower the IOP. Laser trabeculoplasty rarely lowers the pressure and can result promptly in increased pressure. We do not perform laser treatment unless the patient is a candidate for filtration surgery and has an additional condition, such as prolapse of the vitreous body into the anterior chamber, that increases the risk of surgical complications. Our reluctance to perform laser surgery is based on experiences in which a quiet eye with glaucoma has been transformed by laser into an inflamed eye with markedly elevated pressure that then requires surgery.

STEROID-INDUCED PRESSURE ELEVATION

Eliminating corticosteroid use, if possible, is the best treatment for steroid-induced glaucoma. If this is not possible, steroid-induced glaucoma from steroids used for nonocular conditions responds to medical, laser, and surgical therapy, much as does POAG. If the steroids are used for ocular inflammation, the prognosis and treatment depend on the primary disease.

CHRONIC ANGLE CLOSURE GLAUCOMA

Primary chronic angle closure glaucoma usually presents as an asymptomatic pressure elevation. If the pressure decreases markedly after iridectomy, chronic management resembles that of acute angle closure glaucoma after iridectomy (Chapter 8)). In this circumstance, even if manifest glaucoma is present, the new intraocular pressure may generally be observed without treatment to determine whether it causes progressive glaucomatous damage.

If iridectomy does not alter the IOP significantly, the initial management and subsequent follow-up of chronic angle closure glaucoma differs little from that of open-angle pressure elevation. The patient should have regular gonioscopic examinations to rule out angle narrowing related to anterior lens movement. Laser trabeculoplasty treatment is useful only in open areas of the angle.

IRIDOCORNEAL ENDOTHELIAL SYNDROMES

The glaucoma associated with the iridocorneal endothelial syndromes is very difficult to treat and generally results in significant visual loss. There is no known treatment to halt the pathologic process, and the angle gradually closes. Suppressants of aqueous humor formation are more successful than use of miotics. Laser trabeculoplasty is not effective, and many patients require surgery, which has a poor prognosis.

STRONG FAMILY HISTORY OF OPEN-ANGLE GLAUCOMA

A normotensive adult with a family history of severe glaucoma but no abnormal findings should have a yearly examination. We also obtain disc photographs as a baseline record because the nerve appearance is less likely to change from a nonglaucomatous cause than is the field. If the pressure rises or the nerve appears to change, then we manage the condition by the routine guidelines in Chapters 2 through 5.

LARGE BUT APPARENTLY PHYSIOLOGIC CUPS

Sometimes a patient has large but healthy looking cups—perhaps with large nerve heads—that do not appear glaucomatous and do not seem to warrant a major evaluation for normal tension glaucoma. The clinician should obtain photographs and a diagnostic field. If both are normal, reexamine the patient in 6 months and, if unchanged, at routine intervals determined by the patient's age thereafter.

Index

R

S

T